FOGSI
Handbook of
Antenatal Care

FOGSI
Handbook of
Antenatal Care

Series Editors

Nandita Palshetkar MD FCPS FICOG FRCOG (UK)
Professor Emeritus in Obstetrics and Gynecology
DY Patil School of Medicine
Navi Mumbai, Maharashtra, India
Scientific Director and Co-Founder, Bloom IVF
Scientific Director and Co-Founder
Baufici Genetics
President, AMOGS
President, ISAR
Past President, FOGSI, IAGE, MOGS and MSR

Rohan Palshetkar MS (Obs & Gyne) FRM
Associate Professor
DY Patil School of Medicine
Navi Mumbai, Maharashtra, India
2nd Joint Secretary, AMOGS
Managing Committee Member, MSR, MOGS

Editors

Sadhana Gupta
MS (Obs & Gyne) MNAMS FICOG FICMU FICMCH
Senior Consultant in Obstetrician and Gynecologist
Jeevan Jyoti Hospital and Medical Research Centre
Jeevan Jyoti Test Tube Baby Centre
Gorakhpur, Uttar Pradesh, India
Organizing Chairperson, FOGSI Saving Mothers
Conference 2016, 2019
Vice President, FOGSI (2016)
FOGSI Representative, SAFOG (2018–2020)
Corresponding National Editor Jr Obs Gyn India
(2017–2019)

Pratima Mittal
MD FICOG FICMCH
Ex-Professor and HOD
Department of Obstetrics and Gynecology
Vardhman Mahavir Medical College and
Safdarjung Hospital
New Delhi, India

Ruchika Garg
MD MRCOG1 FICOG FICMCH FMAS MAMS CIMP
Professor
Department of Obstetrics and Gynecology
SN Medical College, Agra, Uttar Pradesh, India
Joint Editor, Journal of SAFOG
Associate Editor, Journal of Midlife Health

Foreword
CN Purandare

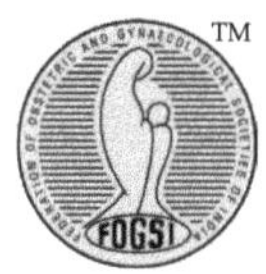

Federation of Obstetric and Gynaecological Societies of India (FOGSI)

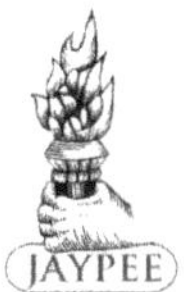

JAYPEE BROTHERS MEDICAL PUBLISHERS
The Health Sciences Publisher
New Delhi | London

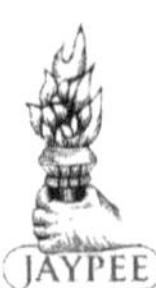 **Jaypee Brothers Medical Publishers (P) Ltd**

Headquarters

Jaypee Brothers Medical Publishers (P) Ltd
EMCA House, 23/23-B
Ansari Road, Daryaganj
New Delhi 110 002, India
Landline: +91-11-23272143, +91-11-23272703
+91-11-23282021, +91-11-23245672
Email: jaypee@jaypeebrothers.com

Corporate Office

Jaypee Brothers Medical Publishers (P) Ltd
4838/24, Ansari Road, Daryaganj
New Delhi 110 002, India
Phone: +91-11-43574357
Fax: +91-11-43574314
Email: jaypee@jaypeebrothers.com

Overseas Office

JP Medical Ltd
83 Victoria Street, London
SW1H 0HW (UK)
Phone: +44 20 3170 8910
Fax: +44 (0)20 3008 6180
Email: info@jpmedpub.com

Website: www.jaypeebrothers.com
Website: www.jaypeedigital.com

FOGSI Handbook of Antenatal Care

First Edition: **2022**

ISBN: 978-93-89188-79-0

Printed at:

Dedication
*To all Practitioner who are interested in
learning obstetrics.*

Contributors

Aanchal Sablok
Abha Rani Sinha
Alka Kriplani
Alpesh Gandhi
Ameya Purandare
Anita Kaul
Anuradha Tiberawal
Archana Patil
Arup Kumar Majhi
Asis Kumar Mukhopadhyay
Asmita Kaundal
Aswath Kumar
Baseerat Kaur
Charmila Ayyavoo
Chinmayee Ratha
Fessy Louis T
Garima Kachhawa
Girija Wagh
Gorakh G Mandrupkar
Janki Munjal Pandya
Jayprakash Shah
Jeetika
K Aparna Sharma
Kawita Bapat
Madhuri Chandra
Mala Arora
Mandakini Pradhan
Monika Gupta
Monu Singh
Mousumi Das Ghosh
Nandita Palshetkar

Neha Agarwal
Nidhi Nagar
Parth Shah
Parul Kotdawala
Parvathy T
Phagun Shah
Prabhat Agrawal
Prashant Achari
Pratik Tambe
Pratima Mittal
Preeti Deshpande
Priti Kumar
Rajendra Singh Pardeshi
Reshma Joy
Richa Singh
Rohan Palshetkar
Ruchika Garg
Sadhana Gupta
Sarita Agrawal
Saroj Singh
Sebanti Goswami
Seema Hakim
Semanti Bose
Shelly Agarwal
Shobha N Gudi
Sneha Bhuriyar
Sumitra Bachani
Susheela Rani
Tushar Kar
Urvashi Verma
Vidya Thobbi

Editorial Message

The health of women and children is an unfinished agenda and a global challenge. The importance of antenatal care (ANC) cannot be underestimated. The ANC in our country is lacking in many areas. In order to reach the Sustainable Development Goals (SDGs), efforts are needed to increase ANC at every level.

This is a comprehensive handbook covering all aspects of ANC—starting history of ANC to changing pyramid of ANC. Current recommendations for screening and imaging of ANC have been covered in a very comprehensive manner. From the management of common pregnancy ailments to high-risk conditions, all have been discussed taking in account current guidelines and latest treatment strategies. Preventive ANC is a very important aspect of antenatal care. Vaccination in pregnancy and screening for various conditions have been described in a very lucid style. Supporting images will be of great help to the readers. We have brought out this handbook to help postgraduate students, consultants, and busy practitioners to keep abreast with the newer recommendations for the ANC. We congratulate all the authors for bringing out the best and contributing for this book.

We are very happy to release this Handbook at the FOGSI Saving Mothers Conference, Gorakhpur, Uttar Pradesh, India.

Happy reading!

Nandita Palshetkar
Rohan Palshetkar
Sadhana Gupta
Pratima Mittal
Ruchika Garg

President's Message

We have to bear in mind that we are all debtors to the world and world does not owe us anything. It is a great privilege for all of us to be allowed to do anything for the world. In helping the world, we really help ourselves.

Do not look back–forward, infinite energy, infinite enthusiasm, infinite daring, and patience—then alone can great deeds be accomplished.

—Swami Vivekananda

The goal of antenatal care (ANC) package is to prepare for the birth and parenthood and to prevent, detect, and manage pre-existing conditions that worsen during pregnancy. In developed countries, more than 95% women have access to ANC, but it is not so in our country. ANC visits provide opportunities to promote lasting health and offering benefits that continue beyond the pregnancy care. By focusing on this very important issue, we can bring significant improvement in maternal and newborn health. Keeping in spirit with the theme of the year, "We for Stree—safer and stronger".

It gives me intense pleasure to release this *FOGSI Handbook of Antenatal Care* at the Saving Mothers Conference, Gorakhpur, Uttar Pradesh, India. My Co-editors, Former Vice President, FOGSI Dr Sadhana Gupta; Former Vice President, FOGSI Dr Pratima Mittal; and Ruchika Garg have also worked very hard to bring out this handbook with the latest guidelines and current treatment protocols. This handbook will be a great help to the fellow gynecologists to get updated on ANC of pregnant women.

Nandita Palshetkar

Foreword

It is a moment of great pleasure to recommend this *FOGSI Handbook of Antenatal Care* edited by Dr Nandita Palshetkar, Co-editors Dr Sadhana Gupta; Pratima Mittal; and Ruchika Garg. All the stalworths in obstetrics have contributed to this handbook. This handbook covers all aspects of antenatal care (ANC) from screening, imaging, and management of common ailments to promotive ANC covering nutrition and vaccination in pregnancy. Prescribing in pregnancy covers principles of prescribing during pregnancy. High-risk obstetrics such as hypertension and Rh-negative pregnancy have been discussed with the newer developments. Chapters on birth preparedness and respectful maternity care are the newer dimension in obstetrics. It is a must book with latest guidelines and recommendations for all the practicing obstetricians, who want to keep themselves abreast. The images and illustrations will be very helpful to the readers.

It is a ready reckoner for our fellow colleagues.

CN Purandare

Every Clinician caring for pregnant mother encounters women with many common situations for managing antenatal cases. We congratulate all authors who have contributed and have written all the latest recommendations and are very experienced in their fields.

This book is an easy-to-use, and ready reference guide. All the chapters reflect current evidence to support management strategies for medical disorders in pregnancy. This book will help postgraduate students and practitioners as it fuels an interest and thirst for knowledge in the field of obstetrics. It is a must guide for midwives, obstetricians and trainees preparing for MRCOG Part 2, DNB part 2, NEET PG etc. Many multiple choice questions have been added.

We are happy to recommend this book in all libraries and currently this book is one of the best and latest book on Antenatal situations. Readers will definitely be benefitted from this book and will not have to search internet for any other query related to this.

Nandita Palshetkar
Rohan Palshetkar
Sadhana Gupta
Pratima Mittal
Ruchika Garg

Acknowledgments

We are extremely thankful to Shri Jitendar P Vij (Group Chairman), Mr Ankit Vij (Managing Director), Mr MS Mani (Group President), Ms Chetna Malhotra (Senior Director – Professional Publishing, Marketing and Business Development), Ms Pooja Bhandari (Production Head), and Ms Kritika Dua (Senior Development Editor) of M/s Jaypee Brothers Medical Publishers (P) Ltd, New Delhi, India, for giving the go-ahead at the very beginning and helping us in every way possible to bring out this book.

Contents

Section 8: Social Obstetrics

Section 9: 21st Century Antenatal Care: Special Issues in Special Times

Changing Times in Antenatal Care

Changing Trends of Antenatal Care

Richa Singh

INTRODUCTION

Today, the form of healthcare in the world is changing from therapeutic to preventive. Antenatal care (ANC) is a type of preventive healthcare for mother. Now, it is being proved that the health, genetics, and constitution of baby are determined from health status and mental health of mother at the time of conception. So, the importance of prenatal care evolved in present century.

This is in absolute contrast to what happened many years ago in the times of our great-great-grandparents when giving birth was a natural phenomenon, which did not require any medical assistance. The local Dais acted as traditional birth attendant and it was passed as a skill down the generations. No practices of sterilization were followed. Intrapartum complications such as malpresentation, prolonged labor, and postpartum complications such as retained placenta and postpartum hemorrhage were dealt by these dais in their own manner resulting in high maternal and perinatal mortality.

India may be the only country where motherhood and mother is valued as power, eternal force, and service of life. "Ayurveda", the oldest system of medicine in India, defines obstetrics as a separate branch and advises precisely about diet, nutrition, rest, daily routine, and precautions in pregnancy. Many scripts of Vedic period tell the story of empowered and healthy mother of many children. Scripts from 12th to 15th century show a decline in women's status and health.

With the emergence of East India Company came the changes in medicine to form an organized medical system. Many radical acts and rules for women empowerment were made with initiative of visionary leaders in Indian renaissance such as Raja Ram Mohan Roy, Gopal Krishna Gokhale, and Mahatma Gandhi.

Before independence, initiatives taken for ANC for Indian women were:
- Establishment of Dufferin hospitals to provide medical care to pregnant women in 1885.
- Lady Hardinge Medical School was set up train female health visitors in 1918.

- Lady Chelmsford League was found in India for developing maternal welfare services in 1921.
- In 1946, Bhore Committee gave an important statement for women health that maternal deaths were preventable with the help of organized health services. This was perhaps the beginning of the idea of primary and universal healthcare and primary health centers were set up all over India for this purpose.
- In 1977, multipurpose health workers were made to provide ANC door to door.

Janani Suraksha Yojana launched in 2005 by National Health Mission has brought about a revolutionary change in ANC and institutional deliveries. ASHA (the accredited social health activist) is now working as an effective link between government and poor pregnant women for providing services.

Antenatal care was developed with a vision:
- To promote and maintain maternal health during pregnancy.
- To keep an eye on the development of any high-risk factor and treat it at the earliest.
- To have the aim of reduction of maternal and fetal mortality and morbidity.

The achievement has been shown by decline in maternal mortality rate in India from 254 in 2004–06 to 212 in 2007–09 to 167 in 2011–13 to 130 in 2014–16, according to the sample registration system data released by the office of Registrar General of India.

In today's era with the discovery of a positive pregnancy test begins the journey of safe motherhood by regular consultations with the obstetrician.

The 2016 World Health Organization (WHO) ANC model aims to provide pregnant women with respectful, individualized, person-centered care at every contact and to ensure that each contact delivers effective and integrated clinical practices, provides relevant and timely information, and offers psychosocial and emotional support by practitioners with good clinical and interpersonal skills working in a well-functioning health system.

2016 WHO ANC model:
- *First trimester: Contact 1*: Up to 12 weeks
- *Second trimester*:
    - *Contact 2*: 20 weeks
    - *Contact 3*: 26 weeks
- *Third trimester*:
    - *Contact 4*: 30 weeks
    - *Contact 5*: 34 weeks
    - *Contact 6*: 36 weeks
    - *Contact 7*: 38 weeks
    - *Contact 8*: 40 weeks

Return for delivery at 41 weeks, if not given birth.

■ KEY MESSAGE

The comprehensive antenatal program involves a coordinated approach to provide critical care and psychosocial support to a pregnant woman. It should ideally begin before conception and should extend throughout pregnancy and delivery.

■ SUGGESTED READING

1. Kumari N, Sharma S, Gupta P. Midwifery and gynaecological nursing. Jalandhar, Punjab, India; S Vikas and company (Medical Publishers); 2010.
2. World Health Organization (2006). Jump up the newsletter of the partnership for maternal, newborn and child health. 2nd Jan, 2006. ISSN 1815-9184. [online] Available from: https://www.who.int/pmnch/media/lives/lives_newsletter_2006_2_english.pdf. [Last accessed May, 2020].
3. World Health Organization; USAID; Maternal and Child Survival Program (2018). WHO recommendations on antenatal care for a positive pregnancy experience: Summary. [online] Available from: https://apps.who.int/iris/bitstream/handle/10665/259947/WHO-RHR-18.02-eng.pdf;jsessionid=D70CB40A68DB588F9CD2B696FB59EAD9?sequence=1. [Last accessed May, 2020].

Aim and Structure of Antenatal Care in Developing World

Rohan Palshetkar, Jeetika

◼ INTRODUCTION

Pregnancy and childbirth delivery and menopause are natural and normal events in the life of a woman. Almost around 60–70% of childbirths and pregnancies happen naturally but still there are a few, around 20%, births and pregnancies, which are associated with complications.

A few of these complications may be life threatening for the mother and baby or for both.

Antenatal care (ANC), monitoring, and institutional delivery are of utmost importance in early detection and for appropriate and timely management of such complications. Through various government organizations (National Rural Health Mission/Reproductive and Child Health-II program, policies, and NGOs), India is on verge of best provision of ANC by universal coverage of all births with skilled attendance, both at the institutional and at community level, by providing access to emergency obstetric and neonatal care services for women and newborns, and thereby restrict the number of maternal and newborn deaths in the country.

Maternal death is defined as the death of a woman while pregnant or within 42 days of the termination of pregnancy (delivery or abortion), irrespective of the duration and site of pregnancy, from any cause related to or aggravated by pregnancy or its management, but not due to accidents, trauma, or incidental causes.

The maternal mortality ratio (MMR) is defined as the number of maternal deaths per 100,000 live births, which, in India, is very high. The five major direct obstetric causes of maternal mortality in India are hemorrhage, puerperal sepsis, hypertensive disorders of pregnancy, obstructed labor, and unsafe abortions and contribute to about 70% of maternal deaths in the country. The time of childbirth and the period immediately after birth are particularly critical and very important for maternal, fetal, and neonatal survival and well-being. Fetal and neonatal complications such as preterm birth, birth asphyxia, intrapartum-related neonatal death, and neonatal infections together are responsible for more than 85% of neonatal mortality and morbidity.

Maternal anemia is a major contributor to the "indirect" obstetric causes. While most of these causes cannot be reliably predicted, early detection and timely management can save most of these lives.

Women below the age of 18 years or above 40 years have greater chances of having pregnancy-related complications. Primigravidas and grand multiparas (those who have had four or more pregnancies) are at a higher risk of developing complications during pregnancy and labor.

To combat maternal mortality, few points and measures are to be taken into account such as awareness of the danger signs in pregnancy, early ANC registrations, institutional deliveries, easy accessibility to healthcare services, quick treatment options and provisions, management of emergencies, availability of necessary and lifesaving drugs, blood banks, tertiary care centers, ICU, neonatal intensive care unit (NICU), trained staff and healthcare providers.

The health workers—staff nurses, lady health visitors and auxiliary nurse midwives (ANMs), skilled birth attendant, medical officers—have a very important role to play in reducing the MMR by providing definitive ANC and postnatal care, identifying complications, and referring ANC patients with complications after basic management to tertiary care center for further management.

Antenatal care is the care of the women and fetus in pregnancy before delivery and labor.

A properly devised antenatal follow-up provides necessary care to the mother and helps to identify complications of pregnancy such as anemia, pre-eclampsia, and hypertension, diabetes, etc. in the mother and slow inadequate growth of the fetus.

Antenatal care helps in the timely management of complications by referring patient to tertiary care center for further treatment. It also provides chance and time for making decisions and deciding plan of action, mode of delivery, facilities, and to make necessary arrangements if required.

Primary steps:
- *Early registration within first 3 months of pregnancy:*
  At least four antenatal check-ups (including the first visit for registration)—
  - *1st visit:* Within 12 weeks—preferably as soon as pregnancy is suspected.
  - *2nd visit:* Between 14 and 26 weeks
  - *3rd visit:* Between 28 and 34 weeks
  - *4th visit:* Between 36 weeks and term
- Starting folic acid supplements in first visit
- Administer two doses of tetanus toxoid (TT) injection.

Essential components of every antenatal check-up:
- Take the patient's detailed history, which includes personal details, family history, addiction, medical and surgical history, and any major illness in patient and in family.
- Conduct a physical examination—measure the weight, blood pressure, and respiratory rate and check for pallor and edema. This helps to record

the baseline parameters and which will be easy to compare for further pregnancy care.

- Conduct abdominal palpation for fetal growth, fetal lie, and auscultation of fetal heart sound according to the stage of pregnancy.
- Carry out laboratory investigations such as hemoglobin estimation and urine tests (for sugar and proteins), blood group, including the Rh factor.
- Blood tests for Venereal Disease Research Laboratory/rapid plasma reagin test to rule out syphilis.
- Test for human immunodeficiency virus (HIV), hepatitis B surface antigen (HBsAg), and hepatitis C.
- Check the blood sugar, which includes fasting tests, postprandial test, and glycosylated hemoglobin.
- Counsel the woman to plan and prepare for birth (birth preparedness/ microbirth plan). This should include deciding on the place of delivery and the presence of an attendant at the time of the delivery.
- Awareness about the benefits and necessity of institutional deliveries and risks involved in home deliveries.
- Awareness about the danger and emergency signs not only to the pregnant woman but also to the husband and family members during the antenatal care and where to go if an emergency arises, and how to arrange for transportation, money, and blood donors in case of an emergency.
- Dietary advice, nutrition, antenatal exercise, importance of breastfeeding for both mother and the child, and information on sex during pregnancy.
- Warn against domestic violence (explain the consequences of violence on a pregnant woman and her fetus).
- Provide family planning options and alternatives.

SYMPTOMS DURING PREGNANCY

Women must be asked for following symptoms and we should be able to distinguish between those indicating chances of high-risk pregnancy and complications in pregnancy, which may need necessary intervention.

Symptoms indicating discomfort may include nausea and vomiting, heartburn, constipation, and increased frequency of urination.

Symptoms indicating complications include fever, persistent vomiting, abnormal vaginal discharge/itching, palpitations, easy fatigability, breathlessness at rest/on mild exertion, generalized swelling of the body, puffiness of the face, severe headache, blurring of vision, frequent urination, burning sensation during micturition, vaginal bleeding, decreased or absent fetal movement, and leaking of watery fluid per vaginam.

One should try and gather past and previous pregnancy details such as the number of previous pregnancies and childbirths (birth weight/live births/stillbirth/neonatal mortality and morbidity/NICU admission for the baby/preterm deliveries/cervical encerclage).

Certain women with history of body mass index of greater than 30 kg/m^2, previous gestational diabetes mellitus (GDM), previous macrosomia, family are high risk for development of GDM, history of diabetes mellitus, and ethnicity with a high prevalence of diabetes mellitus.

A systematic review of cohort studies shows that women with hyperglycemia (diabetes mellitus and GDM) detected during pregnancy are at greater risk of adverse pregnancy outcomes, including macrosomia, pre-eclampsia/hypertensive disorders in pregnancy, and shoulder dystocia.

Usually diagnosis is done between 24 and 28 weeks of gestation. The glycosuria at dipstick test along with 2 hour 75 g oral glucose tolerance test is the key diagnostic test for GDM. The management differs according to the gestational age and the levels of sugars. Lifestyle changes (nutritional counseling and exercise) followed by oral blood–glucose-lowering agents or insulin, if necessary, are usually considered as treatment options for patients with GDM. This helps in improving the poor outcomes in the patients.

Mode of delivery along with information on instrumental delivery, obtain information about any obstetric complications and events in the previous pregnancies. Make a note of presence of following complications such as recurrent early abortion, post-abortion complications, hypertension, pre-eclampsia or eclampsia, antepartum hemorrhage, breech or transverse presentation, obstructed labor, including dystocia, perineal injuries/tears, excessive bleeding after delivery, and puerperal sepsis. Ask for a history of blood transfusions and ICU admission plays a very important role.

History of any current medical disorders/past history of illness should be noted. The medical disorders include high blood pressure (hypertension), diabetes, breathlessness on exertion, palpitations (heart disease), chronic cough, blood in the sputum, prolonged fever (tuberculosis), renal disease, convulsions (epilepsy), attacks of breathlessness or asthma, jaundice, malaria, and other illnesses, e.g., reproductive tract infection, sexually transmitted infection and HIV/AIDS, and hepatitis.

▓ IRON AND FOLIC ACID SUPPLEMENTATION

Folic acid plays a very important role in prevention of neural tube defects.

Prophylactic Dose

All pregnant women need to be given one tablet of iron and folic acid (IFA) (100 mg elemental iron and 0.5 mg folic acid) every day for 9 months, starting after the first trimester, at 12–13 weeks of gestation. This is the dose of IFA given to prevent anemia (prophylactic dose). This dosage regimen is to be repeated for 3 months post-partum. If a woman is anemic (hemoglobin < 11 g/dL) or has pallor, she needs two IFA tablets per day. Levels of hemoglobin and iron studies should be done to decide the dosage of iron in pregnancy. Women with severe anemia (hemoglobin of <7 g/dL), or those who have breathlessness and tachycardia (pulse rate of >100 beats per minute) due to anemia should be treated vigorously with parenteral iron preparations and, if required, blood transfusion depending on the gestational age. Proper counseling about the need and importance of iron preparations and about the side effects should be done before starting the supplementations.

CALCIUM SUPPLEMENTATION IN PREGNANT WOMEN

- Dietary counseling of pregnant women should promote adequate calcium intake through locally available, calcium-rich foods should be done.
- The dose of calcium should be divided, which may improve acceptability. The suggested dosage for calcium supplementation is 1.5–2 g daily, with the total dose divided into three doses, preferably after meals.
- Negative interactions between iron and calcium supplements may occur. Therefore, the two supplements should preferably be administered several hours apart rather than concomitantly. There is some evidence of additional benefit of multivitamin supplements containing 13–15 different micronutrients (including iron and folic acid) over IFA supplements alone.

  Pregnant women should be guided that sunlight is the most important source of vitamin D. The amount of time needed in the sun is not known and depends on many variables, such as the amount of skin exposed, the time of day, latitude and season, skin pigmentation (darker skin pigments synthesize less vitamin D than lighter pigments), and sunscreen use. The recommended dose is 200 IU per day in pregnancy, which can be combined with calcium supplements.
- Healthy food and balanced diet are the most important components for the nutrition in pregnancy. Diet counseling plays a very important role during all visits in ANC care.

STRUCTURE OF ANTENATAL CARE

Two doses of TT should be given to all patients in ANC period at 16 weeks and 20 weeks. According to WHO guidelines, first dose of TT should be given at the first visit of patient to the ANC clinic. Women should get the TT, reduced diphtheria toxoid, and acellular pertussis vaccine (T-dap) during each pregnancy. All pregnant women should get a T-dap shot in the third trimester, preferably between 27 and 36 weeks of pregnancy. T-dap can be administered with in 1 week postpartum if not given in ANC (please note that T-dap given postpartum does not provide immunity to child).

Micro-birth planning is very essential component of ANC care in developing countries like India. Note of following points is recommended:

- Registration of pregnant woman, gathering important documents and filling up of the Maternal and Child Protection Card and Janani Suraksha Yojana card/below poverty line certificates/necessary proofs or certificates for the purpose of keeping a record.

- Making chart and card stating the woman about the dates of antenatal visits, schedule for TT injections and the estimated date of delivery (EDD).
- Identifying the place of delivery, mode of delivery, and the person who would conduct the delivery.
- Identifying a referral facility and the mode of referral.
- Taking the necessary steps to arrange for transport of the pregnant women and the attendant.
- Making sure that funds are available to the ANM/ASHA.

First Trimester Care

- Registration of patient with personal details and provide health education and health promotion.
- *History*: Menstrual and contraceptive history, present pregnancy, obstetric history, medical history, surgical and social history, infection history, genetics history, immunization status, addiction, patient safety, and domestic violence.
- Calculate EDD/gestational age by last menstrual period (LMP) and physical examination.
- *Physical examination*: General well-being, vital signs/blood pressure, pulse, conjunctiva, palms, breasts, abdomen, uterine size, extremities, and external genitalia.
- *Basic blood investigations*: Hemoglobin (hemoglobin color scale), urine protein (test strip), syphilis and HIV, hepatitis B (if test strip available), hepatitis C virus, screening test for thalassemia, and hemoglobinopathies.
- Obstetric ultrasound scan in first trimester on first visit. Prior to 24 weeks (preferably in 1st trimester) when LMP is unknown or uterine size is abnormal for gestational week.
- *Testing at hospital level*: Full blood count, ABO group and Rhesus, urine protein (test strip), syphilis and HIV, hepatitis B (if test strip available), and microscopic urine examination as necessary.

First Trimester Screening

All patients should be offered aneuploidy screening. The main role of first trimester maternal serum screening programs is to identify women at increased risk of having a baby with Down's syndrome, Patau's syndrome, and Edward syndrome defects and those that will benefit from the testing.

First trimester screen is a screening test and not a diagnostic test and it is very important to make a note and explain to patients. This test only indicates whether mother is at risk of carrying a baby with a genetic disorder and whether further genetic (invasive) testing is required. It includes maternal serum-free beta human chorionic gonadotropin (β-hCG) and PAPP-A at 11–12 weeks and then fetal NT/NB scan at 12–14 weeks. It was first reported by Schulte-Valentine and Schindler in 1992. Nuchal traslucency (NT) measures the subcutaneous fluid-filled space between the back of the spine and the skin in the fetal neck. NT increases with gestational age at the rate 17% a week. The translucent area disappears after 14 weeks of gestational age, when the subcutaneous tissue becomes more echogenic. NT is therefore a transient phenomenon. It can show 5% false-positive rate. This sonography should be combined with dual marker blood report to complete the first trimester screening.

In addition, those women identified as high risk for preterm birth would also have first trimester measurement of cervical length, a uterine artery Doppler and mean arterial blood pressure would be used to check for risk of impaired placentation, which are relevant for prediction of both pre-eclampsia and fetal growth restriction.

Dual Marker Test

The test involves two markers in combination with maternal age, specifically PAPP-A, and free β-hCG. Some women whose results show a "high risk" for screening are given options of amniocentesis or chorionic villus sampling (CVS).

High risk for aneuploidy as indicated by one of the following:
- Advanced maternal age (35 years or older at expected time of delivery).
- Previous pregnancy affected with a trisomy.
- Positive conventional prenatal screening test (integrated or PRS).
- Fetal ultrasound findings indicating an elevated risk of aneuploidy.
- Previously identified chromosome 21, 18, or 13 translocation in self or partner.

The Role of Noninvasive Prenatal Testing

The most commonly used test for genetic diagnosis is amniocentesis, but the rate of spontaneous fetal loss related to amniocentesis averages about one in every 200 procedures. Because of this risk, serum analyte testing has become an important, noninvasive first step in detecting patients at risk for congenital abnormalities. Patients at increased risk of aneuploidy can be offered testing with cell-free DNA (also called cell-free fetal DNA, or noninvasive prenatal testing). This technology has approximately 99% sensitivity and specificity with a false-positive rate of less than 0.5%. The screening test provides information on the most common aneuploidies—trisomy 21, 18, and 13. This test can also detect monosomy X and sex chromosome aneuploidies. Because false-positive results can occur, confirmation by amniocentesis or CVS is recommended.

Detailed counseling before and after the cell-free DNA screening test is recommended.
- It is not diagnostic test and has high sensitivity and specificity.
- Positive results should be followed up with an invasive diagnostic test (amniocentesis or CVS).

- Negative ("normal") results do not guarantee a chromosomally normal fetus.
- The test will only screen for the common trisomies and monosomy X. It does not include risk assessment for neural tube defects or for other structural or developmental anomalies.

Second Trimester Screening

The quadruple screen test is a blood test done during pregnancy. It is most accurate between the 16th and 18th weeks. The test measures levels of four pregnancy hormones: α-fetoprotein, hCG, unconjugated estriol (uE3), and inhibin A. The higher value has high risk of chromosomal abnormalities and is indication for the invasive genetic screening.

Invasive diagnostic tests for follow-up of any positive screening result:
- *Chorionic villus sampling*: Women at increased risk for genetic birth defects such as aneuploidy and inherited disorders due to advanced maternal age, family history, or abnormal first trimester screening, and is performed at 10–13 weeks of pregnancy.
- *Amniocentesis*: Women at increased risk for genetic birth defects such as aneuploidy and inherited disorders, neural tube defects due to advanced maternal age, family history, or abnormal first trimester screening and is performed at 15–20 weeks of pregnancy.

Additional testing that may be ordered by the fetal medicine specialist includes:
- *Fluorescence in situ hybridization (FISH)* provides information on chromosomes 21, 18, and 13, sex chromosomes, and specific micro-deletion/duplication syndromes, which may be suspected on certain ultrasound findings.
- *Microarray* detects genomic imbalances that may account for abnormal ultrasound findings that do not follow a specific pattern. Parental studies may be needed to interpret uncertain microarray results.
- *Mendelian disorders testing* may be offered based on a pattern of specific ultrasound findings.

Ultrasound (18–22 Weeks)

The second trimester ultrasound is designed to detect structural anomalies and growth. Structural anomalies should be followed up by a referral for high-resolution ultrasound and/or maternal–fetal medicine consultation by a specialist for confirmation, consultation, and discussion of risks/available testing options/therapeutic options.

Cardiac scan with color Doppler at 22–24 weeks is done for the detailed heart evaluation.

Third Trimester Monitoring

Blood investigation including complete blood counts, liver function tests, kidney function tests, thyroid profile, blood sugars, and urine routine tests is done at 32–34 weeks especially in high-risk cases of eclampsia and pre-eclampsia. Ultrasound with color Doppler and biophysical profile (BPP) are done to see the interval growth, placental position, fetal weight, blood flows, and the presence of resistance.

Role of Biophysical Profile (Table 1)

It consists of nonstress test (NST) combined with four observations made by real-time ultrasonography.

Each of the five areas of the BPP has a possible total score of two points, for a total of 10 points. A score of:

- Eight to ten is usually considered normal.
- Six is considered equivocal (uncertain).
- Four or less is considered abnormal.

TABLE 1: Biophysical profile.		
Fetal variable	*Normal behavior (score = 2)*	*Abnormal behavior (score = 0)*
Fetal breathing movements	One or more episodes of more than 30 seconds duration, within 30 minutes BPP time frame Hiccups count	Completely absent breathing or no sustained episodes Continuous breathing without cessation
Body or limb movements	At least three discrete body or limb movements in 30 minutes Includes fine motor movements, rolling movements, but not REM or mouthing movements	Three or fewer body/limb movements in a 30 minutes observation period
Fetal tone/ posture	One or more episodes of active extension with rapid return to flexion of fetal limbs and brisk repositioning/ truck rotation. Opening and closing of hand, mouth, and kicking	Low-velocity movement only Incomplete flexion, flaccid extremity positions, abnormal fetal posture. Must score = 0 when FM completely absent
Amniotic fluid evaluation	At least one pocket ≥2 cm with no umbilical cord. Also consider criteria for subjectively reduced fluid	No cord-free pocket ≥2 cm, or multiple elements of subjectively reduced amniotic fluid volume definite
Nonstress test (NST)	At least two episodes of fetal acceleration of ≥15 beats/min and of ≥15-second duration. Normal mean variation (computerized FHR interpretation), accelerations associated with maternal palpation of FM (accelerations graded for gestation	Fetal movements and accelerations not coupled Insufficient accelerations, absent accelerations, or decelerative trace. Mean variation <20 on numerical analysis of NST

(BPP: biophysical profile; FHR: fetal heart rate; FM: fetal movement; REM: rapid eye movement)

Mode of Delivery

About 36–38 weeks per vaginal examination of the patient should be done to decide the mode of delivery. Necessary arrangements and referrals should be done according to the need.

SUGGESTED READING

1. American college of Obstetrics & Gynaecologists; Centers for disease control & Prevention. 2019.
2. Dunn J, Guideline Oversight Group. Prenatal Care Guideline. 2018.
3. Güdücü N, Görmüş U, Güner EI, Güzel O, Kavak ZN. Quadruple test parameters in art pregnancies. Int J Clin Exp Med. 2014;7(8):2319-23.
4. Müller F, Dreux S, Lemeur A, Sault C, Desgrès J, Bernard MA, et al. Medically assisted reproduction and second-trimester maternal serum marker screening for Down's syndrome. Prenat Diagn. 2003;23(13):1073-6.
5. National Institute for Health and Care Excellence (2019). Antenatal care for uncomplicated pregnancies Clinical guideline [CG62]. [online] Available from: https://www.nice.org.uk/guidance/cg62. [Last accessed May, 2020].
6. Tunçalp Ö, Were WM, MacLennan C, Oladapo OT, Gülmezoglu AM, Bahl R, et al. Quality of care for pregnant women and newborns—the WHO vision. BJOG. 2015;122(8):1045-9.
7. Wilson RD. Amended Canadian Guideline for prenatal diagnosis (2005) change to 2005—techniques for prenatal diagnosis. SOGC Clinical Practice Guidelines, No. 168, November 2005. J Obstet Gynaecol Can. 2005;27(11):1048-54.
8. World Health Organization (2016). New guidelines on antenatal care for a positive pregnancy experience. [online] Available from: https://www.who.int/reproductivehealth/news/antenatal-care/en/. [Last accessed May, 2020].

Changing Pyramid of Antenatal Care

Monika Gupta, Monu Singh

INTRODUCTION

Antenatal care (ANC) is an essential part of maternal healthcare services. It comprises history taking, screening for maternal illnesses such as hypertensive disorders and anemia, screening, prevention and management of infectious diseases, provision of prophylactic medication and essential health education.[1] ANC has been considered essential for identification and early management of high-risk pregnancies as a means to improve pregnancy outcomes, which later was argued to have little predictive value for reduction of maternal mortality.[2-4] Global attention therefore shifted to emergency obstetric care and skilled care at birth as essential strategies to reduce maternal deaths.[5,6] Currently, however, it is globally accepted that while ANC alone is not sufficient to reduce morbidity and mortality, it remains an essential component in improving maternal and newborn health and well-being.[7,8]

EFFECTIVENESS OF ANTENATAL CARE

A number of studies have been conducted to identify essential interventions and required number of visits for ANC for establishing the evidence of effectiveness of ANC services.

Historically, the traditional ANC service model was developed in the early 1900s. This model assumes that frequent visits and classifying pregnant women into low and high risk by predicting the complications ahead of time are the best way to care for the mother and the fetus. The traditional approach was replaced by *focused antenatal care (FANC)*—a goal-oriented ANC approach, which was recommended by researchers in 2001 and adopted by the World Health Organization (WHO) in 2002.[9]

The FANC, as proposed by WHO, recommended a minimum of four visits for low-risk pregnancies with targeted interventions in each visit. FANC was meant to increase the quality of ANC and to ensure a positive pregnancy outcome. A reduction of the number of visits with targeted interventions in each visit to identify diseases and high-risk factors proved to be equally effective as monthly ANC visits.[10] One of the drawbacks of FANC was that the model was not tested in settings with low coverage of ANC visits and high-mortality ratios.[11] Recently, concerns have been raised that a reduced number of visits are associated with an increase in perinatal mortality.[12]

Current evidence shows that the FANC model is probably associated with more perinatal deaths than models that comprise at least eight ANC visits. Furthermore, literature suggests that more ANC visits, irrespective of the resource setting, are probably associated with greater maternal satisfaction than less ANC visits.

Consequently, the WHO updated their ANC guideline in 2016 aiming to provide women with a positive pregnancy experience and included a recommendation of a minimum of eight contacts.[13] The Guideline Development Group reviewed how ANC should be delivered in terms of both the timing and content of each of the ANC contacts, and arrived at a new model—the 2016 WHO ANC model, which replaces the previous four-visit focused ANC model.[14]

INVERTED PYRAMID OF ANTENATAL CARE: A NEW CONCEPT (FIGS. 1 AND 2)

Traditionally, it has always been believed that most of the problems and life-threatening complications develop during later half of the pregnancy and that is the reason why most of the ANC schedules have increased number of visits during second half of pregnancy. The frequency of visits increases with advancing gestation, reaching to weekly visits from 36 weeks onward. But recently, more importance is being given to maternal and fetal investigations during first trimester of pregnancy.

Professor Kypros Nicolaides from UK had developed a new concept of ANC, which focused on the very early weeks of pregnancy to identify

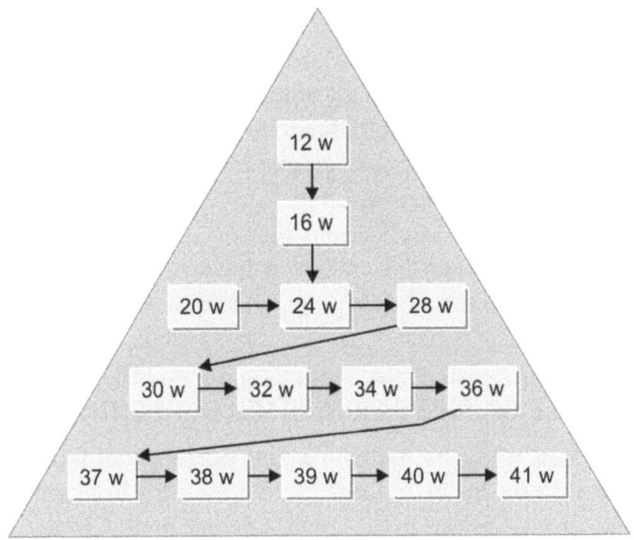

Fig. 1: Traditional pyramid of antenatal care.

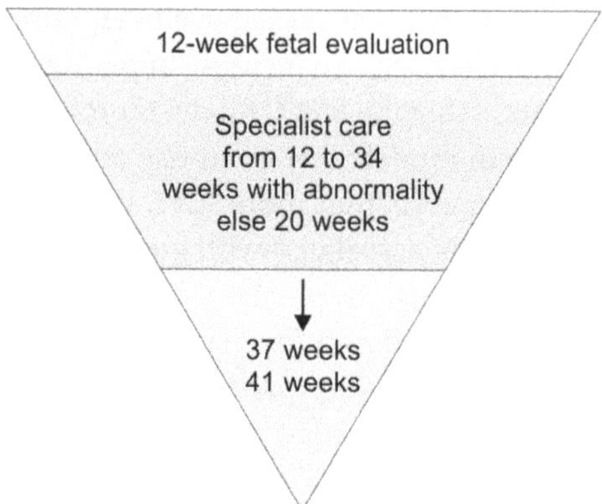

Fig. 2: Newer model of inverted pyramid of antenatal care.[16]
[*Source*: Adapted from Nicolaides KH. Turning the pyramid of prenatal care. Fetal Diagn Ther. 2011;29(3):183-96].

high-risk pregnancies.[15] According to this concept, a prenatal care plan can be developed that is suited to individual patients, by selecting pregnancies that are at the highest risk for complications, which become apparent only later in gestation and by identifying those that are at very low risk.

This inverted pyramid of care enables a much more patient and disease-specific approach of ANC.[16] The women who are identified to be at low risk in the beginning of pregnancy do not need such frequent and specialized ANC.

Thus, it was considered worthwhile to increase the focus of clinical evaluations in early pregnancy, thus, inverting the pyramid of prenatal care. The possibility of early identification of risk factors and detection of complications at 11–13 weeks of pregnancy enables effective treatment or even prevention of a disease.

This was possible due to increased use of ultrasound in the first trimester, which has revealed that many fetal structural problems can already be accurately diagnosed at this point.[17] Maternal serum biochemical screening in first trimester has also gained a lot of importance. Its use has now been expanded from screening of aneuploidies to predict pregnancy complications that become apparent only later on in pregnancy, such as pre-eclampsia (PE) and severe intrauterine growth restriction.[18]

Some very important complications that occur later in pregnancy can be predicted in the first trimester; therefore, it is worthwhile to increase the focus of clinical evaluations in early pregnancy, thus, inverting the pyramid of prenatal care.[19]

IMPORTANCE OF FIRST TRIMESTER SCREENING

The benefit of first trimester screening and diagnosis of fetal anomalies is that parents become aware of these conditions early in pregnancy when they can make their decisions in the greatest degree of privacy and when the treatment or termination is the least expensive and most safe, and also has minimal bearing on the emotional and mental health of the mother. This is also the ideal time for multidisciplinary care providers to intervene with health promotion activities and establish a baseline understanding of the pregnant woman's pre-existing health conditions.[15,20,21]

Fetal Aneuploidy Screening

First trimester screening helps in the diagnosis of fetal aneuploidy by combined screening [maternal age, history, gestational age, nuchal translucency (NT) measurement, and PAPP-A]. The detection rate of major aneuploidies is close to 99.3%, with a false positive rate of 0.11%, using certain maternal characteristics such as previous reproductive history, first trimester screening for aneuploidy, increased NT, the abnormal ductus venosus flow and low level of pregnancy associated plasma protein-A (PAPP-A).[22,23]

Screening the combined test can identify more than 90% of fetuses with trisomy 21. The detection rate of trisomies 18 and 13 is about 95% for the same false-positive rate.[24] The effectiveness of the first trimester combined screen can be further augmented by the addition of other biochemical markers, such as placental growth factor (PGF) and maternal serum α-fetoprotein and fetal markers such as nasal bone evaluation and Doppler evaluations of the ductus venosus and blood flow across the tricuspid valve.[24,25]

These additional ultrasound markers can be either obtained at the time of the combined screen or on a contingent basis. The contingent protocol acts on patients is divided into three categories based on the traditional combined screen—high risk (1:50), intermediate risk (1:51–1:1,000), and low risk (1:1,000). Patients in the high-risk category are offered an invasive procedure, and those in the low-risk category are reassured. Patients in the intermediate category then undergo stage-2 screening using the additional ultrasound markers. If the final risk assessment in this group is 1:100 or greater, an invasive test is offered. Those whose risk is less than 1:100 are reassured. The screening performance of both approaches is similar; the detection rate is approximately 93–96% for a 2.5% false-positive rate.[26]

Detection of Congenital Structural Defects

Even in absence of aneuploidy, it has been proven that an increased NT can be associated with a large variety of genetic syndromes and structural defects, such as diaphragmatic hernia, omphalocele, cleft lip/palate, skeletal defects, congenital adrenal hyperplasia, fetal akinesia deformation sequence, Noonan's syndrome, Smith–Lemli–Opitz syndrome, and spinal muscular atrophy.[27]

This risk increases significantly for fetuses with NT greater than 3.5 mm and reaching up to 50% for fetuses with an NT of 6.5 mm or greater. The overall detection rates of fetal anomalies in the first trimester can be as high as 51% and even higher (62–65%) in cases where both transabdominal and transvaginal ultrasound are used in cases with a thickened NT.[28]

As regards the open neural defects, the detection of anencephaly and spina bifida can be carried out in the first trimester itself by examination and measurements of intracranial translucency and the size of the brainstem in the sagittal section.[21]

Other markers that may prove helpful in detection of open neural tube defects are narrowing of the frontomaxillary angle, biparietal diameter (BPD) measurement less than the fifth percentile, or a small BPD to transabdominal diameter ratio.[29-31]

Markers such as tricuspid regurgitation (TR) and a reversed flow in the ductus venosus in first trimester screening have proved beneficial in predicting major fetal congenital heart defects. A combination of three markers (NT > 99th percentile, TR, and abnormal a-wave in ductus venosus) can result in a detection rate of 52% for congenital heart diseases.[32]

ASSESSMENT OF MULTIPLE GESTATIONS

First trimester screening is helpful in assessment of multiple gestations, detection of chorionicity and prediction of future complications. This allows accurate counseling regarding the risk involved in the pregnancy.

Also, it has been proposed that a significant difference between the NT measurements of the two fetuses in monochorionic twins or the presence of ductus venosus blood flow abnormalities may point toward an increased risk for Twin-to-twin transfusion syndrome.[33]

First trimester ultrasound evaluation in multiple gestations has especially gained importance, as the incidence of twins has increased significantly in the past few decades.

Prediction of other Fetomaternal Complications

The placental architecture and blood flow are well established by the end of first trimester and no further changes occur after 4th month, so complications like fetal growth restriction and PE arising out of poor placentation can be well predicted in advance and treatment and close follow-up can be instituted early. This is important because any treatment to be effective in reducing the risk of complications related to placental dysfunction must be started early in pregnancy before the complete placentation occurs.

Other additional markers, which have been recently extensively studied to predict PE, are—estimation of downstream resistance by measuring the pulsatility index (PI) in the uterine arteries Doppler, maternal blood pressure measurement in the late first trimester, and evaluation of certain placental product levels in maternal serum such as PAPP-A and PGF.[34]

Detection of early PE can be approximately 90% based only on historical factors, maternal blood pressure measurement, and uterine artery PI. The addition of biochemical markers such as PAPP-A and PGF levels increases the detection rates to 96%.[35]

Other Screening Protocols

Combination of markers such as serum PAPP-A, free beta human chorionic gonadotropin (β-hCG), PGF, placental protein 13 (PP13), and a disintegrin and metalloproteinase 12 (ADAM12) along with maternal characteristics can largely identify approximately small for gestational age fetuses, which required to be delivered before term.[36]

Cervical length measured transvaginally in combination with maternal characteristics can prove to be important in identifying high-risk group for preterm delivery that may benefit from close follow-up and possible treatment.[37]

Maternal serum biochemical markers such as adiponectin, sex hormone-binding globulin, and visfatin in combination with maternal characteristics can identify 75% of high-risk pregnancies to develop gestational diabetes mellitus.[38]

Also, increased values of NT measurement, levels of maternal serum free β-hCG and PAPP-A, and a decreased level of adiponectin can largely predict large for gestational age/macrosomic fetuses.[39]

■ CONCLUSION

A more intensive approach in the first trimester itself can be beneficial to detect future maternal and fetal complications and institute early treatment. Hence, an inverted pyramid of ANC was proposed to promote the intensified approach in first trimester.

The importance of ANC cannot be underestimated, it is important to reduce not only maternal mortality but also perinatal mortality. ANC coverage has been used globally to assess the efficiency of various maternal health programs. According to the WHO updated guidelines 2016, it has been changed to a minimum of eight contacts with the pregnant mother starting as early as 8–12 weeks. Emphasis should be laid on the initiation of ANC in the first trimester, which is also referred to as early ANC.

A greater emphasis should be on prevention, early identification, and timely interventions rather than dealing with complications. This philosophy has driven most advances in ANC.

Also, ANC should incorporate health promotion, prevention, screening, and detection of diseases. It should be more of a public health approach with involvement of the community itself. Early pregnancy evaluation not only benefits patients but also investment in data collection and improvement of data collection methods will help to implement a responsible public health policy.

■ FUTURE ASPECTS

With the advancement in medical science, the more appropriate approach would be an extended inverted pyramid for better results in perinatal medicine.[40]

The interventions focusing on the preconception and perimplantation periods are to be researched upon. The therapy can be envisaged to be applied at subcellular and genetic level by applying the latest biotechnological procedures.

REFERENCES

1. WHO; UNICEF; UNFPA; The World Bank and the United Nations Population Division. Trends in Maternal Mortality: 1990 to 2013. Geneva: World Health Organization; 2014.
2. Greenberg RS. The impact of prenatal care in different social groups. Am J Obstet Gynecol. 1983;145(7):797-801.
3. Fiscella K. Does prenatal care improve birth outcomes? A critical review. Obstet Gynecol. 1995;85(3):468-79.
4. Carroli G, Rooney C, Villar J. How effective is antenatal care in preventing maternal mortality and serious morbidity? An overview of the evidence. Paediatr Perinat Epidemiol. 2001;15(Suppl 1):1-42.
5. Yanagisawa S, Oum S, Wakai S. Determinants of skilled birth attendance in rural Cambodia. Trop Med Int Health. 2006;11(2):238-51.
6. Carroli G, Villar J, Piaggio G. WHO systematic review of randomized controlled trials of routine antenatal care. Lancet. 2001;357(9268):1565-70.
7. WHO; UNICEF. Antenatal care in the developing countries: Promises, achievements and missed opportunities. Analysis of trends, levels and differentials 1990-2001. Geneva: WHO; 2003.
8. Villar J, Ba'aqeel H, Piaggio G, Lumbiganon P, Miguel Belizán J, Farnot U, et al. WHO antenatal care randomised trial for the evaluation of a new model of routine antenatal care. Lancet. 2001;357(9268):1551-64.
9. World Health Organization (2002). WHO antenatal care randomized trial: manual for the implementation of the new model. [online] Available from: https://apps.who.int/iris/bitstream/handle/10665/42513/WHO_RHR_01.30.pdf?sequence=1&isAllowed=y. [Last accessed May, 2020].
10. World Health Organization. WHO handbook for guideline development, 2nd edition. Geneva: World Health Organization; 2014. [online] Available from: https://www.who.int/publications/guidelines/handbook_2nd_ed.pdf?ua=1. [Last accessed May, 2020].
11. von Both C, Flessa S, Makuwani A, Mpembeni R, Jahn A. How much time do health services spend on antenatal care? Implications for the introduction of the focused antenatal care model in Tanzania. BMC Pregnancy Childbirth. 2006;6:22.
12. Downe S, Finlayson K, Tunçalp Ö, Gülmezoglu AM. Factors that influence the provision of good quality routine antenatal care services by health staff: a qualitative evidence synthesis. Cochrane Database Syst Rev. 2017;(12):CD012752.
13. World Health Organization. WHO recommendations on antenatal care for a positive pregnancy experience. Geneva, Switzerland; WHO; 2016. [online] Available from: https://apps.who.int/iris/bitstream/handle/10665/250796/9789241549912-eng.pdf?sequence=1. [Last accessed May, 2020].
14. Gurol I, Scheel I. Adoption and implementation of ANC guidelines at large scale. Presentation at ANC guideline development group meeting (21–23 March). Geneva: World Health Organization; 2016.
15. Nicolaides KH. A model for a new pyramid of prenatal care based on the 11 to 13 weeks' assessment. Prenat Diagn. 2011;31(1):3-6.
16. Nicolaides KH. Turning the pyramid of prenatal care. Fetal Diagn Ther. 2011;29(3):183-96.
17. Syngelaki A, Chelemen T, Dagklis T, Allan L, Nicolaides KH. Challenges in the diagnosis of fetal non-chromosomal abnormalities at 11-13 weeks. Prenat Diagn. 2011;31(1):90-102.

18. Sharp AN, Alfirevic Z. First trimester screening can predict adverse pregnancy outcomes. Prenat Diagn. 2014;34(7):660-7.

19. Sonek JD, Kagan KO, Nicolaides KH. Inverted pyramid of care. Clin Lab Med. 2016;36:305-17.

20. Kagan KO, Anderson JM, Anwandter G, Neksasova K, Nicolaides KH. Screening for triploidy by the risk algorithms for trisomies 21, 18 and 13 at 11 weeks to 13 weeks and 6 days of gestation. Prenat Diagn. 2008;28(13):1209-13.

21. Chen FC, Gerhardt J, Entezami M, Chaoui R, Henrich W. Detection of spina bifida by first trimester screening–results of the prospective multicenter Berlin IT-study. Ultraschall in Med. 2017;38(02):151-7.

22. Kagan KO, Hoopmann M, Abele H, Alkier R, Lüthgens K. First-trimester combined screening for trisomy 21 with different combinations of placental growth factor, free b-human chorionic gonadotropin and pregnancy-associated plasma protein-A. Ultrasound Obstet Gynecol. 2012;40(5):530-5.

23. Sonek JD, Cuckle HS. What will be the role of first-trimester ultrasound if cell-free DNA screening for aneuploidy becomes routine? Ultrasound Obstet Gynecol. 2014;44(6):621-30.

24. Wright D, Syngelaki A, Bradbury I, Akolekar R, Nicolaides KH. First-trimester screening for trisomies 21, 18 and 13 by ultrasound and biochemical testing. Fetal Diagn Ther. 2014;35(2):118-26.

25. Maiz N, Wright D, Ferreira AF, Syngelaki A, Nicolaides KH. A mixture model of ductus venosus pulsatility index in screening for aneuploidies at 11-13 weeks' gestation. Fetal Diagn Ther. 2012;31(4):221-9.

26. Abele H, Wagner P, Sonek J, Hoopmann M, Brucker S, Artunc-Ulkumenet B, et al. First trimester ultrasound screening for Down syndrome based on maternal age, fetal nuchal translucency, and different combinations of the additional markers nasal bone, tricuspid and ductus venosus flow. Prenat Diagn. 2015;35(12):1182-6.

27. Timmerman E, Pajkrt E, Maas SM, Hoopmann M, Brucker S, Artunc-Ulkumen B, et al. Enlarged nuchal translucency in chromosomally normal fetuses: strong association with orofacial clefts. Ultrasound Obstet Gynecol. 2010;36(4):427-32.

28. Rossi AC, Prefumo F. Accuracy of ultrasonography at 11-14 weeks of gestation for detection of fetal structural anomalies: a systematic review. Obstet Gynecol. 2013;122(6):1160-7.

29. Lachmann R, Picciarelli G, Moratalla J, Greene N, Nicolaides NH. Frontomaxillary facial angle in fetuses with spina bifida at 11-13 weeks' gestation. Ultrasound Obstet Gynecol. 2010;36(3):268-71.

30. Khalil A, Coates A, Papageorghiou A, Bhide A, Thilaganathan B. Biparietal diameter at 11-13 weeks' gestation in fetuses with open spina bifida. Ultrasound Obstet Gynecol. 2013;42(4):409-15.

31. Simon EG, Arthuis CJ, Haddad G, Bertrand P, Perrotin F. Biparietal/transverse abdominal diameter ratio 1: potential marker for open spina bifida at 11-13-week scan. Ultrasound Obstet Gynecol. 2015;45:267-72.

32. Pereira S, Ganapathy R, Syngelaki A, Maiz N, Nicolaides KH. Contribution of fetal tricuspid regurgitation in first-trimester screening for major cardiac defects. Obstet Gynecol. 2011;117(6):1384-91.

33. Khalil A, Rodgers M, Baschat A, Bhide A, Gratacos E, Hecher K, et al. ISUOG practice guidelines: the role of ultrasound in twin pregnancy. Ultrasound Obstet Gynecol. 2016;47(2):247-63.

34. Velauthar L, Plana MN, Kalidindi M, Zamora J, Thilaganathan B, Illanes SE, et al. First-trimester uterine artery Doppler and adverse pregnancy outcome: a meta-analysis involving 55,974 women. Ultrasound Obstet Gynecol. 2014;43(5):500-7.

35. Park FJ, Leung CH, Poon LC, Williams PF, Rothwell SJ, Hyett JA. Clinical evaluation of a first trimester algorithm predicting the risk of hypertensive disease of pregnancy. Aust N Z J Obstet Gynaecol. 2013;53(6):532-9.

36. Poon LC, Karagiannis G, Staboulidou I, Shafiei A, Nicolaides KH. Reference range of birth weight with gestation and first-trimester prediction of small-for-gestation neonates. Prenat Diagn. 2011;31(1):58-65.

37. Retzke JD, Sonek JD, Lehmann J, Yazdi B, Kagan KO. Comparison of three methods of cervical measurement in the first trimester: single-line, two-line, and tracing. Prenat Diagn. 2013;33(3):262-8.

38. Ferreira AF, Rezende JC, Vaikousi E, Akolekar R, Nicolaides KH. Maternal serum visfatin at 11-13 weeks of gestation in gestational diabetes mellitus. Clin Chem. 2011;57(4):609-13.

39. Poon LC, Karagiannis G, Stratieva V, Akolekar R, Nicolaides KH. First-trimester prediction of macrosomia. Fetal Diagn Ther. 2011;29(2):139-47.

40. Ljubić A. Inverted pyramid of prenatal care – is it enough? Should it be – extended inverted pyramid of prenatal care? J Perinat Med. 2018;46(7):716-20.

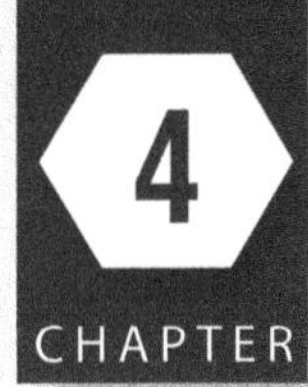

Preconceptional Care: A Review[#]

K Aparna Sharma, Alka Kriplani

INTRODUCTION

Preconceptional care (PCC) provides a window of opportunity to optimize the conditions in which the conception occurs to have a desirable maternal and fetal outcome.

EVIDENCE FOR PRECONCEPTIONAL CARE

Numerous studies reported that PCC substantially reduced the adverse pregnancy outcomes. Two large interventional studies aimed at improving maternal and perinatal care in India, witnessed positive outcomes.

COMPONENTS OF PRECONCEPTIONAL CARE

All the aspects of PCC need to be discussed under the broad categories of: *identify (pre-empt), educate (counsel), and intervene (cure)* **(Fig. 1)**.

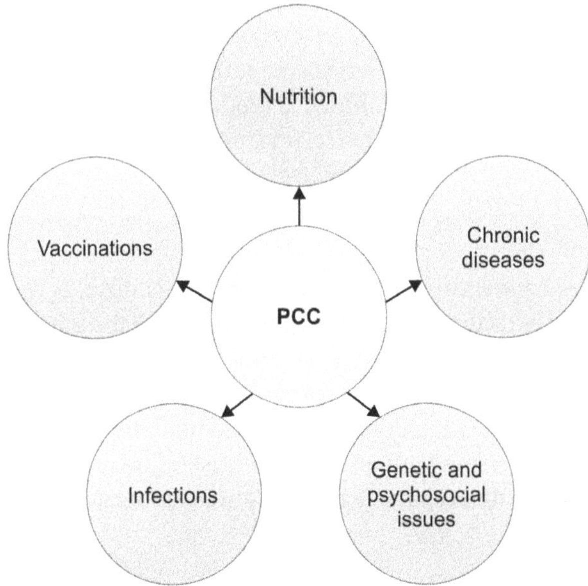

Fig. 1: The whorl of preconceptional care (PCC).

[#]The literature review for this document was conducted as a part of the formulation of FOGSI Good Clinical Practice Guidelines of Preconceptional Care and is available on: https://www.fogsi.org/gcpr-preconception-care/

NUTRITIONAL INTERVENTIONS IN PRECONCEPTIONAL CARE

Role of Folic Acid

Preconceptional folic acid (FA) intake is currently the classical example of a preconceptional intervention, which is known to have a profound impact on the fetal outcomes. Two landmark trials—(1) the Medical Research Council vitamin study and (2) the randomized controlled trial (RCT) by Criezal et al. emphasized on the relationship between folate intake and the neural tube defects (NTDs).

Folate and Other Malformations

A Cochrane meta-analysis did not find any association between folate deficiency and any other birth defects such as cleft palate cleft lip and congenital cardiovascular defects. There was also no association with miscarriages.

Folate and Adverse Pregnancy Outcomes

Although certain studies have shown some beneficial impact of maternal folate on pre-eclampsia, a Cochrane review in 2013 did not find conclusive evidence of benefit.

Folate and Multivitamins

In a study, high-plasma folate was associated with functional indicators of impaired B12 status. In the Cochrane analysis, the protective effect of folate on NTDs was not affected by addition of multivitamins. In some studies, however, multivitamins have shown to reduce heart defects and renal abnormalities, and have shown that fortification with multivitamins reduced heart defects and urinary tract anomalies.

Dosing of Folic Acid

Various studies have used FA, in a 0.4–1.0 mg daily dose, is not known to cause demonstrable harm to the developing fetus or to the pregnant woman.

Presently, there are no RCTs assessing the impact of FA toxicity in preconceptional period, but high dose of FA impact has been studied in a meta-analysis, in which high dose of FA supplementation for mother during pregnancy was associated with an amplified risk of infant asthma, whereas supplementation with a relatively low-dose was associated with a reduced risk of infant asthma.

Folate and MTHFR

Folic acid is converted to 5-methyltetrahydrofolate (5-MTHF) (active form) by the enzyme methylenetetrahydrofolate reductase (MTHFR) in the body. Some people could inherit a natural genetic variation in the *MTHFR* gene, which damages its ability to process folate. However, despite the genetic variation, there are some activities in the enzyme, which can process folate if taken in sufficiently high doses. This variation in the *MTHFR* gene can lead to elevated levels of homocysteine. Hyperhomocysteinemia has been associated with various diseases. In the presence of *MTHFR* gene variation, 5-MTHF could be an alternative for supplementation. It has been found to be at least as effective as FA for supplementation in various trials. Use of 5-MTHF can prevent the masking hematological symptoms of severe vitamin B12 deficiency, which can occur with the excessive use of FA. Also, 5-MTHF has a lower interaction with antifolate drugs such as antimalarials.

The Practice Points

- All women of childbearing age should take FA 0.4/0.5 mg daily for at least 3 months before conception to up to 3 months after conception.
- Women who are at moderate risk of NTDs [e.g., family history of NTD in a first- or second-degree relative, personal positive or family history of other folate-sensitive congenital anomalies, maternal diabetes (type I or II), and malabsorption syndrome] should take FA 1 mg daily for at least 3 months before conception to up to 3 months after conception.
- Women who are at high risk of NTDs (personal or history of NTDs in previous pregnancies) should take a higher dose (4 mg) of folate. FA should be taken in a multivitamin including 2.6 µg/day of vitamin B12.
- The role of other micronutrients is not very clear. Some studies have shown improvement in birth weight, preterm labor, and congenital malformations.
- Methyltetrahydrofolate is at least as affective as folate according to the available trials. It may have an advantage in patients with *MTHFR* gene mutation. However, more evidence needs to be generated.

Iron Supplementation

Iron deficiency anemia is a mammoth problem, which leads to significant maternal morbidity and mortality.

Role of Preconceptional Care in Iron Deficiency Anemia

According to Government of India, the iron supplementation should continue from the early years throughout the reproductive years.

A study by Berger et al. showed that intermittent weekly iron during preconception (60 mg iron and 3.5 mg FA) and pregnancy (120 mg iron and 3.5 mg FA) is effective for prevention of iron deficiency anemia and has been called the Weekly Iron Folic acid Supplementation.

The Practice Points

All women in reproductive age group including those planning conception can be advised to take weekly 100 mg elemental iron and 500 µg of FA.

Along with this, Albendazole (400 mg) tablets for biannual deworming for helminthic control should also be prescribed.

Overweight and Obesity

Optimal weight before pregnancy is a prerequisite for a desirable outcome of pregnancy.

Preconceptional Care in Obesity

In a meta-analysis, weight loss before pregnancy reduced the risk of gestational diabetes and large for gestational age infants. Although a Cochrane review could not find studies on PCC in obese women, another review reported improved outcomes with bariatric surgery.

The Practice Points

Preconceptional care points for overweight and obese women are summarized in **Table 1**.

Underweight

Weight below average is also a high risk for adverse pregnancy outcome. Timely identification and intervention can ameliorate these affects to a certain extent. The preconceptional aspects can be summarized as given in **Table 2**.

◼ CHRONIC ILLNESSES

Diabetes Mellitus

Numerous studies have shown that preconceptional glycemic control can help in improving the pregnancy outcome in these women.

TABLE 1: Preconceptional care points for overweight and obese women.		
Identify	*Educate*	*Intervene*

• *Overweight:* 23–24.9 kg/m^2
 	
• *Obese:* >25 kg/m^2
	• Obese women more likely to have GDM, PE, induction of labor, cesarean section, PPH, thromboembolism, genital tract infection, wound infection, and intrauterine death
	• *Ideal BMI:* 18–23 before conception 5–10% weight loss in 6 months
		• Nutritional modification
		• Aerobic and strength conditioning
		• Individualized according to the patient profile
		• Bariatric surgery:
		  – BMI above 32.5 kg/m^2 with comorbidities
		  – BMI above 37.5 kg/m^2 without comorbidities
		  – Avoid pregnancy for at least 12–18 months after the surgery

(BMI: body mass index; GDM: gestational diabetes mellitus; PE: pulmonary embolism; PPH: postpartum hemorrhage)

TABLE 2: Preconceptional care points for underweight women.

Identify	Educate	Intervene
• Underweight • BMI < 18 kg/m²	• Higher risk of preterm birth (OR: 1.13; 95% CI: 1.01–1.27) • Low birth weight (OR: 1.66; 95% CI: 1.50–1.84) SGA (OR: 1.85; 95% CI: 1.69–2.02)	• Examine the food choices and provide nutritional advice • Screen and treat for eating disorders such as anorexia nervosa and bulimia • Weight gain in pregnancy does not reduce the risks

(BMI: body mass index; CI: confidence interval; OR: odds ratio; SGA: small for gestational age)

TABLE 3: Preconceptional care points for diabetic women.

Identify	Educate	Intervene
Screened all women for diabetes as per following WHO criteria in preconception: • FPG ≥ 126 mg/dL • 2-h ≥ 200 mg/dL	PGDM increases the risk of miscarriages, congenital fetal anomalies macrosomia, stillbirth, preterm delivery, cesarean delivery, and perinatal death	• Counsel on the diabetes self-management skills. Importance of maintaining good glycemic control before and throughout pregnancy • Achieve an HbA1c goal of < 6.5% before conception and a fasting glucose of 60–100 mg/dL • CHC and POP can be used in PGDM without vascular disease and disease of less than 20 years duration. • Even Cu IUDs can be used with caution

[FPG: fasting plasma glucose (glucose after no caloric intake for at least 8–12 hours); PGDM: pregestational diabetes mellitus; CHC: combined hormonal contraceptives; POP: progesterone only contraceptives; IUD: intrauterine device]

The Practice Points

Preconceptional care points for diabetic women are given in **Table 3**.

Thyroid Disorders

Currently, the evidence on universal screening for thyroid dysfunction during preconception is not very clear. Evidence reveals that although more women are diagnosed and treated by universal screening, its impact on maternal and neonatal outcomes is not evident.

Practice Points

The preconceptional care points for women with thyroid disorders are described in **Box 1**.

Heart Disease

Preconception is the ideal time to detect any previously asymptomatic cardiac conditions or optimize the existing known conditions.

BOX 1: Preconceptional care points for women with thyroid disorders.

Identify:
- *Universal screening*: Desirable
- *Case finding*: Alternative for—
  - Symptomatic women
  - Women from an area of known moderate-to-severe iodine insufficiency
  - Those who have a family or personal history of thyroid disease
  - Type 1 or type 2 diabetes
  - History of miscarriage/preterm delivery
  - History of head and neck radiation
  - Morbid obesity (BMI > 40)

Educate:
- Hypothyroidism associated with adverse maternal (gestational hypertension and pre-eclampsia postpartum hemorrhage, abortion, and preterm delivery), fetal and neonatal consequences
- Early identification of hyperthyroidism before pregnancy may allow a woman to optimize the disease condition before planning conception

Intervene:
- *Hypothyroidism:*
  - Women with overt hypothyroidism (TSH > 2.5–3 mIU/L with low FT4 levels or TSH > 10 mIU/L irrespective of FT4) should be treated
  - Women with subclinical hypothyroidism (serum TSH between 2.5 and 10 mIU/L with normal FT4 concentration) detected during preconception should be referred to an endocrinologist for further evaluation and management. Anti-TPO antibodies should be advised and treatment may be offered in their presence
  - Increase in levothyroxine (LT4) dose (by around 30%) at the time of confirmation of pregnancy is recommended for women with hypothyroidism
- *Hyperthyroidism:*
  - Surgery better, if conception planned within 2 years
  - If radioactive iodine: Postpone conception for 6 months
  - *Antithyroid drugs:*
    - PTU in first trimester
    - Methimazole after first trimester

(PTU: propylthiouracil; TSH: thyroid-stimulating hormone; BMI: body mass index)

Practice Points

Preconceptional care points for women with cardiac disorders are summarized in **Box 2**.

Hypertensive Disorders

Practice Points

- Screen all women for hypertensive disorders before pregnancy especially those with previous hypertensive disorders in pregnancy, renal disease, autoimmune disorders (AIDs), or thrombophilias.
- Women with hypertension for several years should be assessed for renal disease, ventricular hypertrophy, and retinopathy.

> **BOX 2:** Preconceptional care points for women with cardiac disorders.
>
> *Identify:*
> - At least a basic clinical cardiac assessment in the preconceptional period for all women referral to a specialist, if required
> - Identify conditions where pregnancy is contraindicated due to unacceptable risk of maternal mortality like:
>   - Severe pulmonary arterial hypertension of any cause
>   - Severe systemic ventricular dysfunction
>   - NYHA III–IV or LVEF < 30%
>   - Previous peripartum cardiomyopathy with any residual impairment of LV function
>   - Severe left heart obstruction
>   - Marfan syndrome with aorta dilated > 40 mm
>   - Aortic dilatation > 50 mm in aortic disease associated with bicuspid aortic valve
>   - Native severe coarctation
>
> *Educate:*
> - Counsel about the consequences of:
>   - Pregnancy on the pre-existing heart condition
>   - Cardiac condition on the mother and the fetus
>   - Implications of drugs used, e.g., anticoagulants
>
> *Intervene:*
> - In a woman with known cardiac condition, detailed cardiac assessment should be carried out to assess the baseline cardiac condition, to review the medications and to evaluate the requirement for corrective surgery
> - Genetic counseling should be offered for women with congenital heart disease
> - Medication review should be done for the mechanical valve replacement patients who are on anticoagulation therapy

- All women with pre-existing hypertension should be advised to achieve a target blood pressure of 150/100 mm Hg in the case of uncomplicated chronic hypertension and below 140/90 mm Hg in the presence of target organ damage.
- Avoid angiotensin-converting enzyme inhibitors and angiotensin II receptor blocker in women planning pregnancy.
- Progestin-only contraception is recommended in patients with chronic hypertension till they are optimized.

Seizure Disorders

Evidence

There are more than 10 million living with epilepsy in India. As reported in a recent review, the odds of spontaneous miscarriage, antepartum hemorrhage, postpartum hemorrhage, hypertensive disorders, induction of labor, cesarean section, any preterm birth, and fetal growth restriction were more in women with epilepsy.

Practice Points

- *Contraception till disease optimization*: Hormonal contraceptive failure may occur at standard doses in the presence of hepatic cytochrome

P-450-inducing antiepileptics such as carbamazepine, phenytoin, phenobarbital, and topiramate. Hence, low-dose pills should be avoided.

- *Titrating the antiepileptic drugs (AEDs)*: All the commonly used AEDs are teratogenic. Drugs like valproate, phenytoin, carbamazepine, phenobarbital, and topiramate have higher baseline rates. Newer drugs such as levetiracetam have a lower risk of major malformations. The general principles of administering AEDs are:
  - They should be administered at the lowest possible dose.
  - Avoid multiple agents especially combinations involving valproate, carbamazepine, and phenobarbital.
  - If there is a family history of NTDs, avoid valproate and carbamazepine.
  - After pregnancy has been confirmed, AEDs should not be changed only to reduce the risk of teratogenicity, as this may precipitate seizures or an overlap of another drug may expose the fetus to additional risk.
  - Woman should be on a stable anticonvulsant regimen for at least 6 months (after dose modification or withdrawal) prior to conception.
- *Preconceptional folic acid*: A higher dose of FA up to 4 mg can be given to women on AEDs, especially those known to cause NTDs such as valproate and carbamazepine.

Autoimmune Disorders

A woman with a known AID should use effective contraception till the disease is optimized. The management of such patients should be a multidisciplinary with active involvement of the concerned physicians. Systemic lupus erythematosus and rheumatoid arthritis are more commonly seen in pregnancy.

The general aspects of preconceptional care are given in **Box 3**.

BOX 3: Preconceptional care points for women with autoimmune disorder (AID).

Identify: Woman with known AID can have an improvement, worsening, or no change when a woman becomes pregnant depending upon her specific autoimmune disease

Educate:
- Pregnancies in women with SLE are at high risk for maternal and fetal complications, including spontaneous abortion and premature delivery, intrauterine growth retardation, and superimposed pre-eclampsia
- There is spontaneous amelioration of RA during pregnancy and an increased risk of flare after delivery

Intervene:
- Women with SLE who wish to get pregnant should be advised to achieve quiescent SLE at least 6 months before conception
- Methotrexate and leflunomide are extremely teratogenic and should be discontinued in women planning a pregnancy

(SLE: systemic lupus erythematosus; RA: rheumatoid arthritis)

◼ INFECTIONS

Universal Screening

Universal screening is advisable for human immunodeficiency virus (HIV), hepatitis B surface antigen (HbsAg), and venereal disease research laboratory. A systematic review reported a median prevalence of treponema pallidum (2.6%), hepatitis B virus (4.3%), and hepatitis C virus to be 2.6%, 4.3%, and 1.4% respectively in the low and middle-income countries. Global prevalence of HIV in women is approximately 16 million.

Once detected, HIV-positive women on antiretroviral therapy (ART) have very low chances of perinatal transmission if the ART is instituted on time **(Box 4)**. With treatment, the rate of transmission has been reported to be as low as 1% in mothers whose viral load was less than 1%. The use of ART in a discordant couple reduces the risk of transmission to the unaffected partner.

High-risk Screening

Screening for certain infections should be offered to the women at high risk of acquiring the infection like tuberculosis, sexually transmitted infections, toxoplasmosis, and cytomegalovirus (CMV).

◼ GENETIC DISORDERS

Having a child born with a disability is like a dream shattered for a couple. Preconception is the ideal time to identify, understand, and prevent genetic disorders in the fetus.

Prevalence

The prevalence of chromosomal, single gene, and multifactorial disorder has been reported to be 0.6%, 0.56%, and 2% respectively at the time of birth. Each year in India, around 5 lakhs babies are born with congenital malformations while 20,000 have Down's syndrome and around 10,000 have thalassemia.

BOX 4: Preconceptional care points for women with human immunodeficiency virus (HIV) infection.

Identify: All couples planning pregnancy should be offered HIV screening and counseling

Educate: All HIV-positive couples should be informed of the risk of transmission to the uninfected partner and the fetus

Intervene:
- Initiation and continuation of combined ART
- Effective contraception until viral loads suppressed below the limits of detection
- For serodiscordant couples, in whom the woman is HIV-positive, it is preferable to attempt home insemination with the partner's sperm during ovulation for 3–6 months before considering other methods. If the male partner is HIV-positive, then a referral to a fertility specialist should be considered and an option of sperm washing with intrauterine insemination should be given

(ART: antiretroviral therapy)

The purpose of preconceptional care is to:

- *Identify couples at high risk of genetic disorders in the fetus*: A thorough family medical history needs to be taken and a complete three-generation family tree including ethnicity information should be constructed during the preconceptional period in order to identify couples who have genetic predisposition to an adverse pregnancy outcome. A history of consanguinity, hereditary disorder in family, advanced parental age, teratogen exposure or infection, birth defects, intellectual disability, and recurrent pregnancy loss are some of the indications for a referral to a geneticist.
- *Provide a detailed overview of the likelihood of affection*: The commonly seen genetic disorders can be—
  - *Single gene disorders*: Fragile X syndrome, muscular dystrophy, hemophilia, and cystic fibrosis
  - Cytogenetic disorders like Down's syndrome
  - *Multifactorial*: Anencephaly and spina bifida
  Depending on the type of disorder, the likelihood of affection in the next pregnancy (e.g., 25% for autosomal recessive disorders like thalassemia) can be predicted and also the impact of the affection of the underlying genetic disorder (degree of disabilities, e.g., Down's syndrome) can be understood.
- *Understand if there is a possibility of modifying the impact or likelihood of occurrence of the disorder* (e.g., prenatal diagnosis and thalassemia).

VACCINATIONS

Some vaccines benefit by preventing the congenital infection, while others are useful in preventing the perinatal transmission.

Strongly Advisable

Measles, Mumps, and Rubella

Measles, mumps, and rubella (MMR) are associated with spontaneous abortion, prematurity, low birth weight (LBW), and other birth defects.

Women in reproductive age group should be screened for rubella immunity and immunized if nonimmune. Some salient features about the vaccination are:

- Serological testing for rubella is not absolutely essential before vaccinating
- MMR preferred over rubella vaccine alone
- Counseled to avoid pregnancy for 3 months after vaccination
- Accidental vaccination in pregnancy does not pose a substantial risk to the fetus.

Hepatitis B Vaccine

This vaccine provides high-protective efficacy (95%) against perinatal transmission. Immunization in prepregnancy at least for those who are at risk, e.g., those having multiple sex partners, those with history of sexually transmitted disease (STDs), or recent or current injection-drug use or those having more than one sex partner during the previous 6 months, been evaluated or treated for an STD, recent or current injection-drug use, or having had an HBsAg-positive sex partner is a practical option.

Desirable

Tetanus, Diphtheria, and Pertussis

There are definite advantages of tetanus, diphtheria, and pertussis (Tdap) vaccine during pregnancy. In a systematic review, there was definite reduction in the neonatal deaths when compared to placebo.

The TdaP should be given in the preconceptional period, if the tetanus vaccination schedule in is not up-to-date (no booster in the last 2 years). Also, even if the woman has been vaccinated in the preconception, the pregnancy schedule should be followed.

Varicella

Infection in pregnancy can cause varying manifestations depending on the gestation of affection. Early pregnancy infection may result in fetal varicella syndrome characterized by fetal scarring of the skin and affected limb(s), limb deformities (hypoplasia), eye damage, LBW, brain atrophy, and mental retardation, sometimes fetal death or spontaneous abortion, while infection in the third trimester leads to chances of neonatal disease.

Practice points: With the availability of varicella vaccine, preconception is a good time to screen for varicella immunity by a history of infection, immunization, or serology. Nonimmune women should receive two doses of varicella vaccine at 4 weeks interval, with a counseling to avoid pregnancy for 3 months.

Influenza

Influenza can be effectively prevented by vaccination up to (70–90%). Vaccination is 70–90% effective in preventing influenza. *Vaccination of pregnant women during influenza season is safe and recommended to reduce the risk to the mother and also for passive protection to the neonate.*

Human Papillomavirus

Women in the preconceptional period should be advised to carry out the routine protocol for vaccination against HPV and preferably complete the vaccination schedule before conception. If they conceive before completing the schedule, the rest of the doses can be given after delivery.

■ PSYCHOSOCIAL ISSUES AND SUBSTANCE ABUSE

Preconceptional care points for dealing with women having psychosocial issues are described in **Box 5.**

BOX 5: Preconceptional care points for dealing with women having psychosocial issues.

Identify:
- Screen for depression and anxiety and other psychotic disorders such as mania and schizophrenia by a personal or family history and presence of other social stressors such as:
  - Income below or near poverty level, difficulty in accessing the primary care services, intimate partner violence and maltreatment (abuse or neglect) as a child or adolescent, unwanted pregnancy, and lack of support system
- Women should be screened for signs of alcohol, tobacco (smoking and smokeless tobacco), and illicit drugs usage dependence

Educate:
- Psychiatric ailments during pregnancy have been associated with poor obstetric outcomes
- Smoking is associated with miscarriage, preterm delivery, LBW and fetal growth restriction, stillbirth, and sudden infant death syndrome
- Heavy alcohol consumption (>10 g/day or more than 3 alcoholic drinks a day) was found to increase the risk of LBW infants, SGA infants, and preterm birth
- Prenatal exposure to illicit drugs such as opiates, marijuana, cocaine, and methamphetamine is associated with an increased risk of pregnancy complications and adverse outcomes

Intervene:
- Appropriate treatment (avoiding teratogenic drugs) for depression, anxiety, bipolar disorder, and schizophrenia should be offered with a multidisciplinary approach
- Those women who show signs of alcohol, tobacco, and illicit drugs usage dependence should be educated about the adverse impact on pregnancy outcomes and efforts should be made to identify programs that would assist them to achieve cessation and long-term abstinence prior to conception

(LBW: low birth weight; SGA: small for gestational age)

▨ SUGGESTED READING

1. Adolescent Division, Ministry of Health and Family Welfare, Government of India. (2013) Guidelines for Control of Iron Deficiency Anemia: National Iron + Intiative. [online] Available from: https://www.nhm.gov.in/images/pdf/programmes/child-health/guidelines/Control-of-Iron-Deficiency-Anaemia.pdf. [Last accessed May, 2020].
2. Agency for Healthcare Research and Quality. Management of chronic hypertension during pregnancy. Evidence Report/Technology Assessment no.14. AHRQ publication no. 00- E011. Rockville, MD: Agency for Healthcare Research and Quality; 2000.
3. American College of Obstetricians and Gynecologists. ACOG educational bulletin: viral hepatitis in pregnancy Number 248, July 1998 (Replaces No. 174, November 1992). Int J Gynaecol Obstet. 1998;63(2):195-202.
4. Anglemyer A, Rutherford GW, Horvath T, Baggaley RC, Egger M, Siegfried N. Antiretroviral therapy for prevention of HIV transmission in HIV-discordant couples. Cochrane Database Syst Rev. 2013;(4):CD009153.
5. Arora N, Kausar H, Jana N, Mandal S, Mukherjee D, Mukherjee R. Congenital heart disease in pregnancy in a low-income country. Int J Gynaecol Obstet. 2015;128(1):30-2.
6. Behnke M, Smith VC. Prenatal substance abuse: short- and long-term effects on the exposed fetus. Pediatrics. 2013;131(3):e1009-24.
7. Berger J, Thanh HT, Cavalli-Sforza T, Smitasiri S, Khan NC, Milani S, et al. Community mobilization and social marketing to promote weekly iron-folic acid supplementation

in women of reproductive age in Vietnam: impact on anemia and iron status. Nutr Rev. 2005;63(12 Pt 2):S95-108.

8. Bhatla N, Lal S, Behera G, Kriplani A, Mittal S, Agarwal N, et al. Cardiac disease in pregnancy. Int J Gynaecol Obstet. 2003;82(2):153-9.

9. Butler NR, Goldstein H, Ross EM. Cigarette smoking in pregnancy: its influence on birth weight and perinatal mortality. Br Med J. 1972;2(5806):127-30.

10. Czeizel AE, Dudas L. Prevention of the first occurrence of neural tube defects by periconceptional vitamin supplementation. N Engl J Med. 1992;327(26):1832-5.

11. Dean SV, Lassi ZS, Imam AM, Bhutta ZA. Preconception care: closing the gap in the continuum of care to accelerate improvements in maternal, newborn and child health. Reprod Health. 2014;11(Suppl 3):S1.

12. De-Regil LM, Peña-Rosas JP, Fernández-Gaxiola AC, Rayco-Solon P. Effects and safety of periconceptional oral folate supplementation for preventing birth defects. Cochrane Database Syst Rev. 2015;(12):CD007950.

13. Dieguez M, Herrero A, Avello N, Suarez P, Delgado E, Menendez E. Prevalence of thyroid dysfunction in women in early pregnancy: does it increase with maternal age? Clin Endocrinol (Oxf). 2016;84(1):121-6.

14. Dornhorst A, Paterson CM, Nicholls JS, Wadsworth J, Chiu DC, Elkeles RS, et al. High prevalence of gestational diabetes in women from ethnic minority groups. Diabet Med. 1992;9(9):820-5.

15. El Baba KA, Azar ST. Thyroid dysfunction in pregnancy. Int J Gen Med. 2012;5:227-30.

16. Elsinga J, de Jong-Potjer LC, van der Pal-de Bruin KM, le Cessie S, Assendelft WJ, Buitendijk SE. The effect of preconception counselling on lifestyle and other behaviour before and during pregnancy. Womens Health Issues. 2008;18(6 Suppl): S117-25.

17. Ezzati MD, Lopez A, Rodgers A, CJL M. Comparative quantification of health risks: Global and regional burden of disease attributable to selected major risk factors. Geneva: World Health Organization; 2004.

18. Ferrer RL, Sibai BM, Mulrow CD, Chiquette E, Stevens KR, Cornell J. Management of mild chronic hypertension during pregnancy: a review. Obstet Gynecol. 2000;96 (5 Pt 2):849-60.

19. Fodinger M, Horl WH, Sunder-Plassmann G. Molecular biology of 5,10-methylenetetrahydrofolate reductase. J Nephrol. 2000;13(1):20-33.

20. Forsum E, Brantsaeter AL, Olafsdottir AS, Olsen SF, Thorsdottir I. Weight loss before conception: A systematic literature review. Food Nutr Res. 2013;57.

21. Geeta MG, Riyaz A. Prevention of mother to child transmission of hepatitis B infection. Indian Peditr. 2013;50(2):189-92.

22. Gelson E, Curry R, Gatzoulis MA, Swan L, Lupton M, Steer P, et al. Effect of maternal heart disease on fetal growth. Obstet Gynecol. 2011;117(4):886-91.

23. Glazer NL, Hendrickson AF, Schellenbaum GD, Mueller BA. Weight change and the risk of gestational diabetes in obese women. Epidemiology. 2004;15(6):733-7.

24. Goh YI, Bollano E, Einarson TR, Koren G. Prenatal multivitamin supplementation and rates of congenital anomalies: a meta-analysis. J Obstet Gynaecol Can. 2006;28(8):680-9.

25. Haddow JE, Palomaki GE, Allan WC, Williams JR, Knight GJ, Gagnon J, et al. Maternal thyroid deficiency during pregnancy and subsequent neuropsychological development of the child. N Engl J Med. 1999;341(8):549-55.

26. Hazes JM, Coulie PG, Geenen V, Vermeire S, Carbonnel F, Louis E, et al. Rheumatoid arthritis and pregnancy: evolution of disease activity and pathophysiological considerations for drug use. Rheumatology (Oxford). 2011;50(11):1955-68.

27. Houghton LA, Sherwood KL, Pawlosky R, Ito S, O'Connor DL. [6S]-5-Methyltetrahydrofolate is at least as effective as folic acid in preventing a decline in blood folate concentrations during lactation. Am J Clin Nutr. 2006;83(4):842-50.

28. Ioannidis JP, Abrams EJ, Ammann A, Bulterys M, Goedert JJ, Gray L, et al. Perinatal transmission of human immunodeficiency virus type 1 by pregnant women with RNA virus loads <1000 copies/ml. J Infect Dis. 2001;183(4):539-45.

29. Kim MW, Hong SC, Choi JS, Han J-Y, Oh MJ, Kim HJ, et al. Homocysteine, folate, and pregnancy outcomes. J Obstet Gynaecol Can. 2012;32(2):520-4.

30. Kjaer MM, Nilas L. Pregnancy after bariatric surgery—a review of benefits and risks. Acta Obstet Gynecol Scand. 2013;92(3):264-71.

31. Kriplani A, Buckshee K, Bhargava VL, Takkar D, Ammini AC. Maternal and perinatal outcome in thyrotoxicosis complicating pregnancy. Eur J Obstet Gynecol Reprod Biol. 1994;54(3):159-63.

32. Kumari P, Gupta M, Kahlon P, Malviya S. Association between high maternal body mass index (BMI) and feto-maternal outcome. J Obes Metab Res. 2014;3:143-4.

33. Lamers Y, Prinz-Langenohl R, Moser R, Pietrzik K. Supplementation with [6S]-5-methyltetrahydrofolate or folic acid equally reduces plasma total homocysteine concentrations in healthy women. Am J Clin Nutr. 2004;79(3):473-8.

34. Lassi ZS, Bhutta ZA. Community-based intervention packages for reducing maternal and neonatal morbidity and mortality and improving neonatal outcomes. Cochrane Database Syst Rev. 2015;(3):CD007754.

35. Lassi ZS, Imam AM, Dean SV, Bhutta ZA. Preconception care: preventing and treating infections. Reprod Health. 2014;11(Suppl 3):S4.

36. Lassi ZS, Salam RA, Haider BA, Bhutta ZA. Folic acid supplementation during pregnancy for maternal health and pregnancy outcomes. Cochrane Database Syst Rev. 2013;(3):CD006896.

37. Lewycka S, Mwansambo C, Rosato M, Kazembe P, Phiri T, Mganga A, et al. Effect of women's groups and volunteer peer counselling on rates of mortality, morbidity, and health behaviours in mothers and children in rural Malawi (MaiMwana): a factorial, cluster-randomised controlled trial. Lancet. 2013;381(9879):1721-35.

38. Li M, Yao Q, Xing A. A clinical analysis of 188 cases of pregnancy complicated with critical heart disease. Zhong Nan Da Xue Xue Bao Yi Xue Ban. 2014;39(11):1145-50.

39. Lone FW, Qureshi RN, Emanuel F. Maternal anaemia and its impact on perinatal outcome. Trop Med Int Health. 2004;9(4):486-90.

40. Luewan S, Chakkabut P, Tongsong T. Outcomes of pregnancy complicated with hyperthyroidism: a cohort study. Arch Gynecol Obstet. 2011;283(2):243-7.

41. McDonald SD, Han Z, Mulla S, Beyene J. Overweight and obesity in mothers and risk of preterm birth and low birth weight infants: systematic review and meta-analyses. BMJ. 2010;341:c3428.

42. Michaan N, Amzallag S, Laskov I, Cohen Y, Fried M, Lessing JB, et al. Maternal and neonatal outcome of pregnant women infected with H1N1 influenza virus (swine flu). J Matern Fetal Neonatal Med. 2012;25(2):130-2.

43. Misra A, Chowbey P, Makkar BM, Vikram NK, Wasir JS, Chadha D, et al. Consensus statement for diagnosis of obesity, abdominal obesity and the metabolic syndrome for Asian Indians and recommendations for physical activity, medical and surgical management. J Assoc Physicians India. 2009;57:163-70.

44. Mitchell EA, Milerad J. Smoking and the sudden infant death syndrome. Rev Environ Health. 2006;21(2):81-103.

45. More NS, Bapat U, Das S, Alcock G, Patil S, Porel M, et al. Community mobilization in Mumbai slums to improve perinatal care and outcomes: a cluster randomized controlled trial. PLoS Med. 2012;9(7):e1001257.

46. MRC Vitamin Study Research Group. Prevention of neural tube defects: results of the Medical Research Council Vitamin Study. Lancet. 1991;338(8760):131-7.

47. Murai U, Nomura K, Kido M, Takeuchi T, Sugimoto M, Rahman M. Pre-pregnancy body mass index as a predictor of low birth weight infants in Japan. Asia Pac J Clin Nutr. 2017;26(3):434-7.

48. Murphy HR, Roland JM, Skinner TC, Simmons D, Gurnell E, Morrish NJ, et al. Effectiveness of a regional prepregnancy care program in women with type 1 and type 2 diabetes: benefits beyond glycemic control. Diabetes Care. 2010;33(12):2514-20.

49. Nathwani D, Maclean A, Conway S, Carrington D. Varicella infections in pregnancy and the newborn. A review prepared for the UK Advisory Group on Chickenpox on behalf of the British Society for the Study of Infection. J Infect. 1998;36(Suppl 1):59-71.
50. National High Blood Pressure Education Program Working Group. Report of the National High Blood Pressure Education Program Working Group on High Blood Pressure in Pregnancy. Am J Obstet Gynecol. 2000;183(1):S1-22.
51. Nduati E, Diriye A, Ommeh S, Mwai L, Kiara S, Masseno V, et al. Effect of folate derivatives on the activity of antifolate drugs used against malaria and cancer. Parasitol Res. 2008;102(6):1227-34.
52. NFHS-3. National Nutrition Monitoring Bureau Survey (NNMBS). 2006.
53. Obeid R, Holzgreve W, Pietrzik K. Is 5-methyltetrahydrofolate an alternative to folic acid for the prevention of neural tube defects? J Perinat Med. 2013;41(5):469-83.
54. Opray N, Grivell RM, Deussen AR, Dodd JM. Directed preconception health programs and interventions for improving pregnancy outcomes for women who are overweight or obese. Cochrane Database Syst Rev. 2015;(7):CD010932.
55. Patra J, Bakker R, Irving H, Jaddoe VW, Malini S, Rehm J. Dose-response relationship between alcohol consumption before and during pregnancy and the risks of low birthweight, preterm birth and small for gestational age (SGA)-a systematic review and meta-analyses. BJOG. 2011;118(12):1411-21.
56. Pierce M, Kurinczuk JJ, Spark P, Brocklehurst P, Knight M. Perinatal outcomes after maternal 2009/H1N1 infection: national cohort study. BMJ. 2011;342:d3214.
57. Pietrzik K, Bailey L, Shane B. Folic acid and L-5-methyltetrahydrofolate: comparison of clinical pharmacokinetics and pharmacodynamics. Clin Pharmacokinet. 2010;49(8):535-48.
58. Rahman MM, Abe SK, Rahman MS, Kanda M, Narita S, Bilano V, et al. Maternal anemia and risk of adverse birth and health outcomes in low- and middle-income countries: systematic review and meta-analysis. Am J Clin Nutr. 2016;103(2):495-504.
59. Rimoin DL, Connor JM, Pyeritz RE, Korf BR. Emery and Rimoin's principles and practice of medical genetics, 5th edition. Edinburgh: Churchill Livingstone Elsevier; 2007.
60. Sahu MT, Das V, Mittal S, Agarwal A, Sahu M. Overt and subclinical thyroid dysfunction among Indian pregnant women and its effect on maternal and fetal outcome. Arch Gynecol Obstet. 2010;281(2):215-20.
61. Schneid-Kofman N, Sheiner E, Levy A. Psychiatric illness and adverse pregnancy outcome. Int J Gynaecol Obstet. 2008;101(1):53-6.
62. Sebire NJ, Jolly M, Harris JP, Wadsworth J, Joffe M, Beard RW, et al. Maternal obesity and pregnancy outcome: a study of 287,213 pregnancies in London. Int J Obes Relat Metab Disord. 2001;25(8):1175-82.
63. Selhub J, Morris MS, Jacques PF. In vitamin B12 deficiency, higher serum folate is associated with increased total homocysteine and methylmalonic acid concentrations. Proc Natl Acad Sci U S A. 2007;104(50):19995-20000.
64. Seshiah V, Balaji V, Balaji MS, Sanjeevi CB, Green A. Gestational diabetes mellitus in India. J Assoc Physicians India. 2004;52:707-11.
65. Simpson JL, Shulman LP, Brown H, Holzgreve W. Closing the folate gap in reproductive-age women. Contemp Ob Gyn. 2010;55:34-40.
66. Singh S, Sedgh G, Hussain R. Unintended pregnancy: worldwide levels, trends, and outcomes, 2010. Stud Fam Plan. 2010;41(4):241-50.
67. Singru SA, Tilak VW, Gandham N, Bhawalkar JS, Jadhav SL, Pandve HT. Study of Susceptibility Towards Varicella by Screening for the Presence of IgG Antibodies Among Nursing and Medical Students of a Tertiary Care Teaching Hospital in Pune, India. J Glob Infect Dis. 2011;3(1):37-41.
68. Smith NM, Bresee JS, Shay DK, Uyeki TM, Cox NJ, Strikas RA. Prevention and control of influenza: recommendations of the Advisory Committee on Immunization Practices (ACIP). MMWR Recomm Rep. 2006;55(RR-10):1-42.

69. Smyth A, Oliveira GH, Lahr BD, Bailey KR, Norby SM, Garovic VD. A systematic review and meta-analysis of pregnancy outcomes in patients with systemic lupus erythematosus and lupus nephritis. Clin J Am Soc Nephrol. 2010;5(11):2060-8.
70. Spencer L, Bubner T, Bain E, Middleton P. Screening and subsequent management for thyroid dysfunction pre-pregnancy and during pregnancy for improving maternal and infant health. Cochrane Database Syst Rev. 2015;(9):CD011263.
71. Sridharan R, Murthy BN. Prevalence and pattern of epilepsy in India. Epilepsia. 1999;40(5):631-6.
72. Sukumaran L, McCarthy NL, Kharbanda EO, McNeil MM, Naleway AL, Klein NP, et al. Association of Tdap vaccination with acute events and adverse birth outcomes among pregnant women with prior tetanus-containing immunizations. JAMA. 2015;314(15):1581-7.
73. Swamy GK, Beigi RH. Maternal benefits of immunization during pregnancy. Vaccine. 2015;33(47):6436-40.
74. Trimmer EE. Methylenetetrahydrofolate reductase: biochemical characterization and medical significance. Curr Pharm Des. 2013;19(14):2574-93.
75. Tripathy P, Nair N, Barnett S, Mahapatra R, Borghi J, Rath S, et al. Effect of a participatory intervention with women's groups on birth outcomes and maternal depression in Jharkhand and Orissa, India: a cluster-randomised controlled trial. Lancet. 2010;375(9721):1182-92.
76. UNAIDS (2010). UNAIDS report on the global AIDS epidemic. [online] Available from: http://www.unaids.org/globalreport/Global_report.htm. [Last accessed May, 2020].
77. Unnikrishnan AG, Kalra S, Sahay RK, Bantwal G, John M, Tewari N. Prevalence of hypothyroidism in adults: an epidemiological study in eight cities of India. Indian J Endocrinol Metab. 2013;17(4):647-52.
78. Varga EA, Sturm AC, Misita CP, Moll S. Cardiology patient pages. Homocysteine and MTHFR mutations: relation to thrombosis and coronary artery disease. Circulation. 2005;111(19):e289-93.
79. Velu PP, Gravett CA, Roberts TK, Wagner TA, Zhang JS, Rubens CE, et al. Epidemiology and aetiology of maternal bacterial and viral infections in low- and middle-income countries. J Glob Health. 2011;1(2):171-88.
80. Verma IC, Puri RD. Global burden of genetic disease and the role of genetic screening. Semin Fetal Neonatal Med. 2015;20(5):354-63.
81. Viale L, Allotey J, Cheong-See F, Arroyo-Manzano D, McCorry D, Bagary M, et al. Epilepsy in pregnancy and reproductive outcomes: a systematic review and meta-analysis. Lancet. 2015;386(10006):1845-52.
82. Villamor E, Cnattingius S. Interpregnancy weight change and risk of adverse pregnancy outcomes: a population-based study. Lancet. 2006;368(9542):1164-70.
83. Wahabi HA, Alzeidan RA, Bawazeer GA, Alansari LA, Esmaeil SA. Preconception care for diabetic women for improving maternal and fetal outcomes: a systematic review and meta-analysis. BMC Pregnancy Childbirth. 2010;10:63.
84. Wahabi HA, Esmaeil SA, Fayed A, Al-Shaikh G, Alzeidan RA. Pre-existing diabetes mellitus and adverse pregnancy outcomes. BMC Res Notes. 2012;5:496.
85. White SJ, Boldt KL, Holditch SJ, Poland GA, Jacobson RM. Measles, mumps, and rubella. Clin Obstet Gynecol. 2012;55(2):550-9.
86. WHO. Meeting to develop a global consensus on preconception care to reduce maternal and childhood mortality and morbidity. Geneva: World Health Organization; 2013.
87. Yang L, Jiang L, Bi M, Jia X, Wang Y, He C, et al. High dose of maternal folic acid supplementation is associated to infant asthma. Food Chem Toxicol. 2015;75:88-93.

Screening in Antenatal Care: Current Recommendations

5

Screening for Anemia and Hemoglobinopathies

Mala Arora, Baseerat Kaur

INTRODUCTION

The word "anemia" is derived from Greek word "anaimía", which means "without blood". Anemia is a global problem despite improved nutrition. World Health Organization (WHO) estimates that one-third of the worlds' population is anemic and majority live in developing countries. India continues to have a high prevalence of anemia. The Government of India recognizes the problem and has rolled out the "National Nutritional Anemia Control Programme" in 1970. Free iron and folic acid tablets are dispensed free through primary health centers to all pregnant women.

Despite this, the National Family Health Survey (NFHS-4), conducted in 2015–16, revealed that 58.5% of children and 50.3% of all pregnant women continue to be anemic. The reasons are manifold. Frequent pregnancies with inadequate spacing are implicated for this high incidence of anemia. The highest incidence is of nutritional anemia consequent to iron-deficiency, although folic acid and vitamin B_{12} deficiency also play a role. A large proportion of population being vegetarian is deficient in vitamin B_{12} with resultant macrocytic anemia. This poses a diagnostic dilemma, as the blood picture is dimorphic. Other causes such as hemoglobinopathies and hemolysis, although less frequent, do contribute to the burden of anemia.

SCREENING

Screening for anemia is mandatory for all pregnant patients at their first visit. It should preferably be done at the prepregnancy counseling clinic or better still in the adolescent age group so that there is ample time to correct it prior to pregnancy. During pregnancy, a serial check of hemoglobin at the start of each trimester is recommended for early detection of anemia.

Complete Blood Count

This is preferable to a hemoglobin check alone, as it provides valuable information on the blood indices like mean corpuscular volume (MCV), mean corpuscular hemoglobin (MCH), and mean corpuscular hemoglobin concentration (MCHC):

- *MCV*: It is defined as the size of RBC and is expressed in femtoliter (fL). The normal value is 87 ± 7 fL.

- *MCH*: It is the quantity of hemoglobin per RBC. The normal value is 29 ± 2 pg (picogram) per cell.
- *MCHC*: It correlates the hemoglobin content with the volume of the cell. The normal value is 34 ± 2 g/dL.
- Variation in the size of red cell (anisocytosis) can be quantified and expressed as red cell distribution width (RDW) or red cell morphology index. The normal value is 13 ± 1.5%.

Besides, it also tells us about platelet count and the white cell count, which is required to be screened during pregnancy.

Peripheral Smear

It is highly sensitive for excessive RBC production and hemolysis. This provides valuable information on red cell morphology such as:
- Micro-/macrocytosis
- Hypochromia
- Aniso-/poikilocytosis
- Spherocytes and ovalocytes
- Target cells and nucleated RBC in hemolytic anemia
- Sickle cell morphology
- Schistocytes and other red cell parasites
- Platelet adequacy
- Abnormal white blood cells.

Since MCV is an average value, so, it can be normal in presence of two different cell populations (e.g., dimorphic anemia); therefore, it is important to examine the peripheral smear in the evaluation of anemia.

Reticulocyte Count

This is an indicator of bone marrow function. The normal reticulocyte count is 0.5–1.5%, which is raised to over 2% in an anemic patient, partly due to the active bone marrow and partly due to the reduced red cell mass. It is an excellent tool to judge, if a prescribed therapy is working to correct anemia. A corrected reticulocyte count of >2% or absolute reticulocyte count of >100 × 10^9/L indicates an adequate marrow response. Reticulocytes are best visualized when blood is stained with a supravital stain.

Bone Marrow Aspiration and Biopsy

It provides direct assessment of RBC precursors. It is only done in following conditions:
- Unexplained anemia
- More than one cell lineage abnormalities (anemia, leukopenia, and thrombocytopenia)
- Suspected primary bone marrow disorder (e.g., leukemia, aplastic anemia, myelodysplastic syndrome, and myelofibrosis)

Based on the result of CBC, we can grade anemia in three categories:

1. Microcytic
2. Normocytic
3. Macrocytic.

▧ MICROCYTIC ANEMIA

The reference range for MCV is 80–95 fL (femtoliter). Microcytic anemia is defined as a MCV < 80 fL in a women with confirmed anemia.

This is by far the most common type of anemia encountered during pregnancy. The causes are:

- Iron-deficiency
- Anemia of chronic disease (ACD)
- Thalassemia trait disorders.

  Further tests required in this subgroup of anemia are as follows.

Serum Iron Studies

The panel of iron studies includes:

- Serum iron—is reduced (normal value 60–170 µg/dL)
- Total iron-binding capacity (TIBC)—is increased (normal 250–400 µg/dL)
- Transferrin saturation—is reduced (normal 16–50%)
- Serum ferritin—is reduced (normal 15–200 µg/L)
- Serum hepcidin—is reduced (normal 17–286 ng/mL)
- Soluble transferrin receptors (sTR)—increased (normal 2.8–8.5 mg/L)
- Reticulocyte hemoglobin content (CHr) is a new and reliable marker of iron-deficiency (normal > 29 pg).

  In a patient with hypochromic and microcytic anemia, serum iron studies are required to:

- Judge the degree of iron-deficiency—this will allow us to decide whether oral iron is sufficient or parenteral iron is required.

  Iron supplementation should be continued for at least 6 months postcorrection of the blood indices to replenish iron stores of the body.
- Differentiate iron-deficiency from ACD. Iron-deficiency may coexist with ACD and the serum ferritin may be spuriously high due to inflammation.
- Differentiate it from beta thalassemia spectrum of hemoglobinopathies. Thalassemia major requires frequent blood transfusions; however, thalassemia minor/trait may often be confused with iron-deficiency anemia.

Confirmatory Tests for Thalassemia

Hemoglobin Electrophoresis or High-performance Liquid Chromatography

This is the confirmatory test for beta thalassemia. Hemoglobin A2 is elevated above 3.5% (3.5–7%) and HbF may be slightly elevated in patients with beta thalassemia.

NESTROFT Test

The "Naked Eye Single Tube Red Cell Osmotic Fragility Test" (NESTROFT) is a cost-effective screening test in a rural setting. In this test, 2 mL of 0.36% buffered saline solution is taken in one tube and 2 mL of distilled water in another tube. A drop of blood is added to each of tube and left undisturbed for 20 minutes. Both tubes are shaken and held against a white line on which a black line drawn. Normally, the line is clearly visible through the distilled water. If the line is clearly visible similarly through the contents of tube with buffer solution, the test is negative. If the line is not clearly visible, the test is considered positive.

This test has a sensitivity of 100% and specificity of 85.4% with a positive predictive value of 66% and negative predictive value of 100%.[1]

Prenatal Screening of Thalassemia

Since thalassemia can be passed on from one generation to another, both partners should undergo thalassemia screening. If the mother is diagnosed to be thalassemia minor, the husband should be screened as well. If both test positive for thalassemia minor, genetic counseling and prenatal testing of the fetus should be advised to diagnose thalassemia major.

In vitro fertilization/intracytoplasmic sperm injection (IVF/ICSI) with a preimplantation genetic diagnosis (PGD) may also be considered in the presence of hemoglobinopathies in both partners so that a homozygous or compound heterozygous pregnancy can be avoided (Evidence level 3 or 4).[2]

Egg and sperm donors in IVF should be screened for hemoglobinopathies.

Thalassemia major poses multiple risk factors:
- Women with thalassemia have a higher incidence of diabetes. Those with established diabetes mellitus should have serum fructosamine concentrations of <300 nmol/L. HbA1c is not a reliable marker of glycemic control in this subgroup, as this is diluted by transfused blood and results in an underestimation; hence, serum fructosamine is preferred for monitoring.[3]
- Thyroid function should be determined, as hypothyroidism is frequently found in patients with thalassemia.[4]
- *Cardiac assessment*: Echocardiogram and electrocardiogram (ECG) should be performed to assess cardiac status, which may be compromised due to myocardial iron overload.
- Liver and gallbladder ultrasound should be used to detect cholelithiasis and evidence of liver cirrhosis due to iron overload or transfusion-related viral hepatitis.

Distinguishing features between iron-deficiency anemia and thalassemia are mentioned in **Table 1**. We often utilize the:
- *Mentzer index* = MCV/RBC

  In thalassemia, it is < 13 while in IDA it is > 13.
- *England and Fraser index* = MCV – (5 × Hb) is < 0 in beta thalassemia and > 0 in IDA.

TABLE 1: Distinguishing features in types of microcytic anemia.

Indicator	IDA	BT	ACD
Hemoglobin	Decreased	Normal/decreased	Decreased
Ferritin	Decreased	Normal/increased	Normal/increased
Serum iron	Decreased	Normal/increased	Normal/decreased
TIBC	Increased	Normal	Slightly decreased
TS	Decreased	Normal/increased	Normal/slightly decreased
sTfR in severe IDA	Increased	>100 mg/L	Normal
FEP	Increased	Normal	Increased
MCV	Decreased	Decreased	Normal/decreased
RDW	Increased	Normal/increased	Normal
Reticulocytes	Decreased		Normal/decreased
Mentzer index	Increased	Decreased (<13)	

(ACI: anemia of chronic disease; BT: β-thalassemia; IDA: iron-deficiency anemia; FEP: free erythrocyte protoporphyrin; MCV: mean corpuscular volume; RDW: red cell distribution width; SA: sideroblastic anemia; sTfR: soluble transferrin receptor; TIBC: total iron-binding capacity; TS: transferrin saturation).

MACROCYTIC ANEMIA

The reference range for MCV is 80–95 fL (femtoliter). Macrocytic anemia is defined as a MCV > 95 fL in a women with confirmed anemia.

The causes are:
- Vitamin B_{12} deficiency
- Folic acid deficiency
- Hypothyroidism
- Liver diseases
- Drug-induced hemolytic anemia (zidovudine)
- Ethanol abuse.

Peripheral Blood Smear

This will show:
- Macrocytes
- Moderate to marked anisopoikilocytosis
- Macro-ovalocytes, which are diagnostic
- Nucleated RBCs
- Basophilic stippling
- Cabot ring
- Howell–Jolly bodies
- Hypersegmented neutrophils—5% of neutrophils with five or more lobes or even a single nutrophil with six or more lobe. This is the first manifestation of megaloblastic anemia.
  Serum unconjugated bilirubin and serum LDH levels also rise.

Serum Folate Assays

Fasting folate and RBC folate levels are more specific for diagnosis. Serum folate < 2 ng/mL suggests folate deficiency anemia. Fasting folate level < 6 µg/L and RBC folate < 165 µg/L are diagnostic of folate deficiency.

Serum Vitamin B_{12} Assays

Serum vitamin B_{12} level < 100 pg/mL suggests vitamin B_{12} deficiency (normal levels are 160–760 ng/L); radioimmunoassay is sensitive and rapid.

Estimation of intrinsic factor (IF) by Schilling test will diagnose pernicious anemia.

Homocysteine Levels

These are a surrogate marker and are raised (>15) in both B_{12} and folate deficiency as well as in methyltetrahydrofolate reductase (*MTHFR*) gene mutation.

Bone Marrow

It shows megaloblastic erythroid hyperplasia with normal or increased iron stores.

◼ NORMOCYTIC ANEMIA

The causes of normocytic anemia are:
1. *Hemolytic anemias—inherited*:
   - Membrane defects, e.g., hereditary spherocytosis (HS)
   - Globin defects, e.g., sickle cell disease (SCD)
   - Metabolic disorder—glucose-6-phosphate dehydrogenase (G6PD) deficiency.
2. *Acquired*:
   - Protein calorie malnutrition
   - Anemia of chronic disease
   - *Anemia associated with chronic kidney disease*: Hypoplastic anemia
   - Marrow infiltration: Leukemia, myeloma, myelofibrosis, and metastasis.

Biochemical and hormonal tests for above conditions are performed and lastly a bone marrow aspirate to look for abnormal cells.

Hereditary Spherocytosis

- *Complete blood count*: Besides low levels of Hb, it shows low MCV and low MCHC. This is the only condition with raised MCHC, raised RDW, and raised reticulocyte count.
- Peripheral smear shows spherocytes, microspherocytes, acanthocytes, and pincered (mushroom shaped) cells.

- Osmotic fragility test is a laboratory test, which is sensitive but less specific. The test measures in vitro lysis of RBCs suspended in solutions of decreasing osmolarity. Spherocytes are characterized by membrane loss and less capacity to withstand hemolysis. It is normal in 10–20% of cases of HS.[5] The test may also be normal in the presence of iron-deficiency, obstructive jaundice, and in the recovery phase from aplastic crisis when reticulocyte count is increased.[6] A positive test can also be seen in hereditary elliptocytes and hemolysis.
- Direct antiglobulin test is usually negative, which differentiates it from autoimmune hemolytic anemia.
- Evidence of hemolysis is present such as raised bilirubin, jaundice, gallstones, splenomegaly, and reticulocytosis.
- Flow cytometry analysis will confirm sperocytosis.[7]

Sickle Cell Disease

Women and men with SCD should be encouraged to have the hemoglobinopathy status of their partner before they embark on pregnancy. If identified as an "at risk", couple should receive counseling and advice about reproductive options (RCOG green top guideline No 61, Evidence level 3 or 4).[8]

The methods and risk of prenatal diagnosis and termination of pregnancy should be discussed with the couple.[9]

Sperm donors should also be screened for hemoglobinopathies for couples considering in vitro fertilization.

If the woman has not been seen preconceptually, she should be offered partner testing. If the partner is a carrier, appropriate counseling should be offered—ideally by 10 weeks of gestation—to allow the option of first trimester diagnosis and termination, if that is the woman's choice (Evidence level 3 or 4).

Blood pressure and urinalysis should be performed at each visit, as they have an increased risk of pregnancy-induced hypertension.[10] Midstream urine—routine and culture sensitivity at each visit due to increased risk of urinary tract infection and asymptomatic bacteriuria in anemic women.[11] Retinal, renal, and cardiac assessment should be done. Baseline renal function test, urine protein/creatinine ratio. Liver function test and ferritin should be performed.

Glucose-6-Phosphate Dehydrogenase Deficiency

Screening for G6PD deficiency is indicated in patients with suggestive family history or in geographical areas with a high prevalence of the disorder. It is an X-linked recessive disorder that results in hemolysis triggered by infections, stress, medications, and certain food items like fava beans.[12]

Phenotypic Assays

Phenotypic assays include quantitative tests; these are able to detect G6PD activity for all individuals, from those with severe G6PD deficiency (<10% normal) to those with high G6PD activity (>100% normal). The spectrophotometric assay in a leukocyte-depleted sample is standard quantitative test.

Qualitative tests: These can be used to determine whether an individual is above or below a threshold predetermined by the diagnostic test for G6PD activity (30–40% of normal activity). The most commonly used test is fluorescent spot test (FST). It is positive, if the blood spot fails to fluoresce under ultraviolet light.

Genotyping Assays

The G6PD deficiency is usually caused by mutation in the G6PD gene that results in below normal G6PD activity. Polymerase chain reaction (PCR)-based single nucleotide polymorphism (SNP) analysis is most commonly used, but it is limited to identify presence or absence of known genotype; therefore, it may not correctly identify G6PD deficiency in patients with mutation not included in the panel. The other method, DNA sequencing, can identify all mutations in an individual's *G6PD* gene. Both are expensive and technically complex.

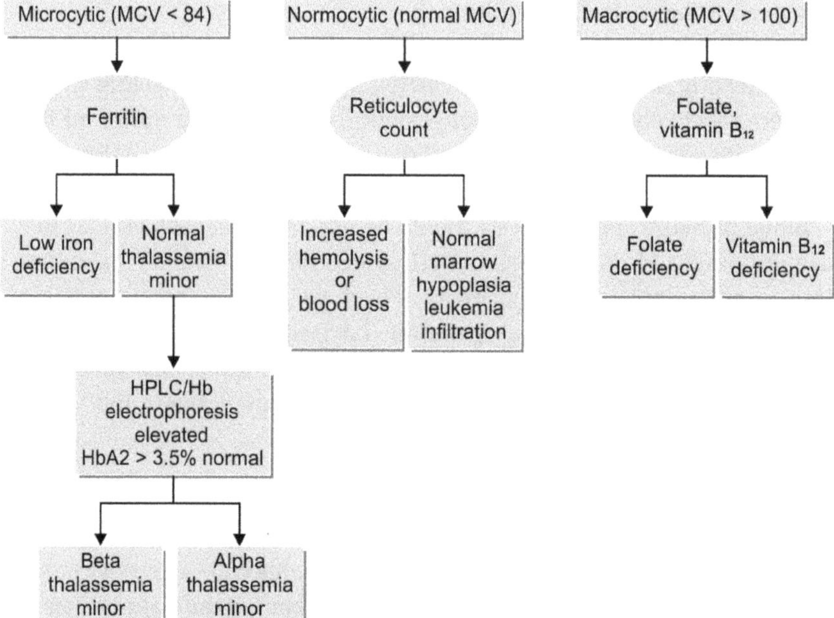

Flowchart 1: Flowchart for screening of anemia and hemoglobinopathies.

(Hb: hemoglobin; HbA2: hemoglobin A2; HPLC: high-performance liquid chromatography; MCV: mean corpuscular volume).

CONCLUSION

Preliminary screening for anemia should always include a complete blood count and a peripheral smear. This, itself, will often hint at the diagnosis. It is useful to classify them according to red cell size as that will direct the further investigative tract (*see* **Flowchart 1**). Confirmatory tests are required to confirm as well as quantify the deficiency states as well as diagnose hemoglobinopathies. A bone marrow examination is the final check to decide about the marrow responsiveness as well its malfunction in cases of leukemia. However, it is rarely required in iron-deficiency anemia. The tests should proceed in a stepwise manner to be cost-effective and arrive at a definitive diagnosis in the shortest possible time.

REFERENCES

1. Piplani S, MananR, Lalit M, Manjari M, Bhasin T, Bawa J, et al. Nestroft a valuable cost effective screening test for beta thalassemia trait in north Indian Punjabi population. J Clin Diagn Res. 2013;7(12):2784-7.
2. Royal College of Obstetrician and Gynecologist (2014). Thalassemia in Pregnancy, management of beta. RCOG green top guideline No 66. [online] Available from: https://www.rcog.org.uk/globalassets/documents/guidelines/gtg_66_thalassaemia.pdf. [Last accessed May, 2020].
3. Spencer DH, Grossman BJ, Scott MG. Red cell transfusion decreases haemoglobin A1c in patient with diabetes. Clin Chem. 2011;57(2):344-6.
4. Abalovich M, Amino N, Barbour LA, Cobin RH, De Groot LJ, Glinoer D, et al. Management of thyroid dysfunction during pregnancy and postpartum: an Endocrine Society Clinical Practice Guideline. J Clin Endocrinol Metab. 2007;92(Suppl):S1-47.
5. Dacie JV, Lewis SM, Luzatto L. Investigation of the hereditary hemolytic anaemia: membrane and enzyme abnormalities. In: Dacie JV, Lewis SM. Practical Haematology. Edinburgh: Churchill Livingstone; 1991. pp. 195-225.
6. Korones D, Pearson HA. Normal erythrocyte osmotic fragility in hereditary spherocytosis. J Paediatr. 1989;114(2):264-6.
7. Bolton–Maggs P, Langer JC, Iolascon A, Paul T, King MJ, General Haematology Task Force of the British Committee for Standards in Haematology. Guidelines for diagnosis & management of hereditary spherocytosis. Br J Haematol. 2012;156(1):37-49.
8. Royal College of Obstetrician and Gynecologist (2011). Management of Sickle cell disease in pregnancy RCOG green top guideline No 61. [online] Available from: https://www.rcog.org.uk/globalassets/documents/guidelines/gtg_61.pdf. [Last accessed May, 2020].
9. Royal College of Obstetricians and Gynaecologists. Amniocentesis and chorionic villous sampling. Green-top Guideline No. 8. London: RCOG; 2010.
10. Tuck SM, Studd JW, White JM. Pregnancy in sickle cell disease in the UK. Br J Obstet Gynaecol. 1983;90:112-7.
11. Villers MS, Jamison MG, De Castro LM, James AH. Morbidity associated with sickle cell disease in pregnancy. Am J Obstet Gynaecol. 2008;199:125.e1-5.
12. National Organisation for rare diseases (NORD) (2017). Glucose 6 phosphate dehydrogenase deficiency. [online] Available from: https://rarediseases.org/rare-diseases/glucose-6-phosphate-dehydrogenase-deficiency/#:~:text=Glucose%2D6%2Dphosphate%20dehydrogenase%20(,break%20down%20prematurely%20(hemolysis). [Last accessed May, 2020].

Screening for Diabetes Mellitus

Priti Kumar, Phagun Shah

■ INTRODUCTION

Hyperglycemia in pregnancy (HIP) is defined as carbohydrate intolerance with recognition or onset during pregnancy, irrespective of treatment with diet or insulin whether or not condition persists after pregnancy. HIP is further classified as pregestational (Type 1, Type 2, and others) or gestational diabetes mellitus (GDM). GDM is the window of opportunity to improve maternal and child health and slow down the diabetes pandemic. It is therefore important to detect the condition as early as possible during pregnancy thereby decreasing the short-term and long-term complications in both mother and child. The prevalence of GDM in India ranges from 4 to 21%. The difference is due to different diagnostic methods and vast topographical locations.

We need a screening method, which can double up as diagnostic test as well in our country because Asian females are at higher risk of developing diabetes mellitus.

We practice "Universal Screening" using single step test. All pregnant women should be screened universally. "DIPSI method" (Diabetes in Pregnancy Study group in India) is now accepted as a method to screening and testing in pregnant ladies.

■ ADVANTAGES OF "DIPSI" TEST

- Fasting state is not needed.
- It can be performed at the first antenatal visit.
- Second visit is not needed for the glucose testing.
- It is found to be equally reliable when compared to the criteria followed by World Health Organization (WHO), American Diabetes Association (ADA), etc.
- It is very simple to perform and effective.
- It is economical.

■ METHOD

- Single step testing using 75 g oral glucose and measuring blood sugar 2 hours after ingestion.
- 75 g glucose is to be given orally after dissolving in approximately 300 mL of water whether the pregnant women comes in fasting or

TABLE 1: Evaluation of blood sugar.

2-h Plasma glucose	
>200 mg/dL	Diabetes
>140–199 mg/dL	GDM
120–139 mg/dL	GGI
<120 mg/dL	Normal

(GDM: gestational diabetes mellitus; GGI: gestational glucose intolerance)

nonfasting state, irrespective of the last meal. The intake of the solution has to be completed within 5–10 minutes.

- A plasma-standardized glucometer should be used to evaluate blood sugar 2 hours after the oral glucose load **(Table 1)**.
- If vomiting occurs within 30 minutes of oral glucose intake, the test has to be repeated the next day, or else refer to a facility. If vomiting occurs after 30 minutes, the test continues.
- *The threshold blood sugar level of ≥140 mg/dL (more than or equal to 140) is taken as cut off for diagnosis of GDM.*

PROTOCOL FOR INVESTIGATION (FLOWCHART 1)

- Testing for GDM is recommended twice during ANC.
- The first testing should be done during first antenatal contact as early as possible in pregnancy.
- The second testing should be done during 24–28 weeks of pregnancy, if the first test is negative. It is important to ensure second test as many pregnant women develop blood sugar intolerance during this period (24–28 weeks). Moreover, only one-third of GDM-positive women are detected during first trimester. If it could not be done during this time, then it can be done any time after 24 weeks of pregnancy.
- There should be at least 4-week gap between the two tests.
- The test is to be conducted for all pregnant women even if she comes late in pregnancy for ANC at the time of first contact.
- If she presents beyond 28 weeks of pregnancy, only one test is to be done at the first point of contact.

Though Government of India advocates testing twice for "gestational diabetes" during 9 months of "pregnancy", but one-third of GDM patients are detected in the third trimester pregnancy. So, it is advisable that all pregnant patient should be tested once also in the third trimester (32–34 weeks of pregnancy).

If a pregnant female has a blood sugar of ≥ 140 mg/dL, the follow-up test should be done with fasting and postprandial blood sugars. The subsequent test should not be done with 75 g glucose load.

- *Expected maintenance reports of glucose*:
- Mean glucose level = 105 mg/dL
- Fasting blood sugar (FBS) = 90 mg/dL
- PP2BS = 120 mg/dL

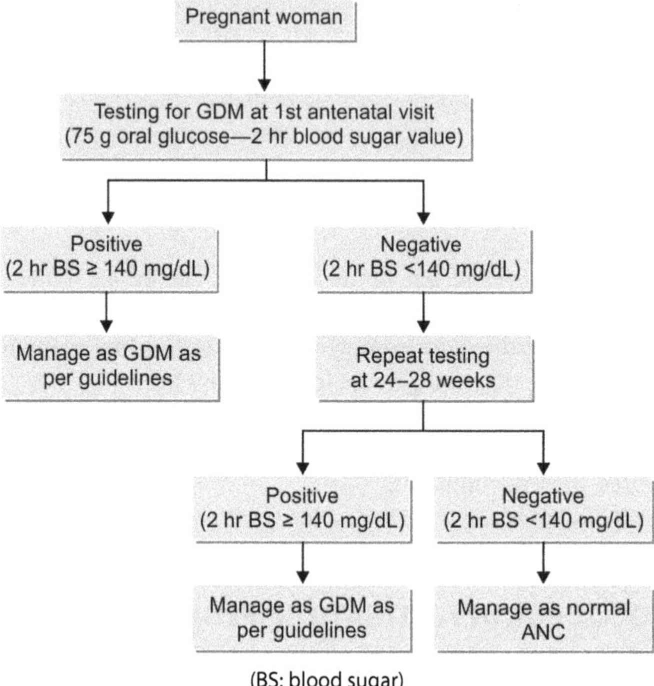

Flowchart 1: Universal testing for gestational diabetes mellitus (GDM).

TABLE 2: Correlation of HbA1c with malformations.	
HbA1c (%)	*Rate of malformations (%)*
<7.9	6.9
8.0–10	19.0
>10	31

Note: Not very useful for monitoring sugar control during pregnancy
(HbA1c: hemoglobin A1c)

ROLE OF HBA1C

Hemoglobin A1c (HbA1c) will differentiate between the pregestational diabetes and GDM in very early pregnancy. It is not found to be sensitive enough to monitor blood sugar control during pregnancy **(Table 2)**.

High HbA1c is not an indication for termination of pregnancy. It helps in counseling regarding the incidence of malformation in fetus, if sugar levels are uncontrolled.

So, to conclude, "DIPSI" is a simple and effective method used for screening and diagnosing GDM.

As Indian women stand (11%) more chance of developing GDM, it becomes very helpful in picking up GDM at early onset and thus preventing maternal and fetal complications during the pregnancy and long-term consequences of developing Type II DM in the women and offspring.

Screening Thyroid Disorders during Pregnancy

Gorakh G Mandrupkar

"To screen or not to screen thyroid disorder...That is the question!"

INTRODUCTION

Thyroid disorders during pregnancy, especially hypothyroidism, have drawn more attention of researchers in last few decades. Thyroid disorders in pregnancy constitute second most common endocrine disorder during pregnancy after diabetes mellitus. Pregnancy affects the functioning of thyroid gland and vice-versa.

Thyroid disorders, especially the untreated hypothyroidism, are associated with early pregnancy loss, pre-eclampsia, preterm labor, and abruptio placenta. Fetal complications such as prematurity, stillbirth, low birth weight babies, and perinatal death are also seen in such cases. Attention deficits, hyperactive child syndrome, and defects in intellectual development are reported in children born to untreated hypothyroid women.

GESTATIONAL HYPOTHYROIDISM

A new insight and a terminology I want to introduce here in the form of gestational hypothyroidism.

We all agree that pregnancy affects the functioning of thyroid gland. It causes 10–40% increase in size of the thyroid gland as well as 50% increase in the production of thyroid hormones namely thyroxine (T4) and triiodothyronine (T3).

The pregnant women who are initially euthyroid but having limited thyroid reserve and/or with iodine deficiency can become hypothyroid during the later stages of pregnancy.

Same is true about the pregnant euthyroid women who are thyroid autoantibody positive (TAb+), as they have increased propensity to develop hypothyroidism later on due to destruction of gland tissue due to autoantibodies.

All such women will require thyroid-stimulating hormone (TSH) monitoring during pregnancy.

Accepted cut-off levels of TSH during pregnancy:
- *First trimester:* 0.1–2.5 mIU/L
- *Second trimester:* 0.2–3.0 mIU/L
- *Third trimester:* 0.3–3.5 mIU/L

Definition

- *Primary maternal hypothyroidism* is defined as increased serum TSH levels during pregnancy.
  Depending upon free T4 (FT4) levels, it can be further classified as:
  - *Subclinical hypothyroidism*: Normal FT4 and high TSH (>2.5–10)
  - *Overt hypothyroidism (OH)*: Low FT4 and high TSH
  The TSH more than 10 with normal FT4 is also considered as overt hypothyroidism.
  These are independent of thyroid antibody levels.
- *Primary maternal hyperthyroidism* is defined as decreased serum TSH levels during pregnancy.
  Depending upon free T4 (FT4) levels, it can be further classified as:
  - *Subclinical hyperthyroidism*: Normal FT4 and low TSH (<2.5)
  - *Overt hyperthyroidism*: High FT4 and low TSH.

Prevalence

There is a great worldwide variation in the prevalence of thyroid disorders in pregnancy.

- Western literature shows a prevalence of hypothyroidism in pregnancy of 2.5% and hyperthyroidism in pregnancy has prevalence of 0.1–0.4%.[1] Studies have demonstrated 60% risk of fetal loss and 22% risk of gestational hypertension with untreated OH. The miscarriage rate in subchorionic hematoma (SCH) is 6% versus 3.6% in euthyroid women.
- Pathological overt hyperthyroidism, usually due to Graves' disease, occurs with a frequency of approximately 0.2%; however, previously treated maternal Graves' disease prior to pregnancy is more common and can occur prior to 1% of pregnancies.[2] Gestational thyrotoxicosis (suppressed TSH and elevated FT4) mainly through excess human chorionic gonadotropin (hCG) and usually associated with hyperemesis gravidarum occurs in up to 3% of pregnancies.[2]

Indian National Evidence

Prevalence of hypothyroidism in pregnancy in the Indian population is 4.8–11%.[3-5]

Thyroid peroxidase (TPO) antibodies are positive in around 50% pregnant women in SCH, as compared to 7% in euthyroid pregnant women.

Incidence of hypothyroidism in women with first trimester recurrent pregnancy loss is up to 4.1–16.6%. The miscarriage rate in SCH is 12–21%; while in OH, it is 21%. The rate of stillbirth is 0–16.6% for SCH and 4.2% for OH. The incidence of pre-eclampsia has been reported as 16% for OH and 22% for SCH. Intrauterine growth restriction prevalence is 25% in OH and 8% in SCH; while the incidence of preterm delivery, it is 33% with OH and 11% with SCH.

Screening in Pregnancy

Though thyroid disorders, especially hypothyroidism, are associated with so many complications when question of routine screening comes, there are two schools of thoughts.

1. Not "for" as well as not "against" the screening for thyroid disorders in pregnancy and screening in women with specific high-risk factors.[6,7]
2. Routine screening of all pregnant women for thyroid disorders.[8]

INTERNATIONAL CONSENSUS

All women trying for pregnancy and pregnant women with any of the following risk factors should be screened using TSH levels.[6]

- A history of hypothyroidism/hyperthyroidism or current symptoms/signs of thyroid dysfunction
- Known thyroid antibody positivity or presence of a goiter
- History of head or neck radiation or prior thyroid surgery
- Age > 30 years
- Type 1 diabetes or other autoimmune disorders
- History of pregnancy loss, preterm delivery, or infertility
- Multiple prior pregnancies
- Family history of autoimmune thyroid disease or thyroid dysfunction
- Morbid obesity (BMI $\geq$ 40 kg/m^2)
- Use of amiodarone or lithium, or recent administration of iodinated radiologic contrast
- Residing in an area of known moderate-to-severe iodine insufficiency.

INDIAN CONSENSUS

National guidelines of India for screening of hypothyroidism in pregnancy have also accepted the high-risk based approach of screening. The only change from that of international consensus is change in body mass index (BMI) cut-off value of 30 instead of 40.[8]

Only Indian Thyroid Society recommends the universal screening of all pregnant women.[8]

AUTHOR'S CONCLUSION

- Though all are in favor of risk-based screening approach, the message from the study of Vaidya et al.[9] and Horacek et al.[10] should also be given due consideration, who commented that almost 30–50% will remain undetected with this screening. This is similar to the Indian study in which 40% of the hypothyroid and 45% of TPOAb-positive patients did not have above-mentioned high-risk characteristics but found to have thyroid dysfunction during pregnancy.[3] Approximately, 60% of the hypothyroid or TPOAb-positive pregnant women could have been missed by targeted case finding.

- Recent studies have shown increase in overall prevalence of hypothyroidism during pregnancy along with its influence on fetal and maternal outcome.[11]
- As there is definite increase in early miscarriages, preterm labor, preeclampsia, and neonatal intellectual defects in overt as well as subclinical hypothyroidism which warrants the attention for further studies.
- For time being, universal screening for thyroid disorders during pregnancy should be the policy in India till further conclusive research findings.

REFERENCES

1. LeBeau SO, Mandel SJ. Thyroid disorders during pregnancy. Endocrinol Metab Clin North Am. 2006;35:117-36.
2. Cooper DS, Laurberg P. Hyperthyroidism in pregnancy. Lancet Diabetes Endocrinol 2013;1:238-49.
3. Nambiar V, Jagtap VS, Sarathi V, Lila AR, Kamalanathan S, Bandgar TR, et al. Prevalence and impact of thyroid disorders on maternal outcome in Asian-Indian pregnant women. J Thyroid Res. 2011;2011:4290-7.
4. Sahu MT, Das V, Mittal S, Agarwal A, Sahu M. Overt and subclinical thyroid dysfunction among Indian pregnant women and its effect on maternal and fetal outcome. Arch Gynecol Obstet. 2010;281:215-20.
5. Pahwa S, Mangat S. Prevalence of thyroid disorders in pregnancy. Int J Reprod Contracept Obstet Gynecol. 2018;7(9):3493-6.
6. Alexander EK, Pearce EN, Brent GA, Brown RS, Chen H, Dosiou C, et al. 2017 Guidelines of the American Thyroid Association for the Diagnosis and Management of Thyroid Disease During Pregnancy and the Postpartum. Thyroid. 2017;27:315-89.
7. Abalovich M, Amino N, Barbour LA, Cobin RH, De Groot LJ, Glinoer D, et al. Green. management of thyroid dysfunction during pregnancy and postpartum: an endocrine society clinical practice guideline. J Clin Endocrinol Metab. 2007; 92(8 Suppl):S1-47.
8. Maternal Health Division; Ministry of Health and Family Welfare (2014). National guidelines for 'Screening of Hypothyroidism in pregnancy'. [online] Available from: https://nhm.gov.in/images/pdf/programmes/maternal-health/guidelines/National_Guidelines_for_Screening_of_Hypothyroidism_during_Pregnancy.pdf. [Last accessed June, 2020].
9. Vaidya B, Anthony S, Bilous M, Shields B, Drury J, Hutchison S, et al. Detection of thyroid dysfunction in early pregnancy: universal screening or targeted high-risk case finding? J Clin Endocrinol Metab. 2007;92(1):203-7.
10. Horacek J, Spitalnikova S, Dlabalova B, Malirova E, Vizda J, Svilias I, et al. Universal screening detects two-times more thyroid disorders in early pregnancy than targeted high-risk case finding. Eur J Endocrinol. 2010;163(4):645-50.
11. Ajmani SN, Aggarwal D, Bhatia P, Sharma M, Sarabhai V, Paul M. Prevalence of overt and subclinical thyroid dysfunction among pregnant women and its effect on maternal and fetal outcome. J Obstet Gynecol India. 2014;64(2):105-10.

Screening for Sexually Transmitted Infections in Pregnancy

Sarita Agrawal, Anuradha Tiberawal

INTRODUCTION

The terms, sexually transmitted diseases/infections (STDs/STIs), refer to a variety of clinical syndromes and infections caused by pathogens that can be acquired and transmitted through sexual activity. The Centers for Disease Control and Prevention (CDC), American College of Obstetricians and Gynecologists (ACOG), and many other international bodies recommend routine screening for some STIs at the first prenatal visit and then in subsequent visits depending upon prevalence in the community.

MAGNITUDE OF PROBLEM

Sexually transmitted infections rank among the top five conditions for which sexually active adults seek healthcare in the developing countries. There are more than 30 different sexually transmissible bacteria, viruses, and parasites. However, the common STIs, which are known to have significant implications in pregnancy, are syphilis, *Neisseria gonorrhoeae, Chlamydia trachomatis,* human papilloma virus (HPV), herpes simplex virus (HSV), HIV, *Trichomonas vaginalis,* and bacterial vaginosis (BV). According to World Health Organization (WHO), >1 million people acquire an STI every day globally and 500 million new cases of one of four curable STIs (Chlamydia, gonorrhea, syphilis, and trichomoniasis) occur each year worldwide. A community-based STI/reproductive tract infection (RTI) prevalence study conducted during 2002–03 by the Indian Council of Medical Research (ICMR) has shown that 6% of the adult population in India has one or more STI/RTI. This amounts to occurrence of about 30–35 million episodes of STI/RTI every year in the country.

RATIONALE OF SCREENING FOR SEXUALLY TRANSMITTED INFECTIONS IN PREGNANCY

Some of the most important STI/RTI-related problems in pregnancy including postabortion and postpartum infections are not technically difficult or expensive to manage or prevent altogether. Simple improvements in service delivery with use of available technology—such as same-day, on-site early identification by screening in antenatal clinics—can lead to dramatic improvements in pregnancy and neonatal outcome.

TABLE 1: Common sexually transmitted infections and their effects on pregnancy.

Infection	Risks to mother	Risks to baby	Perinatal transmission risk
Bacterial infections			
Syphilis	• Primary syphilis—chancre • Secondary syphilis—rashes and fever • Tertiary syphilis—condylomata lata	• Second trimester abortion, macerated stillbirth, fresh stillbirth, active congenital syphilis in newborn in successive pregnancy in that order • Other manifestations—congenital syphilis, hydrops fetalis deafness, neurologic impairment, bone and tooth abnormalities, LBW	15 and 36%
Gonorrhea	• Infertility • Ectopic pregnancies • PID, pelvic abscess • Bartholin's abscess • Chorioamnionitis • PROM • Postpartum sepsis • Spontaneous, septic abortion	• IUGR • Premature birth (13–67%) • Stillbirth • Ophthalmia neonatorum • Sepsis	30–40% of cases of maternal cervical infection
Chlamydia	• Infertility • Ectopic pregnancies • PID • Postpartum or postabortion endometritis and salpingitis • Preterm delivery • PROM	• Infections to the mucous membranes of the eye, oropharynx, urogenital tract, and rectum • LBW • Ophthalmia neonatorum, blindness • Pneumonia	50% reported to be as high as 60–70%
Trichomoniasis	• Can cause fallopian tube damage • Vaginitis	• Premature birth • Low birth weight • PROM	
Chancroid *Haemophilus ducreyi*	• Is a cofactor for HIV infection	• Neonates can acquire the infection from the mother	
Bacterial vaginosis	• Chorioamnionitis • Miscarriage • Postpartum endometritis • Preterm labor • PROM	• Neonatal infections • LBW and prematurity	

Contd...

Contd...

Infection	Risks to mother	Risks to baby	Perinatal transmission risk
Viral infections			
Human papillomavirus (HPV)	• Genital cancer warts in birth canal can cause complications during delivery • Cesarean delivery	• Warts in the baby's throat • Recurrent respiratory papillomatosis—juvenile laryngeal papillomatosis common benign laryngeal tumor in children due HPV 6, 11 infection at the time of delivery	
Hepatitis B	• The immunological changes during pregnancy and the postpartum period have been associated with hepatitis flares (including hepatic decompensation)	• Intrauterine growth restriction, intrauterine infection, premature delivery, and intrauterine fetal demise • Unless treated within an hour of birth, 90% of babies will be a carrier for life and at risk for liver disease and liver cancer	• Infection in early preg-nancy—10% and in late pregnancy up to 60%
Hepatitis C	• Asymptomatic • Hepatitis in pregnancy		• 5% infants exposed become infected, most often during or near delivery • Breastfeeding does not seem to transmit HCV
Herpes simplex	• Cesarean delivery, if there are prodromes or active lesions when the woman goes into labor	• Severe outbreak in the first trimester can result in miscarriage • Acquires infection from mother; rates are highest when herpes is acquired near time of delivery • Eye infections • Severe disseminated or CNS infection resulting in mental retardation or death	• In primary infec-tion— 40–60%, in nonpri-mary—33%, in recurrent infection—5%, and in asym-ptomatic shedding—1%

Contd...

Contd...

Infection	Risks to mother	Risks to baby	Perinatal transmission risk
Human immuno-deficiency virus (HIV)	• Exacerbation of disease?	• HIV infection in neonate major burden • IUGR, LBW, and PTD—reported in developing countries	• About 20–45% in untreated group 2/3rd of transmission occurs during labor and delivery and 1/3rd occur in antenatal period in non-breastfeeding • Additional risk of 15–20% occurs during breastfeeding

(IUGR: intrauterine growth restriction; LBW: low birth weight; PROM: premature rupture of membrane; PTD: preterm delivery; PID: pelvic inflammatory disease)

SCREENING, PREVENTION, AND CONTROL OF SEXUALLY TRANSMITTED INFECTIONS

The prevention and control of STDs are based upon five major strategies:

1. Accurate risk assessment and education and counseling of persons at risk on ways to avoid STDs through changes in sexual behaviors and use of recommended prevention services.
2. Pre-exposure vaccination of persons at risk for vaccine preventable STDs.
3. Identification of asymptomatically infected persons and persons with symptoms associated with STDs.
4. Effective diagnosis, treatment, counseling, and follow-up of infected persons.
5. Evaluation, treatment, and counseling of sex partners of persons who are infected with an STD.

Assessment of Behavioral Risk

In general, clinicians should determine a pregnant woman's risk status using the same risk factors as for nonpregnant women performing an assessment of behavioral risk, which includes—obtain a thorough sexual history including *4 P's*: (1) *Partners* (any new sexual partner, history of multiple sexual partners, and sexual partners with concomitant partners); (2) *Practices* (history of sexual intercourse with trauma, anatomic sites of exposure); (3) *Protection from STIs* (frequency of condom use); (4) *Past history of STIs* (the history should be straightforward and nonjudgmental with appropriate counseling regarding risk-taking behaviors, as necessary); (5) Prevalence of disease in the geographic area to women belongs to is also taken in consideration while assessing the risks.

TABLE 2: World Health Organization (WHO) antenatal care (ANC) model.

Reason for visit: Pregnancy	*Initial assessment* ↓	*Follow-up antenatal visit* ↓	*Labor and delivery* ↓	*Postpartum* ↓
	Assess STI/RTI symptoms and history of spontaneous abortion or preterm delivery ↓ Provide syphilis screening, treatment, and partner treatment ↓	Assess STI/RTI symptoms ↓ Repeat syphilis screening in late pregnancy ↓ Discuss prevention of mother-to-child transmission, if HIV positive ↓	Assess for STI/RTI symptoms: rule out active herpes ↓ Review syphilis results, consider treatment of newborn ↓ Consider and discuss prevention of MTCT, if HIV positive ↓	Assess for STI/RTI symptoms: rule out postpartum infection ↓ Discuss prevention of MTCT, if HIV positive; consider substitute feeding plan Discuss STI/RTI protection and contraception
	Test for bacterial vaginosis and trichomoniasis, if history of spontaneous abortion or preterm delivery ↓ Offer counseling and testing for HIV ↓ Discuss STI/RTI protection ↓ Discuss birth plan and postpartum FP ↓	Discuss STI/RTI protection ↓ Review birth plan	Provide neonatal eye prophylaxis	

(FV: family planning; MTCT: mother-to-child transmission; RTI: reproductive tract infection; STI: sexually transmitted infection)

Assessment of Clinical Presentations

Identification of asymptomatically infected persons (recommendations for screening)—most of the time even when asymptomatic STIs are associated with fetal and neonatal risk, which depends upon many factors.

Recommendations to screen pregnant women for STDs are based on disease severity and sequelae, prevalence in the population, costs, medicolegal considerations (e.g., state laws), and other factors.

■ SYPHILIS

Universal antepartum screening is widely recommended because screening followed by treatment with appropriate antibiotics usually prevents adverse outcomes in the mother and child.

- A serologic test for syphilis should be performed for all pregnant women at the first prenatal visit.
- When access to prenatal care is not optimal, rapid plasma reagin (RPR) card test screening (and treatment, if that test is reactive) should be performed at the time that a pregnancy is confirmed.
- Women who are at high risk for syphilis or live in areas of high syphilis morbidity should be screened again early in the third trimester approximately at 28–32 weeks and again at delivery.
- Some states require all women to be screened at delivery. Neonates should not be discharged from the hospital unless the syphilis serologic status of the mother has been determined at least one time during pregnancy and preferably again at delivery, if at risk. Any woman who delivers a stillborn infant should be tested for syphilis.
- *Screening test*: Screening is performed using a serologic test either a treponemal or nontreponemal test, and all of have similar sensitivity and specificity, so preference is based on other factors (e.g., cost, time, and personnel requirements).
- Rapid point of care tests are less accurate than standard nontreponemal and treponemal tests; however, these can be helpful in guiding initial treatment decisions in women who may be less likely to return for follow-up. Due to biologic false-positive nontreponemal and treponemal results are relatively common in pregnant women, confirmatory testing of positive tests is recommended and interpretation needs to be as per WHO algorithm.
- *Diagnostic test*: The definitive diagnosis of early-stage lesions is made using dark field examination and direct fluorescent antibody testing of lesion exudates. Confirmatory tests in secondary and late syphilis are fluorescent treponemal antibody absorption tests (FTA-ABS), the microhemagglutination assay for antibodies to *Treponema pallidum* (MHA-TP), or the *Treponema pallidum* passive particle agglutination (TP-PA) test.

Polymerase chain reaction (PCR) is specific for detection of *Treponema pallidum* in amniotic fluid, and treponemal DNA has been found in 40% of pregnancies infected before 20 weeks. Although prenatal diagnosis can be made by funipuncture or amniocentesis, its clinical utility is not yet clear. Postnatally, examination of placenta (large and pale) is done.

TABLE 3: Comparison of screening recommendations for sexually transmitted infections in pregnant women.

Infection	US Preventive Services Task Force	Centers for Disease Control and Prevention	American Academy of Family Physicians	American Congress of Obstetricians and Gynecologists
Chlamydia	Screen women of age 24 years and younger, and older women at increased risk	Screen women of age 24 years and younger, and older women at increased risk	Screen women of age 24 years and younger, and older women at increased risk	Screen women of age 24 years and younger, and older women at increased risk
Gonorrhea	Screen women of age 24 years and younger, and older women at increased risk	Screen women of age 24 years and younger, and older women at increased risk	Screen women of age 24 years and younger, and older women at increased risk	Screen women of age 24 years and younger, and older women at increased risk
Hepatitis B virus	Screen all	Screen all	Screen all	Screen all
HSV	Do not screen	Evidence does not support routine HSV-2 serologic screening in asymptomatic pregnant women. However, type-specific serologic testing may be useful for identifying pregnant women at risk of HSV infection, and for guiding counseling about the risk of acquiring genital herpes during pregnancy	Do not screen	Evidence does not support routine HSV-2 serologic screening in asymptomatic pregnant women. However, type-specific serologic testing may be useful for identifying pregnant women at risk of HSV infection, and for guiding counseling about the risk of acquiring genital herpes during pregnancy
Human immuno-deficiency virus	Screen all	Screen all	Screen all	Screen all
Syphilis	Screen all	Screen all	Screen all	Screen all

(HSV: herpes simplex virus)

Microscopically (decreased number of villous, loss of arborization, and endarteritis), spirochetes may be detected in almost 90% using silver and immunofluorescent staining.

▇ GONORRHEA

- *Screening*: Pregnant women with risk factors for gonorrhea or living in an area where the prevalence of *Neisseria gonorrhoeae* is high are screened for gonorrhea, in agreement with American College of Obstetricians and Gynecologists (ACOG) and CDC guidelines.
- *Screening test: Nucleic acid amplification test (NAAT) (>96% sensitivity) is the preferred test for microbiologic diagnosis because of its superior accuracy. Endocervical and vaginal swabs are of equivalent sensitivity.* False positives may occur. However, confirmatory culture for gonococcus is essential to allow antimicrobial sensitivity testing, which is of paramount importance given increasing antibiotic resistance. Pregnant women who test positive are treated immediately and retested in 3 months.
- Pregnant women who remain at high risk for gonococcal infection also should be retested during the third trimester to prevent maternal postnatal complications and gonococcal infection in the neonate.
- *Routine screening for gonorrhea is not recommended as per Indian guidelines.*

▇ *CHLAMYDIA TRACHOMATIS*

- *Screening*: In United States, routine screening for *Chlamydia trachomatis* during the first prenatal visit is also done in all pregnant women aged <25 years and older women at increased risk for infection (e.g., those in polygamous relations).
- Women at increased risk for *Chlamydia* also should be retested during the third trimester to prevent maternal postnatal complications and chlamydial infection in the neonate.
- Pregnant women found to have Chlamydial infection should have a test-of-cure to document Chlamydial eradication (preferably by NAAT) 3–4 weeks after treatment and then retested within 3 months.
- *In India, supportive evidence for such routine screening for Chlamydia is lacking.*

▇ HUMAN IMMUNODEFICIENCY VIRUS

The HIV screening recommendations:
- HIV testing services (HTS) as early as possible during each new pregnancy enables pregnant women to reduce HIV transmission.
- Screening should be conducted after the woman is notified of the need to be screened for HIV as part of the routine panel of prenatal tests.
- *Partner testing is recommended for all.*

- *Repeat testing (retesting)* is recommended in the third trimester, or during labor, or shortly after delivery in high-prevalence settings and high-risk populations to catch up the women in window period.
- In all settings, HTS should be recommended to all women of unknown HIV status presenting directly in labor or delivery, if that is not feasible, as soon as possible after delivery.
- As per National AIDS Control Organization (NACO) PPTCT guidelines based on single initial positive test result, antiretroviral treatment may be started once for women presenting in labor directly, the confirmatory test may be done subsequently.
- *Screening of neonate*: *Early infant diagnosis (EID)*—infant is tested for HIV DNA PCR at 6 weeks, repeat testing at 6 months, 12 months and 6 weeks after cessation of all breastfeeding. The test recommended for EID is by dry blood spot (DBS). If the DBS sample is positive for HIV DNA PCR, then a repeat sample is tested for HIV DNA PCR through whole blood collection. The HEI, who is confirmed HIV positive through two DNA PCR test, is initiated on lifelong ART at the earliest irrespective of CD4 count.
- *Screening tests and their interpretations (WHO, 2015)*: If initial screening test is positive, confirmation of diagnosis is done usually based upon three tests positive (A1, A2, and A3), which should include three different serological assays that do not share the same false reactivity (i.e., test with different antigens or different principle of test).
- All specimens are first tested with one assay (A1), and specimens that are nonreactive (A1–) are considered HIV-negative and reported as such. A1 should be the most sensitive assay available.
- Any specimens that are reactive on the first assay (A1+) should be reflexed (tested again). For specimens that are reactive both on the first-line assay and the second-line assay (A1+ and A2+), in high-prevalence settings (prevalence >5%), a diagnosis of HIV-positive should be issued to people with two sequential reactive tests. In low-prevalence settings (in settings where prevalence <5%), a diagnosis of HIV-positive should be issued to people with three sequential reactive tests.
- All individuals that are diagnosed HIV-positive should be confirmed with third assay, prior to starting ART to verify their HIV-positive status.
- The test selected should have highest sensitivity (clinical, analytical, and seroconversion) for first-line assay, and highest specificity for second- and third-line assays, irrespective of format. HIV testing services may use combinations of RDTs (rapid diagnostic tests) or combinations of RDTs/EIAs/supplemental assays rather than EIA/Western blot combinations.
- Whichever commercial kit is selected, it should be ensured that it detects antibodies against HIV-1, HIV-2, and their subtypes.

HEPATITIS B

Screening recommendations:

- All pregnant women should be routinely tested for hepatitis B surface antigen (HBsAg) at the first prenatal visit even if they have been previously vaccinated or tested.
- Women who were not screened prenatally, those who engage in behaviors that put them at high risk and those with clinical hepatitis should be retested at the time of admission to the hospital for delivery.
- Pregnant women at risk for HBV infection also should be vaccinated. To avoid misinterpreting a transient positive HBsAg result during the 21 days after vaccination, HBsAg testing should be performed before vaccine administration.
- All laboratories that conduct HBsAg tests should test initially reactive specimens with a licensed neutralizing confirmatory test.
- When pregnant women are tested for HBsAg at the time of admission for delivery, shortened testing protocols can be used, and initially reactive results should prompt expedited administration of immunoprophylaxis to neonates.
- In addition, household and sex contacts of women who are HBsAg positive should be vaccinated.
- Women who are HBsAg positive should be provided with, or referred for, appropriate counseling and medical management.

HEPATITIS C

- Routine screening for HCV infection is not recommended for all pregnant women. Pregnant women with a known risk factor for HCV infection should be offered screening.
- Testing for HCV infection should include use of an FDA-cleared test for antibody to HCV (i.e., immunoassay, EIA, or enhanced chemiluminescence immunoassay, and, if recommended, a supplemental antibody test, followed by NAAT to detect HCV RNA for those with a positive antibody result. Persons with HIV infection with low CD4-positive cell count might require further testing by NAAT because of the potential for a false-negative antibody assay. Evaluate (by referral or consultation, if appropriate) for the presence of acute infection—presence, severity, or development of chronic liver disease (CLD) and eligibility for treatment. Nucleic acid testing, including reverse transcriptase polymerase chain reaction (RT-PCR) to detect HCV RNA, is necessary to confirm the diagnosis of current HCV infection, and testing of liver function (alanine aminotransferase level) provides biochemical evidence of CLD.
- All persons with HIV infection should undergo serologic screening for HCV at initial evaluation.

- Infants born to mothers with HCV infection should be tested for HCV infection, because maternal antibody is present for the first 18 months of life and before the infant mounts an immunologic response, nucleic acid testing is recommended.

HERPES SIMPLEX

Recommendations for Screening

Most expert panels do not support routine HSV-2 serologic screening among asymptomatic pregnant women as available evidence indicates that screening for HSV would not meet usual criteria for an effective preventive strategy, as has been demonstrated in other infections, such as HIV and hepatitis B virus. However, some couples may choose to be screened. If testing is performed, type-specific glycoprotein G (IgG)-based assays for HSV antibodies should be requested [HSV-specific glycoprotein G2 for diagnosis of herpes simplex virus type 2 (HSV-2) and glycoprotein G1 for diagnosis of herpes simplex virus type 1 (HSV-1)]. Low index values (1.1–3.5) with certain commercial assays frequently represent false-positive results; in such cases, the presence of HSV antibody should be confirmed with a different serologic assay. In the absence of lesions during the third trimester, routine serial cultures for HSV are not indicated for women in the third trimester who have a history of recurrent genital herpes.

HUMAN PAPILLOMAVIRUS

Routine screening is not recommended.

BACTERIAL VAGINOSIS AND TRICHOMONIASIS

Bacterial Vaginosis

While there is no evidence to support screening for BV in pregnant women at high risk for preterm delivery, symptomatic women should be evaluated and treated. There are no known direct effects of BV on the newborn.

- *Screening*: Evidence does not support routine screening for BV and *Trichomonas vaginalis* in asymptomatic pregnant women. Systematic reviews from developed countries of antibiotic treatment for these conditions in asymptomatic pregnant women show no significant reductions in adverse pregnancy outcomes. However, antibiotic treatment for BV may reduce the risk of low birth weight and preterm rupture of the membranes among pregnant women with previous preterm deliveries.

CONCLUSION

It is particularly important during the third trimester of pregnancy when an active STD infection can cause the greatest consequences to both the mother and the baby. Screening, identification, education, and treatment should be an important component of prenatal care for women who are increased risk

TABLE 4: Screening recommendations and preferred tests.

Condition	Screening recommended	Preferred test
Chlamydia	Yes: All pregnant women	NAAT
Gonorrhea	Yes: Women who are at risk or living in a high-prevalence area	NAAT or culture on Thayer–Martin media
Hepatitis B	Yes: All pregnant women	HBsAg serology
Hepatitis C	Yes: Women who are at high risk	Anti-HCV
HIV	Yes: All pregnant women	Combo assay, HIV-1/2, antibody differentiation immunoassay, HIV-1 NAT
Syphilis	Yes: All pregnant women	RPR or VDRL

(HBsAg: hepatitis B surface antigen; HCV: hepatitis C virus; NAAT: nucleic acid amplification test; RPR: rapid plasma reagin; VDRL: Venereal Disease Research Laboratory)
Note: "Yes" indicates screening is recommended at the first prenatal visit, with repeat screening in the third trimester for those at risk.

for theses common infections. Most of the international and national bodies recommend universal screening for HIV, HBsAg, and syphilis with repeat testing in late pregnancy for high-risk groups. Screening for *Chlamydia*, gonorrhea, and HCV is recommended in high-risk groups only and they recommend against for routine screening for BV and trichomoniasis. Incorporation of screening for STIs and appropriate treatment has shown impact on reducing STI and HIV-related morbidity and mortality.

SUGGESTED READING

1. ACOG Committee on Practice Bulletins. ACOG Practice Bulletin. Clinical management guidelines for obstetrician-gynecologists. No. 82. June 2007. Management of herpes in pregnancy. Obstet Gynecol. 2007;109(6):1489-98. Reaffirmed 2018.
2. American Academy of Family Physicians. Recommendations by topic: infectious disease. [online] Available from: https://www.aafp.org/patient-care/clinical-recommendations/infectious.html. [Last accessed June, 2020].
3. American Academy of Pediatrics Committee on Fetus and Newborn; American College of Obstetricians and Gynecologists Committee on Obstetric Practice. In: Kilpatrick SJ, Papile L (Eds). Guidelines for Perinatal Care, 8th edition; 2017. [online] Available from: https://shop.aap.org/guidelines-for-perinatal-care-8th-edition-paperback/. [Last accessed June, 2020].
4. American Congress of Obstetricians and Gynecologists. Ages 19–39 years: laboratory and other tests. [online] Available from: http://www.acog.org/About-ACOG/ACOG-Departments/Annual-Womens-Health-Care/Well-Woman-Recommendations/laboratory-testing-Ages-19-39-Years. [Last accessed June, 2020].
5. British HIV Association. Guidelines for the management of HIV infection in pregnant women, 2012. London: British HIV Association; 2012.
6. Centers for Disease Control and Prevention. (2015). 2015 Sexually transmitted diseases treatment guidelines. Screening recommendations referenced in treatment guidelines and original recommendation sources. [online] Available from: http://www.cdc.gov/std/tg2015/screening-recommendations.htm. [Last accessed June, 2020].
7. Centre for Disease Control and Prevention. (2011). Sexually Transmitted Disease. [online] Available from: https://www.cdc.gov/std/treatment/2010/pdf/2011-Booklet-Whole-Press.pdf. [Last accessed June, 2020].

8. Centre for Disease Control and Prevention. A guide to taking a sexual history. Atlanta, GA: US Department of Health and Human Services. [online] Available from: https://www.cdc.gov/std/treatment/sexualhistory.pdf. [Last accessed June, 2020].

9. Centre for Disease Control and Prevention. STDs during Pregnancy—CDC Fact Sheet. [online] Available from: https://www.cdc.gov/std/pregnancy/stdfact-pregnancy-detailed.htm. [Last accessed June, 2020].

10. Hammerschlag MR, Weisman LE, Edwards MD, Arms C. (2018). Chlamydia trachomatis infections in the newborn. [online] Available from: https://www.uptodate.com/contents/chlamydia-trachomatis-infections-in-the-newborn?topicRef=4983&source=see_link. [Last accessed June, 2020].

11. Mullick S, Watson-Jones D, Beksinska M, Mabey D. Sexually transmitted infections in pregnancy: prevalence, impact on pregnancy outcomes, and approach to treatment in developing countries. Sex Transm Infect. 2005;81(4):294-302.

12. National Aids Control Organisation. (2013). NACO: Updated Guidelines for PPTCT of HIV using Multidrug Anti Retroviral Regimen in India, December 2013. [online] Available from: http://naco.gov.in/upload/NACP%20%20IV/18022014%20BSD/National_Guidelines_for_PPTCT.pdf. [Last accessed June, 2020].

13. National Health Portal. (2016). Sexually transmitted infections (STIs). [online] Available from: https://www.nhp.gov.in/disease/reproductive-system/sexually-transmitted-infections-stis. [Last accessed June, 2020].

14. Rogozińska E, Kara-Newton L, Zamora JR, Khan KS. On-site test to detect syphilis in pregnancy: a systematic review of test accuracy studies. BJOG. 2017;124(5):734-41.

15. Romorena M, Velauthapillaib M, Rahmanc M, Sundbyd J, Kloumane E, Hjortdahld P. Trichomoniasis and bacterial vaginosis in pregnancy: inadequately managed with the syndromic approach. [online] Available from: https://www.who.int/bulletin/volumes/85/4/06-031922/en/. [Last accessed June, 2020].

16. Teasdale CA, Abrams EJ, Chiasson MA, Justman J, Blanchard K, Jones HE. Incidence of sexually transmitted infections during pregnancy. PLoS One. 2018;13(5):e0197696.

17. Trepo C, Chan HL, Lok A. Hepatitis B virus infection. Lancet. 2014;384(9959):2053-63.

18. US Preventive Services Task Force, Bibbins-Domingo K, Grossman DC, Curry SJ, Davidson KW, Epling JW Jr, García FAR, et al. Serologic Screening for Genital Herpes Infection: US Preventive Services Task Force Recommendation Statement. JAMA. 2016;316(23):2525-30.

19. Workowski KA, Bolan GA; Centers for Disease Control and Prevention. Sexually transmitted diseases treatment guidelines, 2015. MMWR Recomm Rep. 2015; 64(RR-03):1-137.

20. World Health Organization. (2013). WHO Consolidated Guidelines on the Use of Antiretroviral Drugs for Treating and Preventing HIV Infection, Recommendations for a Public Health Approach. [online] Available from: http://www.who.int/hiv/pub/guidelines/arv2013/download/en/. [Last accessed June, 2020].

21. World Health Organization. (2014). WHO Hepatitis B fact sheet no. 204. [online] Available from: http://www.who.int/medicenter/factsheet/fs204/e4/. [Last accessed June, 2020].

22. World Health Organization. (2015). WHO Consolidated Guidelines for HIV Testing services. [online] Available from: http://apps.who.int/iris/bitstream/10665/179870/1/9789241508926_eng.pdf?ua=1. [Last accessed June, 2020].

23. World Health Organization. (2019). Sexually transmitted infections (STIs). [online] Available from: https://www.who.int/news-room/fact-sheets/detail/sexually-transmitted-infections-(stis). [Last accessed June, 2020].

24. World Health Organization. WHO antenatal randomized trial: manual for the implementation of the new model. Geneva: World Health Organization; 2002. [online] Available from: https://hetv.org/resources/reproductive-health/rtis_gep/rtis_gep.pdf. [Last accessed June, 2020].

Second Trimester Aneuploidy Screening: Continues to have a Place in India

Aanchal Sablok, Anita Kaul

INTRODUCTION

With an ever-increasing population rate of India and with women conceiving at a later age, there is an increase in the burden of genetic disorders and chromosomal abnormalities. Globally, at least 7.6 million children are born annually with severe genetic or congenital malformations; 90% of these are born in middle- and low-income countries.[1] Unfortunately, because of the lack of resources and lack of recent advances, even the common genetic disorders and congenital malformations with a high-prevalence rate are commonly diagnosed at the time of birth or in infancy.

Down syndrome, which is the most common cause of developmental delay and accounts for 15–30% of individuals with intellectual disabilities,[2] is still not screened for in many parts of the country. The recent data suggest that in India, 21,400 children with Down syndrome are born every year[3] and the birth prevalence is reported to vary from one in 1,230 to one in 1,361.[4]

Though the major structural abnormalities can be detected in the first trimester ultrasonography, it is still not realistic that all major structural abnormalities detectable in the second trimester would be visible in the first trimester. Thus, first trimester screening should not replace second trimester anatomical evaluation (American College of Obstetricians and Gynecologists, 2016).

SECOND TRIMESTER SCREENING

Biochemical Screening

The reliability of quadruple test as compared to triple test in the screening of Down syndrome is well-established.

Quadruple test is also known to be abnormal in 96% of fetuses with triploidy, in 75% fetuses with turner syndrome, in 44% with trisomy 13, and in more than 40% of those with major chromosomal abnormalities.[5] Although Quadruple test is a screening test and cannot replace diagnostic test but still can be very useful in women considering amniocentesis.

However, quadruple test offers no benefit over first trimester screening when it comes to screening for trisomy 21 and trisomy 18 and should not replace it. But, in a country like India where women do not begin care until the second trimester, it can be used as a standalone test.

Hence, "triple test" which is now considered to be an obsolete test but is still being used as a second trimester screening tool in many parts of India, a practice which needs to be abandoned.

Apart from screening of Down syndrome or other common aneuploidies like trisomy 13 and trisomy 18, these maternal biochemical parameters can be employed to screen for genetic syndromes and other pregnancy-associated conditions.

Similarly, a high beta human chorionic gonadotropin (β-hCG) level can be an indicative of multiple pregnancy, molar pregnancy, placental cysts, and placental lakes apart from its association with Down syndrome.

Hence, in a developing country like India, where first trimester screening is often missed, second trimester maternal serum screening itself can lead to a diagnosis of multiple conditions.

Role of Second Trimester Ultrasonography

It is recommended that sonography be routinely offered to all pregnant women between the gestational age group of 18 and 22 weeks (American College of Obstetricians and Gynecologists, 2016). However in India, due to Pre-Conception and Pre-Natal Diagnostic Technique (PCPNDT) law, this scan is done between 18 and 20 weeks.

This time period allows the appropriate assessment of the gestational age, fetal anatomy, placental localization, and the cervical length. In a pregnancy at high risk, the fetal anatomy can be evaluated prior to this gestation at 16–18 weeks.

Second Trimester Soft Markers

It has been now well known that certain features detected in an anomaly scan done at 18–20 weeks, which is the most important and routinely performed scan in India, are common to a fetus with aneuploidy, the most common aneuploidy being trisomy 21, which reaches this gestational age. The most widely examined markers are lateral cerebral ventriculomegaly, absent or hypoplastic nasal bone, increased nuchal fold thickness, intracardiac hyperechogenic focus, aberrant right subclavian artery (ARSA), hyperechogenic bowel, mild hydronephrosis, and shortening of the femur or humerus. Agathokoleous et al., in 2013, summarized the accumulated data on the screening performance of second trimester sonographic markers for fetal Trisomy 21 by meta-analysis **(Figs. 1A to E)**.[6]

The pooled estimates of positive and negative likelihood ratio (LR) of various soft markers studied are given in **Table 1**.

Other minor markers or soft signs indicative of trisomy 21 include brachycephaly, shortened ear length, single transverse palmar crease, clinodactyly (hypoplasia of the 5th digit middle phalanx), single umbilical artery, widened iliac angle, and sandal gap deformity **(Fig. 2)**. These soft markers although known to be associated with trisomy 21 can be identified by an expert ultrasonologist and should be looked for whenever there is a suspicion.

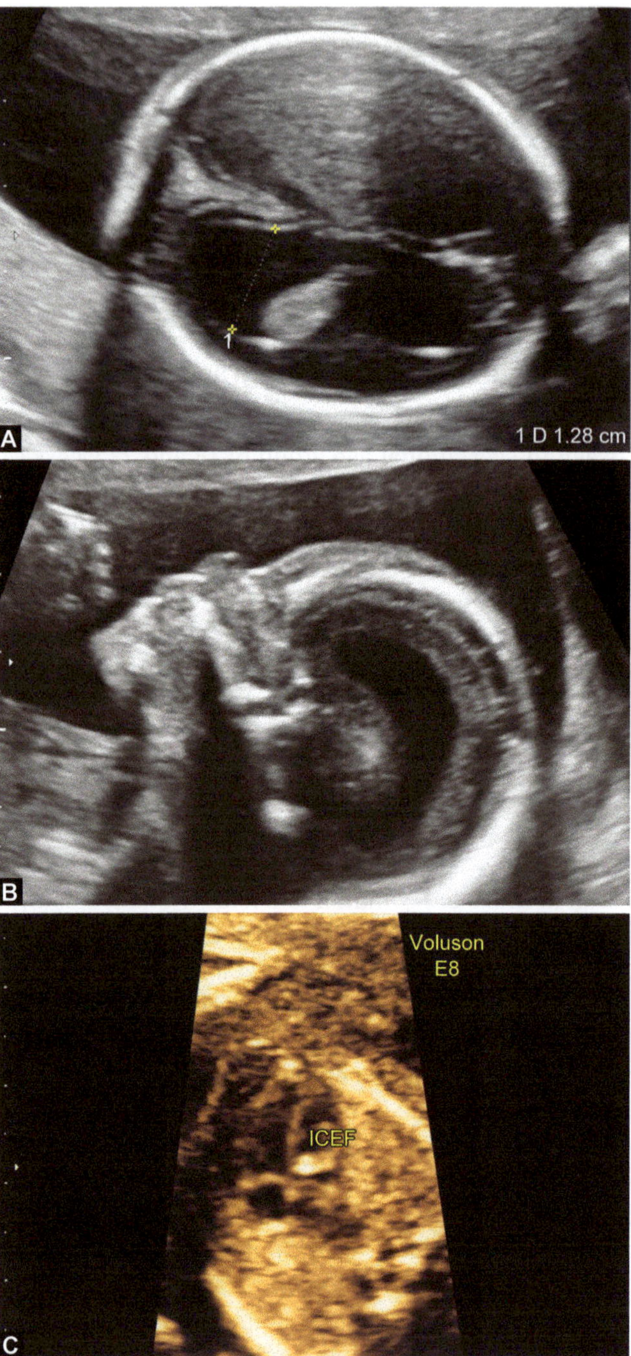

Figs. 1A to C

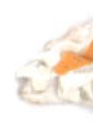

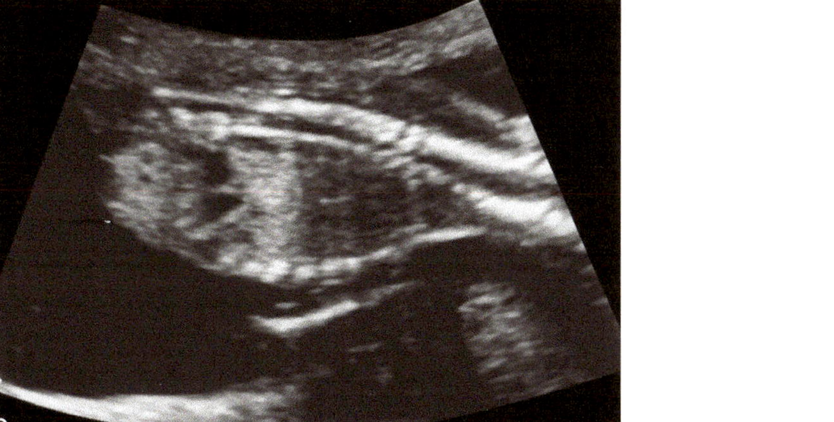

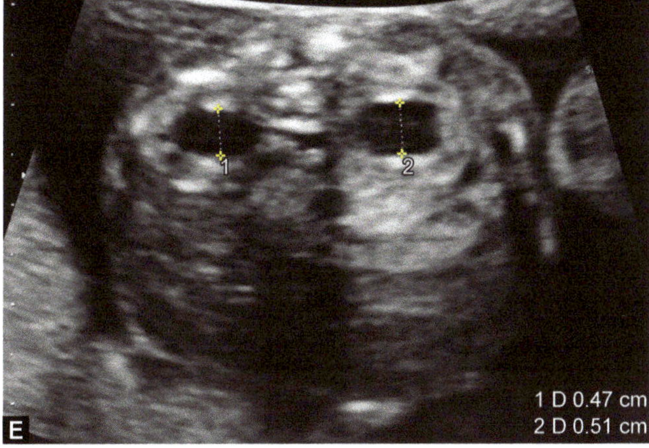

Figs. 1D and E

Figs. 1A to E: Trisomy 21 soft markers. (A) Ventriculomegaly; (B) Absent nasal bone; (C) Intracardiac echogenic focus (ICEF); (D) Echogenic bowel; (E) Hydronephrosis.

The ultrasonographic features when present are not only suggestive of fetal aneuploidy but can also be present in a variety of structural/chromosomal abnormalities.

Absent/Hypoplastic Nasal Bone

Absent nasal bone is a very strong marker of trisomy 21. Hypoplastic nasal bone is defined, if the length of the nasal bone is <2.5 mm (perinatalogy.com) and, when present, calls for a definitive diagnosis by amniocentesis.

Increased Nuchal Fold

Increased nuchal fold is defined as the nuchal fold measurement >6 mm at 18–24 weeks of gestation. It is measured in the transcerebellar plane from outer to outer edge of the skin fold. This finding when present confers a tenfold increased risk of having a fetus with Down syndrome.

TABLE 1: Pooled estimates of positive and negative likelihood ratio (LR) of various soft markers studied.

Marker	DR (95% CI)(%)	FPR (95% CI) (%)	LR+ (95% CI)	LR– (95% CI)	LR isolated marker*
Intracardiac echogenic focus	24.4 (20.9–28.2)	3.9 (3 .4–4.5)	5.83 (5.02–6.77)	0.80 (0.75–0.86)	0.95
Ventriculomegaly	7.5 (4.2–12.9)	0.2 (0. 1–0.4)	27.52 (13.6 1–55.68)	0.94 (0.91–0.98)	3.81
Increased nuchal fold	26.0 (20.3–32.9)	1.0 (0.5–1.9)	23.30 (14.35–37.83)	0.80 (0.74–0.85)	3.79
Echogenic bowel	16.7 (13.4–20.7)	1.1 (0.8–1.5)	11.44 (9.05–14.47)	0.90 (0.86–0.94)	1.65
Mild hydronephrosis	13.9 (11.2–1 7.2)	1.7 (1.4–2.0)	7.63 (6 .11–9.51)	0.92 (0.89–0.96)	1.08
Short humerus	30.3 (17.1–47.9)	4.6 (2.8 - 7.4)	4.81 (3 .49–6.62)	0.74 (0.63–0.88)	0.78
Short femur	27.7 (19.3–38.1)	6.4 (4.7–8.8)	3.72 (2.79–4.97)	0.80 (0.73–0.88)	0.61
ARSA	30.7 (17.8–47.4)	1.5 (1.0–2.1)	21.48 (11.48–40.19)	0.71 (0.57–0.88)	3.94
Absent or hypoplastic NB	59.8 (48.9–69.9)	2.8 (1.9–4.0)	23.27 (14.23–38.06)	0.46 (0.36–0.58)	6.58

Note: *Derived by multiplying the positive LR for the given marker by the negative LR of each of all other markers, except for short humerus. (ARSA: aberrant right subclavian artery; NB: nasal bone).

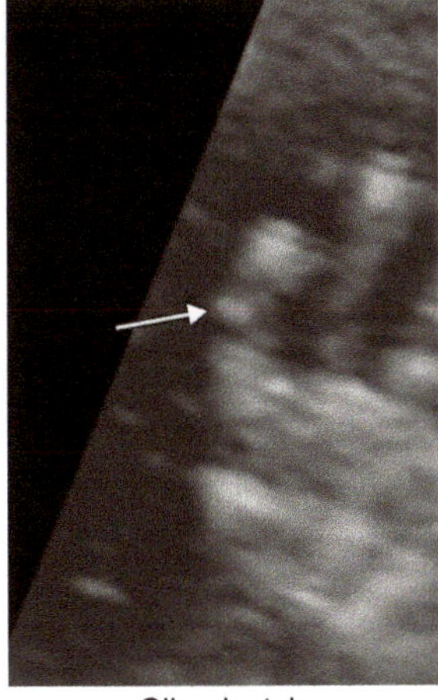
Clinodactyly

Fig. 2: Minor marker.

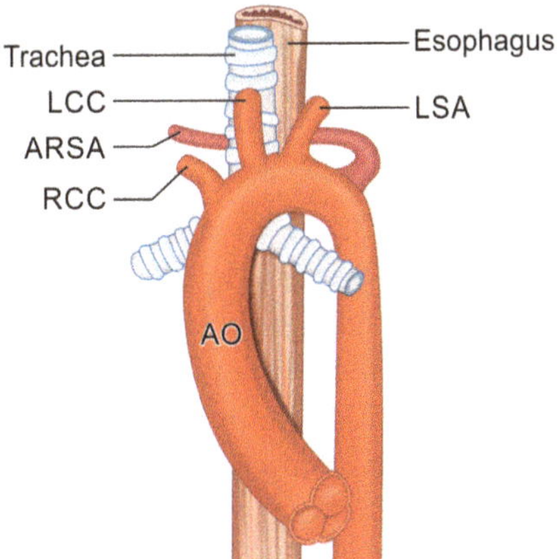

Fig. 3: Aberrant right subclavian artery (ARSA). (LCC: left common carotid artery; LSA: left subclavian artery; RCC: right common carotid artery).

Intracardiac Echogenic Focus

An intracardiac echogenic focus is a papillary muscle calcification, which is most commonly seen in left ventricle. It is present in 8% of normal Asian population and does not affect the function and morphology of the fetal heart.

Aberrant Right Subclavian Artery (Fig. 3)

Aberrant right subclavian artery is demonstrated on Doppler USG rather than on simple 2D scale. The three-vessel tracheal view is most optimal for the diagnosis where the ARSA is demonstrated from the junction of the artic arch and the ductus arteriosus with a course behind the trachea toward the right clavicle and shoulder.

> **BOX 1:** Adverse outcomes associated with echogenic bowel.
>
> - Aneuploidies, particularly Down syndrome
> - Cystic fibrosis
> - Congenital infection, particularly CMV
> - Growth restriction and fetal demise
> - Gastrointestinal obstruction
>
> (CMV: cytomegalovirus).

The observation of ARSA with trisomy 21 fetuses was first reported by Chaoui et al.[7] and the association of ARSA with trisomy 21 fetuses in the range of 14–30% was later confirmed in several studies.[7,8]

Echogenic Bowel

The adverse outcomes associated with echogenic bowel includes as given in **Box 1**.

Hydronephrosis

Hydronephrosis is commonly seen at 18–20 weeks of pregnancy. It is found in about 1% of fetuses. It may be due to ureteric obstruction or reflux, which can require surgery, but most likely, it is functional and resolves spontaneously. In the presence of isolated hydronephrosis and the combined risk of trisomy 21 being low, a follow-up scan at 32 weeks is recommended, and depending on the findings, the pediatrician needs to be informed postnatally to arrange further investigations and to consider prophylactic antibiotics.

Hydronephrosis is also considered to be a soft marker for Down syndrome and the presence of which can mildly increase the risk of trisomy 21, likelihood ration being 1.08 as reported in the meta-analysis.

Short Humerus and Femur

Down syndrome individuals are known to be short statured when they grow up. Nevertheless, in the fetal life, they have short humerus and short femur. The humerus and femur are considered short, if they are less than 2.5 percentile.

Apart from being a soft marker for trisomy 21, short humerus and femur are present in a number of skeletal dysplasias, the most common being achondroplasia.

■ COUNSELING

Whenever, on ultrasonography, a fetus is diagnosed to have a soft marker, the fetal patient should be then referred to a fetal medicine expert. A detailed anomaly scan should be done to rule out the presence of other markers. Risk reassessment is done on the basis of the presence of soft markers and the risk is then combined with the quadruple test to give the final risk score. The sensitivity of the quadruple test plus the anomaly scan is approximately 80%.

Integrated screening can be done by combining the result of the first trimester combined screening with quadruple test with the final risk score of soft markers. The integrated screening has been known to have the highest sensitivity of 94–96% with a false positive rate of 5% (ISPD, 2015).

■ REFERENCES

1. Kaur A, Singh JR. Chromosomal Abnormalities. Genetic Disease Burden in India. Int J Hum Genet. 2010;1-3:1-14.
2. Aggarwal S, Bogula VR, Mandal K, Kumar R, Phadke SR. Aetiologic spectrum of mental retardation and developmental delay in India. Indian J Med Res. 2012; 136:436-44.
3. Verma IC, Saxena R, Kohli S. Past, present and future scenario of thalassaemic care and control in India. Indian J Med Res. 2011;134:507-21.
4. Jaikrishan G, Sudheer KR, Andrews VJ, Koya PK, Madhusoodhanan M, Jagadeesan CK, et al. Study of stillbirth and major congenital anomaly among newborns in the high-level natural radiation areas of Kerala. India J Community Genet. 2013;4:21-31.
5. Kazerouni N, Robert J, Flessel M, Goldman S, Hennigan S, Hodgkinson C, et al. Detection rate of quadruple-marker screening determined by clinical follow-up and registry data in the statewide California program, July 2007 to February 2009. Prenat Diagn. 2011;31:901-6.
6. Agathokleous M, Chaveeva P, Poon L, Kosinski P, Nicolaides KH. Meta-analysis of second-trimester markers for trisomy 21. Ultrasound Obstet Gynecol. 2013;41:247-61.
7. Chaoui R, Rake A, Heling KS. Aortic arch with four vessels: aberrant right subclavian artery. Ultrasound Obstet Gynecol. 2008;31(1):115-7.
8. Vibert-Guigue C, Fredouille C, Gricorescu R. Donn_ees foetopathologiques sur une serie de fœtus trisomique 21. Rev Prat Gynecol Obstet. 2006;103:35-40.

Imaging in Antenatal Care

Ultrasound in Nine Months: Why, When, and How?

Rajendra Singh Pardeshi, Archana Patil

INTRODUCTION

Ultrasound is the best diagnostic and prognostic tool when used but in right hand and for right purpose so as to reduce neonatal, maternal morbidity, and mortality so as to improve perinatal outcome.

Ultrasound can be used as surveillance tool due to easy availability and can be applied to mass population because of its low cost against the benefits concerned, despite of some due limitations. Total number of ultrasound scans cannot be fixed as numbers of examinations depend upon the requirement.

Ultrasound examinations required to care a dormant according to standard protocol in total 9 months duration can be categorized into:

- *First trimester scan*:
  - Early pregnancy scan ($8{-}10{+}^6$)
  - First trimester screening ($11{-}13{+}^6$)
- Targeted imaging for fetal anomalies (TIFFA)(18–20)
- Fetal well-being scan (16/28)
- Limited scans
- Specialized scans.

As far as ultrasound in 9 months is concerned, three questions will arise why, when, and how?

1. **Why?**
- Antepartum surveillance:[1]
  - To determine the structural morphology of developing fetus
  - To determine the actual growth potential of fetus inside womb
- To determine any need of lung maturation supplements:
  - To determine the exact gestational age of fetus and give the recommended steroids and $MgSO_4$ when needed to avoid morbidities resulting from prematurity
- To plan the timing of early termination/delivery:
  - To plan early termination, if any lethal congenital malformation diagnosed (at NT scan or at TIFFA) so as to reduce the social and financial burden
  - To plan delivery in fetuses diagnosed with fetal growth restriction (FGR) (major cause of perinatal morbidity and mortality).

Who should perform?

- Trained in the use of diagnostic ultrasonography and related safety issues
- Regularly perform fetal ultrasound scans[2]
- Participate in continuing medical education activities
- Have established appropriate referral patterns for suspicious or abnormal findings
- Routinely undertake quality assurance and control measures.

Ultrasonographic equipment should be used:[2]

- Real time and gray scale ultrasound capabilities
- Transabdominal and transvaginal ultrasound transducers
- Adjustable acoustic power output controls with output display standards
- Freeze, frame, and zoom capabilities
- Electronic calipers
- Capacity to print/store images
- Regular maintenance and servicing.

Safety:

ALARA (As Low As Reasonably Achievable) principle should be followed, which means that ultrasound exposure time should be set at lowest **(Flowchart 1).**[3]

2. When?

Antepartum surveillance starts in first trimester at booking visit of antenatal care (ANC).

Each and every pregnant woman deserves to offer first trimester scan at 11–13[+6] even earlier in presence of valid indication as:[2]

- History of bleeding per vaginam
- Pain in abdomen
- Mode of conception is ART (2.1% incidence of ectopic)[4]
- History of pregnancy failure in first trimester (BOH)
- Adjunct to invasive procedures (CVS and fetal reduction) planned
- Localization and removal of misplaced intrauterine contraceptive device (IUCD)
- Discrepancy between size of uterus and gestational period

Flowchart 1: As Low As Reasonably Achievable (ALARA) principle.

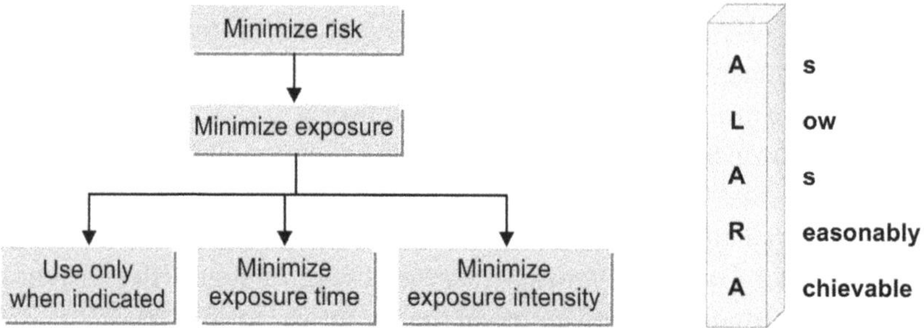

- To diagnose suspected molar pregnancy
- Evaluation of suspected ectopic gestation.

Aim of first trimester scan:[2]
- Assessment of viability:
  - Defining fetal viability (presence of cardiac activity)
  - To determine site of gestation (intrauterine/ectopic)
- To define numbers of fetuses (chorionicity in multiple gestations)
- Assessment of gestational age to determine accurate dating
- Assessment of gross fetal anatomy
- Suspected chromosomal abnormality
- Screening for pre-eclampsia
- Assessment of intra-and extrauterine structures:
  - Placental localization
  - Adnexal pathology.

Methodology of first trimester scan:
- Crown-rump length (CRL) measurement by transabdominal sonography (TAS)/transvaginal sonography (TVS) ultrasound
- Nuchal translucency (NT), IT measurement in midsagittal plane.
  After measuring the CRL, expected date of delivery is calculated. Once it is determined, it should not be changed.

Suggested anatomical planes:[2]
- *Head*: Present—
  - Cranial bones
  - Midline falx
  - Choroid—plexus-filled ventricles
- *Neck*: Normal appearance—
  - Nuchal translucency thickness
    (If accepted after informed consent and trained/certified operator available)
- *Face*: Eyes with lenses—
  - Nasal bone
  - Normal profile/mandible*
  - Intact lips*

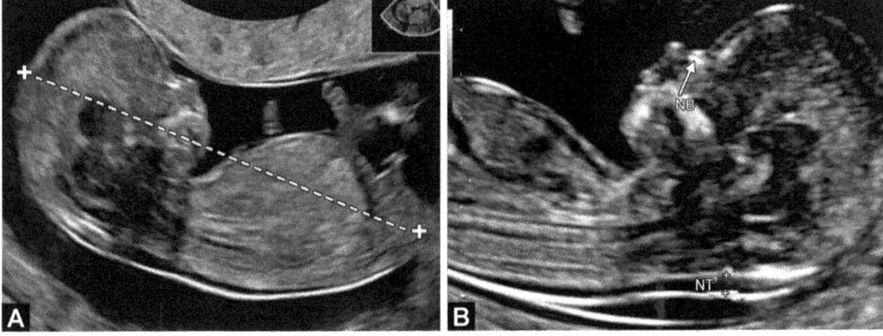

Figs. 1A and B: Nuchal translucency.

- *Spine*: Vertebrae (longitudinal and axial)—
  - Intact overlying skin*
- *Chest*: Symmetrical lung fields—
  - No effusion or masses
- *Heart*: Cardiac regular activity—
  - Four symmetrical chambers*
- *Abdomen*: Stomach present in left upper quadrant, bladder, and kidneys*
- *Abdominal wall*: Normal cord insertion—
  - No umbilical defects
- *Extremities*: Four limbs each with three segments—
  - Hands and feet with normal orientation*
- *Placenta*: Size and texture
- *Cord*: Three vessel cord*

(*Note*: *Optional structure).

Fetal well-being scan can be done at 16 weeks with due indications as:
- Structural survey not possible at first trimester screening due to high BMI
- Absent nasal bone in FTS (as in Asian population, nasal bone ossification is delayed)
- Missed FTS for quadruple screening test
- Monochorionic twin pregnancy follow-up scan for growth.

Based on history, patients are categorized according to maternal medical condition and history of risk factors as low-risk and high-risk mothers.

All pregnant women irrespective of risk deserve to offer routine mid-trimester fetal ultrasound scan at 18–20 weeks of gestation.

As in India, the upper limit for termination of pregnancy is 20 weeks.

The lower limits are same but upper limits are different in different countries.

Aim of mid-trimester scan (TIFFA):[5]
- To determine fetal viability
- To offer optimized antenatal care to ensure best maternal and fetal outcome (singleton and multiple gestations)
- To offer screening for pre-eclampsia, also should be done early detection of growth restriction which may evident in third trimester
- Detection of congenital malformation by means of detailed structural survey of fetus
- Placental localization and appearance
- Cervical assessment.

Methodology of mid-trimester scan:
Parameters used for estimation of gestational age and determination of fetal size are:
- Biparietal diameter (BPD)
- Head circumference (HC)

- Abdominal circumference (AC)
- Femur length (FL).

Suggested anatomical planes:[5]
- *Head*: Intact cranium—
  - Cavum septi pellucid
  - Midline falx
  - Thalami
  - Cerebral ventricles
  - Cerebellum
  - Cisterna magna
- *Face*: Both orbits present—
  - Median facial profile*
  - Mouth present
  - Upper lip intact
- *Neck*: Absence of masses
- *Chest/heart*: Normal appearing shape/size of chest and lungs—
  - Heart activity present
  - Four chamber view of heart in normal position
  - Aortic and pulmonary outflow tracts*
  - No evidence of diaphragmatic hernia
- *Abdomen*: Stomach in normal position—
  - Bowel not dilated
  - Both kidneys present
  - Cord insertion site
- *Skeletal*: No spinal defects (transverse and sagittal views)—
  - Arms and hands present, normal relationship
  - Legs and feet present, normal relationship
- *Placenta*: Position—
  - No masses present
  - Accessory lobe
- *Umbilical cord*: Three-vessel cord—

(*Note*: *Optional structures).

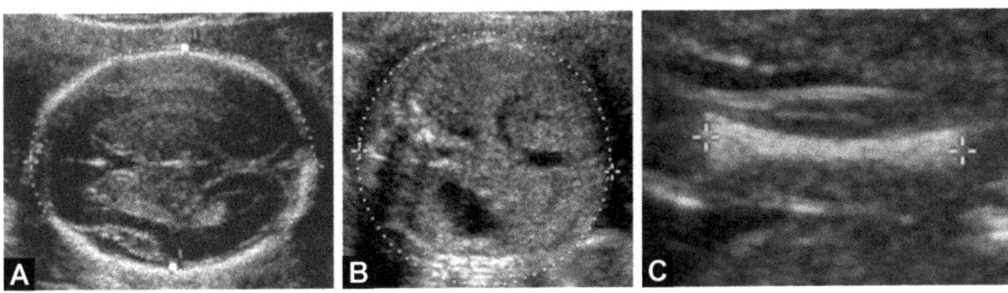

Figs. 2A to C: (A) BPD; (B) Abdominal circumference; (C) Femur length.

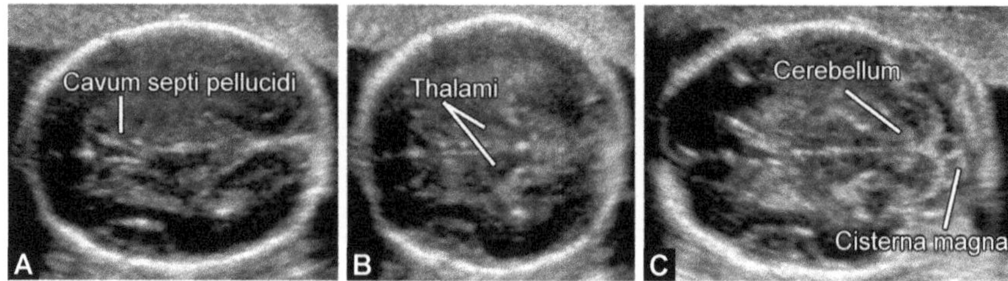

Figs. 3A to C: Cranial abnormalities.

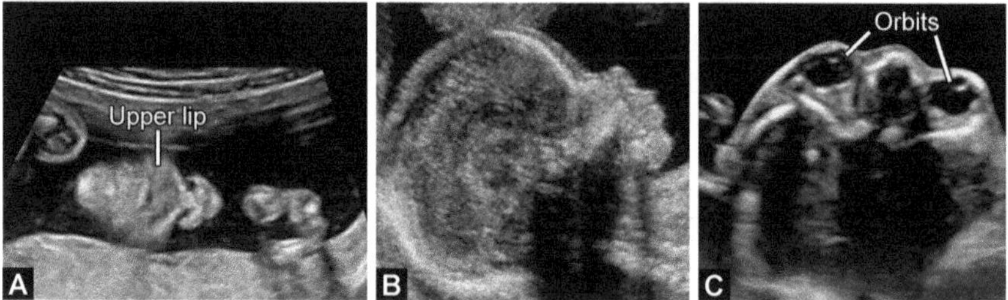

Figs. 4A to C: Facial abnormalities.

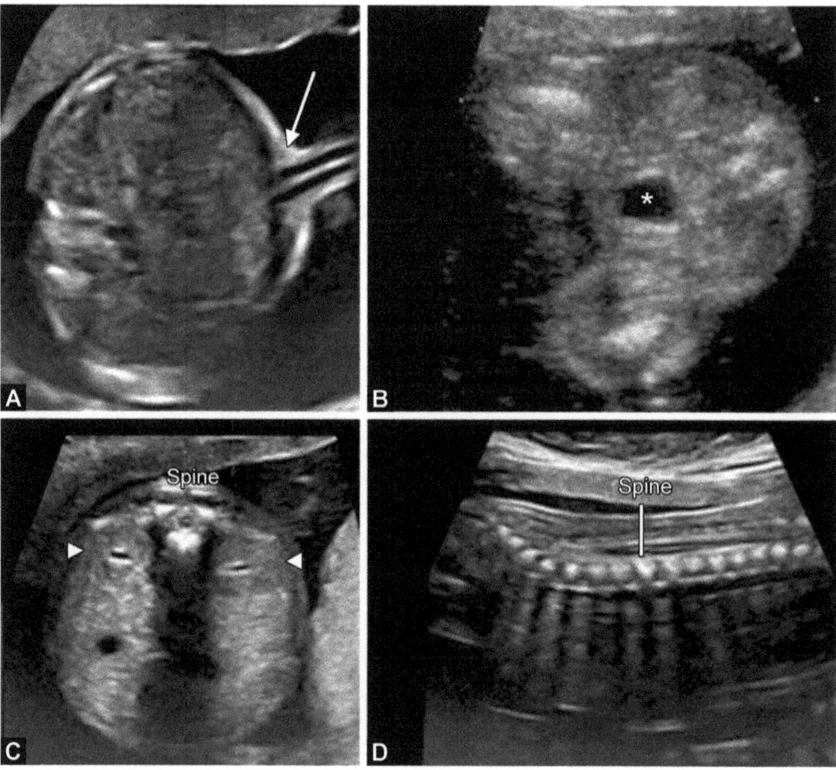

Figs. 5A to D

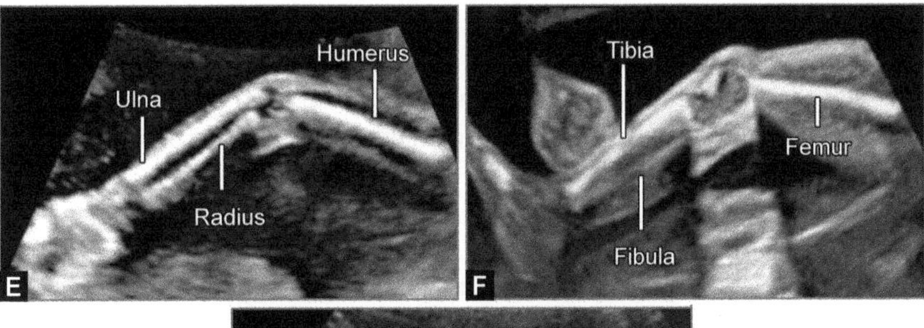

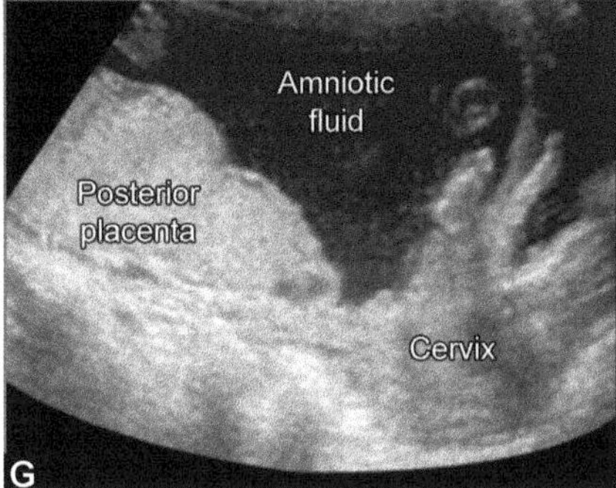

Figs. 5E to G
Figs. 5A to G: Anomalies scan.

Third trimester scans:
Objectives of third trimester ultrasound are:
- To assess fetal growth and fetal well-being
- To study and manage the impact of past and present maternal medical conditions affecting the intrauterine milieu and vice-versa
- To follow and manage the fetuses suspected and diagnosed to be at risk.

Indications for third trimester scans including but not limited to:[6,7]
- To denote cardiac activity
- To determine numbers of fetuses
- To determine fetal presentation
- Placental localization
- To determine liquor status
- To determine growth pattern and potential (SGA, FGR, and LGA) suspected on clinical examination
- To follow the fetuses suspected high risk depending upon first and second trimester scans
- Premature rupture of membrane and or preterm labor
- Complicated obstetric history in last pregnancy
- Maternal medical conditions (acute and chronic) imposing fetus to risk
- Adjunct to external cephalic version
- Suspected fetal death
- Advanced maternal age
- High BMI

- Postdated pregnancies
- Decreased fetal movements
- Evaluation of fetal condition in late registrants for prenatal care.

As far as fetal well-being's scans are concerned, detailed structural survey of the fetus is indicated.

First trimester and mid-trimester scans recommended for all pregnant women.

Third trimester scans indicated in low- as well as high-risk population, but high-risk population may require serial scans to ensure good perinatal outcome.[8]

Application and timings of scan depend upon several factors.

Several studies avail to state the timings for third trimester ultrasound in low-risk patients. Studies recommend that in low-risk patients, fetal well-being scan is to be done at 36 weeks of gestational age.

But, by the experience, we recommend fetal well-being scan should be done at 28–32 weeks of gestational age irrespective of risk factors and factors influencing modification of proposed condition.

The biometric parameters used are:
- Biparietal diameter (BPD)
- Head circumference (HC)
- Abdominal circumference (AC)
- Femoral length (FL).

Methodology of performing scan:[9]
- *Cardiac activity*: Fetal heart rate documentation—
  - Note the rhythmic pattern
- *Placentation*: Position of placenta with respect to cervix is to be mentioned:
  - Cord attachment should be documented
  - In patients with history of previous CS placental
  - Assessment is done in detail to rule out placental adherence
  - Placental thickness and any placental lesion should be looked for.
- *Liquor status*: In gestational age <28 weeks, liquor is documented in terms—
  - *Single vertical pocket, if <2 cm*: Oligohydramnios
  - *If >8 cm*: Polyhydramnios
  - At/after 28 weeks, sum of four quadrants is to be considered [*amniotic fluid index* (AFI)] to document liquor
- *Presentation*: Presentation/lie
- *Fetal movements*: Normal/abnormal—
  - If >28 weeks, consider reporting BPP (biophysical profile)
- *Fetal anatomical survey*: The structural survey should be done once in the third trimester to look for the evolving lesions
- *Brain*: Cavum septum pellucidum (CSP) and normal midline structures—
  - Lateral ventricles and posterior fossa

TABLE 1: Guidelines for redating based on ultrasonography.

Gestational age range*	Method of measurement	Discrepancy between ultrasound dating and LMP dating that supports redating
≤13 6/7 wk • ≤8 6/7 wk • 9 0/7 wk to 13 6/7 wk	CRL	> 5d > 7d
14 0/7 wk to 15 6/7 wk	BPD, HC, AC, FL	> 7d
16 0/7 wk to 21 6/7 wk	BPD, HC, AC, FL	> 10d
22 0/7 wk to 27 6/7 wk	BPD, HC, AC, FL	> 14d
28 0/7 wk and beyond†	BPD, HC, AC, FL	> 21d

(AC: abdominal circumference; BPD: biparietal diameter; CRL: crown-rump length; FL: femur length; HC: head circumference; LMP: last menstrual period).
* Based on LMP.
Note: † Because of the risk of redating a small fetus that may be growth restricted, management decisions based on third trimester ultrasonography alone are especially problematic and need to be guided by careful consideration of the entire clinical picture and close surveillance

- *Heart*: Cardiac size and axis—
  - Apical four-chamber view
  - Outflow tracts
- *Chest*: Lung echogenicity—
  - Lung lesions (CDH, CHAOS, and PS)
- *Abdomen*: Stomach, bladder in coronal view—
  - Kidneys in axial view
  - Bowel
- *Spine*: Sagittal, if possible in coronal and axial view
- *Umbilical cord*: If patient registered in late gestation first time reporting for ultrasound.

All the measurements should be done by standard protocol; accurate age estimation is the mainstay of follow-up scans so as to diagnose growth-restricted and/or large for gestational age fetuses who need further careful evaluation **(Table 1)**.[10]

LIMITED SCANS

These scans are performed under specific indication to do follow-up of a particular condition/pathology:[11]

- *Multivessel fetal Doppler*: For follow-up of the fetuses with growth restriction so as to optimize timing of delivery based on Doppler findings.
- *Middle cerebral artery (MCA) Doppler*: In Rh isoimmunized pregnancies, it is a gold standard noninvasive method for prediction of fetal anemia.

MCA PSV is used to monitor the fetuses of Rh isoimmunized mother for prediction of fetal anemia.

- *Fetal mechanical PR interval*: In patients of systemic lupus erythematosus (SLE), anti-RO and anti-LA positive cases are followed with follow-up scans for measuring PR interval to predict and manage congenital heart blocks.
- *Cervical length*: Previous history of preterm labor and short cervix (<25 mm) observed in TIFFA scan needs cervical surveillance.
- *Placental localization*: If complaints of bleeding PV in third trimester, history of previous low-lying placenta diagnosed at TIFFA scan.
- *Retained products of conception (RPOC)*: Follow-up cases of abortion or cases with previously diagnosed normal intrauterine pregnancy with history of spontaneous expulsion of products of conception.
- *Presentation*: In obese patients, it is sometimes difficult to judge the fetal presentation to plan the delivery.
- *Amniotic fluid index/single vertical pocket (SVP)*: In term pregnancies to monitor liquor amount so as to take decision of induction in cases diagnosed with oligohydramnios/polyhydramnios.
- *Biophysical profile*: Modified BPP can be used as to assess the fetal well-being with advantages of easy to perform and need less time.
- *Estimated fetal weight (EFW)*: It is most frequently performed scan, but should be performed when indicated; in term patients, the accuracy of scan is affected due to fetal position and presentation.

SPECIALIZED ULTRASOUND EXAMINATION

A detailed anatomic examination is performed for women at risk for fetal anatomic or karyotypic abnormalities (advanced maternal age, maternal medical complications of pregnancy, or pregnancy after assisted reproductive technology) or when an anomaly is suspected on the basis of history, abnormal biochemical markers, or the results of either the limited or standard scan.[12]

Fetal Echocardiography

The incidence of CHD is around 8–9 per 1,000 live births, the suspicion for CHD during a routine ultrasound is a risk factor with the highest yield for CHD (40–50%).

Indications for Fetal Echocardiography[13]

- *Maternal*:
  - Maternal metabolic disease (PGDM and phenylketonuria)
  - Maternal autoimmune disease (anti-Ro and anti-La)
  - Maternal infection with a risk of fetal myocarditis

- *Maternal teratogen exposure*: Anticonvulsants, angiotensin-converting enzyme (ACE) inhibitors, retinoic acid, nonsteroidal anti-inflammatory drugs (NSAIDs), selective serotonin reuptake inhibitors (SSRIs), and alcohol
  - Assisted reproduction technology
  - CHD or syndromes associated with CHD in first-degree relatives.
- *Fetal*:
  - Fetal cardiac abnormality suspected on obstetrical ultrasound
  - Fetal extracardiac abnormality suspected on obstetrical ultrasound
  - Fetal karyotype abnormality and abnormal noninvasive prenatal testing (NIPT)
  - Persistent fetal arrhythmias
  - Fetal increased nuchal translucency
  - Fetal hydrops or effusion
  - Monochorionic placentation.

Advanced Neurosonogram

Dedicated fetal neurosonogram has a potential in evaluating the complex CNS malformations, but has to be performed by the expert in field.[14] Transvaginal approach has the added advantage of higher frequency. Advanced neurosonogram consists of transfrontal, transcaudate, transthalamic, transcerebellar—coronal planes and two sagittal planes, i.e., midsagittal and parasagittal. Spinal examination is also important aspect of this examination, which consists of examining the spine in axial, coronal, and sagittal planes.

Sonographic Fetal Micturating Cystourethrogram

The fetal urinary bladder can be visualized from 12 weeks of gestational age. It is a study of entire act of fetal micturition by using ultrasound to diagnose the urethral abnormalities.[15]

As the fetal medicine is developing science, one can expect more advances as far as ultrasound is concerned.

DOCUMENTATION

It is the most crucial part of ultrasound examination.

The American Institute of Ultrasound in Medicine (AIUM) guidelines have suggested standard documentation of ultrasound examination.

Guidelines recommend permanent record of both the images and interpretation of ultrasound should be recorded in a retrievable format. It should be kept as per relevant requirements of local legal and healthcare facilities.

American Institute of Ultrasound in Medicine suggests the documentation should consist of patient's name, identification number, medical record number, date of ultrasound examination, image orientation on all recorded images, in addition to its healthcare provider's name, type of ultrasound examination, and identification of the sonographer/sonologist should be included on the accompanying report. Final report should be included in the patient's medical record, it should also include limitations of examination, biometric data, including variations from normal size, should be accompanied by measurements, and final report should be completed and transmitted to the patient's healthcare provider; according to situation, the result may need to be directly conveyed to the patient's referring healthcare provider and documentation of the communication is recommended.[16]

CONCLUSION

- Ultrasonography constitutes the cornerstone of modern obstetric care.
- Though a well-developed technique, it has its own limitations.
- It can be applied as a screening tool to mass populations due to salient features the system possess.
- First trimester scan and fetal anomaly scan should be subjected to all categories of patients.
- Fetal well-being scans to be performed by the person having at least 6 months of exposure to the field of obstetrics.
- Fetal well-being scans should be performed in-between 28 and 32 weeks of gestational age, which will generate better outcome.
- Updates in the field should be make avail to each and every individual performing ultrasound in the form of continuous education.
- The report document has medicolegal significance and all the criteria to be fulfilled.

REFERENCES

1. Fetal Medicine Foundation (FMF). Guidelines of Antepartum Surveillance.
2. Salomon LJ, Alfirevic Z, Bilardo CM, Chalouhi GE, Ghi T, Kagan KO, et al. ISUOG Practice Guidelines: Performance of First-trimester Fetal Ultrasound Scan. Ultrasound Obstet Gynecol. 2013;41(1):102-13.
3. American Institute of Ultrasound in Medicine. AIUM Practice Guideline for the performance of an ultrasound examination. J Ultrasound Med. 2003;22(10):1116-25.
4. Clayton HB, Schieve LA, Peterson HB, Jamieson DJ, Reynolds MA, Wright VC. Ectopic pregnancy risk with assisted reproductive technology procedures. Obstet Gynecol. 2006;107(3):595-604.
5. Salomon LJ, Alfirevic Z, Berghella V, Bilardo C, Hernandez-Andrade E, Johnsen SL, et al. Practice guidelines for performance of the routine mid-trimester fetal ultrasound scan. Ultrasound Obstet Gynecol. 2011;37(1):116-26.
6. Toward Optimized Prctice (2017). Third Trimester Fetal Well-Being Studies: Criteria & Managing Results. Clinical Practice Guidelines.[online] Available from: https://www.mypureform.com/pdfs/Third-Trimester-Fetal-Well-Being-Studies-Criteria-And-Managing-Results-Clinical-Practice-Guideline-2017.pdf. [Last accessed July, 2020].
7. National Institutes of Health. Diagnostic Ultrasound Imaging in Pregnancy: Report of a Consensus. Washington, DC: US Government Printing Office: NIH Publication; 1984. pp. 84-667.

8. Balogun OA, Sibai BM, Pedroza C, Blackwell SC, Barrett TL, Chauhan SP. Serial third-trimester ultrasonography compared with routine care in uncomplicated pregnancies: a randomized controlled trial. Obstet Gynecol. 2018;132(6):1358-67.

9. Accelerating Change Transformation Team, Alberta Medical Association (2017). Third Trimester Fetal Well-Being Studies: Criteria & Managing Results. Clinical Practice Guidelines. [online] Available from: https://actt.albertadoctors.org/CPGs/Lists/CPGDocumentList/Third-Trimester-Fetal-Well-Being-Studies.pdf. [Last accessed July, 2020].

10. The American College of Obstetricians and Gynecologists. Methods for estimating the due date. Committee Opinion No. 700. Obstet Gynecol. 2017;129(5):e150-4.

11. American Institute of Ultrasound in Medicine (2014). Limited Obstetric Ultrasound. [online] Available from: http://www.aium.org/officialStatements/19. [Last accessed July, 2020].

12. Wax J, Minkoff H, Johnson A, Coleman B, Levine D, Helfgott A, et al. Consensus report on the detailed fetal anatomic ultrasound examination: indications, components, and qualifications. J Ultrasound Med. 2014;33(2):189-95.

13. Abuhamad A, Chaoui R. A Practical Guide to Fetal Echocardiography, 2nd edition. Philadelphia, PA: Lippincott Williams & Wilkins; 2009. pp.1-8.

14. International Society of Ultrasound in Obstetrics & Gynecology Education Committee. Sonographic Examination of the Fetal Central Nervous System: Guidelines for Performing the 'Basic Examination' and the 'Fetal Neurosonogram'. Ultrasound Obstet Gynecol. 2007;29(1);109-16.

15. Boopathy VS. Sonography of fetal micturition. Ultrasound Obstet Gynecol. 2004;24(6):659-63.

16. Kurjak A, Chervenak FA. Chapter 5. Donald School Textbook of Ultrasound in Obstetrics & Gynecology, 4th edition. New Delhi: Jaypee Brothers Medical Publisher (P) Ltd. 2017. p. 54.

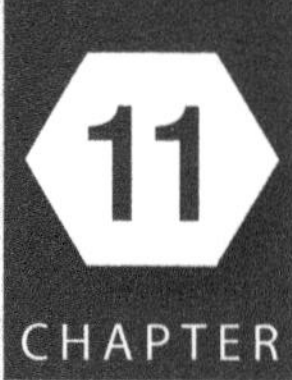

Anomaly Scan: Technique and Communication

Jayprakash Shah, Parth Shah, Prashant Achari

■ INTRODUCTION

Ultrasonography has become integral part of obstetrics and gynecology. It has almost become part of routine clinical examination in day-to-day practice. Almost all gynecology outpatient departments (OPDs) are now equipped with at least basic ultrasound machines. Initially, it was considered to be domain of radiologists but today, nearly 50% of obstetricians in Gujarat are doing obstetrics and gynecology scan routinely on their own and scenario is rapidly changing in other parts of country as well.

With the introduction of real-time ultrasound, one can identify external and internal fetal structures precisely. One can measure different parts of fetus and based on biometry charts, which has been prepared by many researchers using huge statistical data of normal fetuses, one can estimate fetal growth accurately. Apart from that, we can look at certain chromosomal markers, which categorize scanned population in high-risk and low-risk population so that we can offer invasive testing to high-risk group and minimize risk of abortion with high-detection rate. Defining number of fetus, anomaly, growth problems, placental localization, cervical incompetence, detection of unruptured ectopic pregnancies and mass lesions of uterus and adnexa with pregnancy all these had reduced maternal and neonatal morbidity and mortality. When obstetricians are doing malformations screening on their own, it has become equally necessary to do it precisely. Simple trick for all anomaly scan is to follow the guidelines for it, which has been published by different organizations and to go for additional sections of fetus to confirm the abnormal finding and to reach to the diagnosis precisely. In this Chapter, we will discuss this technique.

For anomaly scan, we need to refresh certain additional knowledge, which we have learned in our undergraduate study as is shown in **Box 1**. Before starting ultrasound, certain basic information we must enter in the machine as per **Box 2** and history of patient is necessary as per **Box 3**.

For fetal anomaly scan, we must follow systemic methods. First comfortable position for patient and examiner shall be managed. Screen shall be in line of eye and position of patient, examiners, and machine shall be having orthogonal compliance.

BOX 1: Anomaly scanning.

- Physics of ultrasound and Doppler
- Settings of machine for better 2D image and color Doppler
- Anatomy of fetus and how it appears on sonography
- Embryology
- Pitfalls and artifact in ultrasound images

BOX 2: Basic information of patient.

- Patient name
- Birth date
- Type of ultrasound and indication
- Referring doctor
- Sonographer
- Height and weight (optional)
- Obstetric history (optional)

BOX 3: History of patient before scanning.

- LMP
- History of (H/O) malformation or H/O malformation in family
- Consanguinity
- Ethnicity
- History of genetic disorders of metabolic disorders in family of both sides
- Rh status
- History of exposure to drug and radiation
- Profession
- Medical disorders and diseases in pregnancy

TABLE 1: Steps to be followed for fetal anomaly scan.

- Overall survey	- Abdomen
- Biometry	- Spine
- Head	- All four limbs
- Face	- Placenta and cord
- Chest	- Cervix
- Heart	- Uterus and adnexa

Start systematically with application of abundant gel, moving from symphysis pubis to fundus and from side to side looking at screen to note number of fetuses, cardiac activity, position of fetus, amount of amniotic fluid (AF) and any gross malformation. Follow steps as show in **Table 1**.

FETAL BIOMETRY AND GROWTH

- Measurement of biparietal diameter (BPD) and head circumference (HC) at transthalamic or transventricular view [cavum septum pellucidum (CSP), thalami, and bilateral symmetry]
- Abdominal circumference (AC) at AC view (trans-section with spine stomach, UV turning to right, and part of ribs visible with exclusion of lungs and kidneys)

- Femur length (FL) (only diaphysis to be measured with both epiphyses in view)
- Estimated fetal weight (EFW) (calculated from biometry)
- Amniotic fluid assessment [amniotic fluid index (AFI)/deepest pocket/ visual criteria]
- Fetal movement.

Multifetal Pregnancy

- Defining chorionicity and amnionicity:
  - Lambda sign/"T" sign or twin peak sign
  - Number of placenta
  - Thickness of membrane (two layers/four layers)
- Estimation and comparison of growth
- Fetus to be given number—near the internal OS is fetus 1 and then start in clockwise direction and give fetus number in clockwise direction.

▮ FETAL ANATOMY SURVEY

Head

In head, three/two sections are to be seen and four things are to be observed.

Sections

1. *Transthalamic view (Fig. 1)*: This view is not mandatory as per International Society of Ultrasound in Obstetrics and Gynecology (ISUOG) and Fetal Medicine Foundation (FMF) or Royal College of Obsthetricians and Gynaecologists (RCOG) guidelines. American College of Obstetricians and Gynecologists (ACOG) and many other non-European Societies suggest that this is scan plane, which, as name suggests, passes through

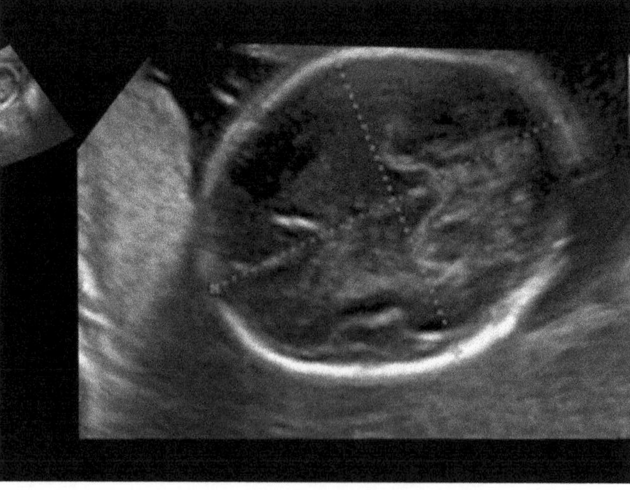

Fig. 1: Transthalamic view.

thalamus. Ideal transthalamic plane shows central falx line interrupted only by CSP; in center of falx, thin slit like third ventricle may be visible. On both sides of third ventricular slit, there are paired thalami. On both sides of CSP, frontal horns of lateral ventricle brace CSP forming its lateral wall. Anterior to CSP, thick black curved line is visible—genu of corpus callosum. BPD is to be measured from outer border of calvarium to inner border of calvarium passing through middle of falx line. OFD is to be measured from anterior border of frontal bone to inner border of occiput. HC is to be measured at outer border of calvarium.

2. *Transventricular view (Fig. 2)*: Apart from all findings visible at transthalamic view, toward occiput in both cerebrums, occipital horn of lateral ventricle marked by medial and lateral wall with choroid plexus within is noted. LV is to be measured at level of parieto-occipital sulcus from inner to inner perpendicular to long-axis of LV as shown in photograph.

3. *Transcerebellar view (Fig. 3)*: Apart from all findings visible at transthalamic view, posteriorly ball-like cerebellum with echogenic border and hypoechoic center with echogenic vermis lying in-between two cerebellums are visible. Transcerebellar diameter is measured from outer to outer cerebellar margin. CM is space between posterior borders of vermis and inner border of calvarium. Nuchal fold is to be measured from outer border of calvarium to outer border of skin in true transcerebellar view **(Fig. 4)**.

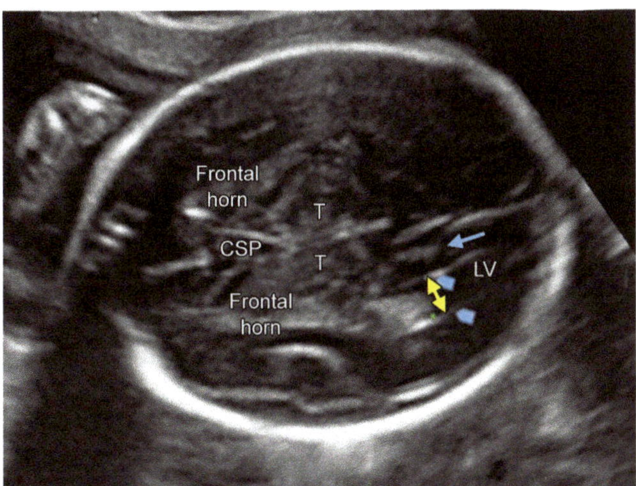

Fig. 2: Transventricular view: Section of brain passing through both thalamus with central falx line in middle with bilateral symmetry. Notice a triangular cavity in front at junction of one-third from anterior and two-third from posterior occipital region marked as CSP is cavum septum pellucidum. Both frontal horns are forming lateral wall. Arrow is pointed to parieto-occipital sulcus. Arrow head pointing to medial and lateral wall of lateral ventricle. Measurement of LV at atrium is done.

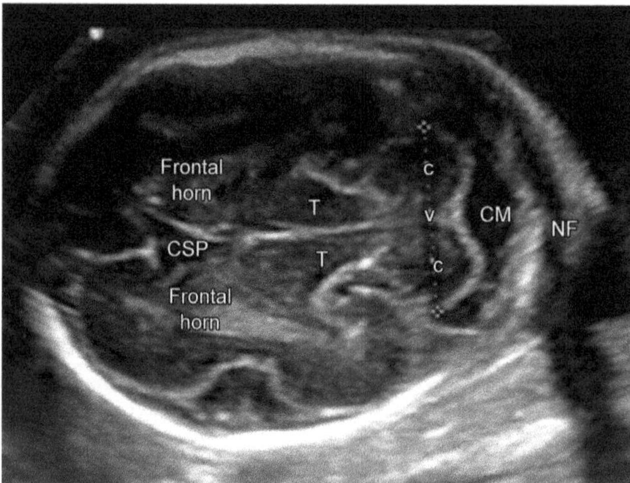

Fig. 3: Transcerebellar view: Section of brain passing through both thalamus with central falx line in middle with bilateral symmetry. Notice a triangular cavity in front at junction of one-third from anterior and two-third from posterior occipital region marked as CSP is cavum septum pellucidum. Both cerebellums are visible as rounded structure marked "C" and vermis is marked as "V". (CM: cisterna magna; NF: Nuchal fold).

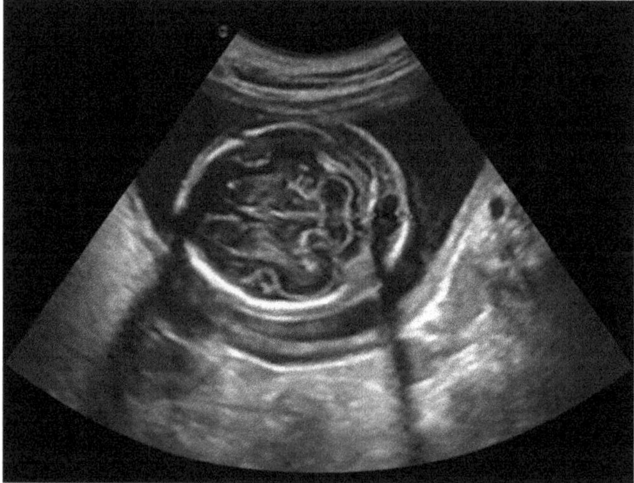

Fig. 4: High Nuchal fold (NF) at transcerebellar view.

4. *Additional views*:
   - Coronal view
   - Midsagittal view **(Fig. 5)**
   - Parasagittal view
   - Base of skull for circle of villus **(Fig. 6)**.

In transventricular and transcerebellar view, malformations listed in **Table 2** can be diagnosed.

In head, the findings mentioned in **Box 4** shall be noted.

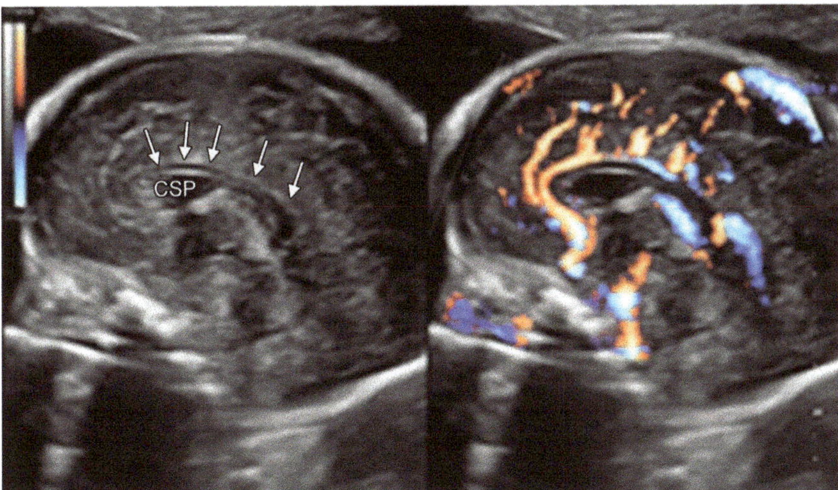

Fig. 5: Note cavum septum pellucidum (CSP). Multiple arrows pointing to black line is corpus callosum. Pericallosal artery in color can be identified as running parallel to corpus callosum.

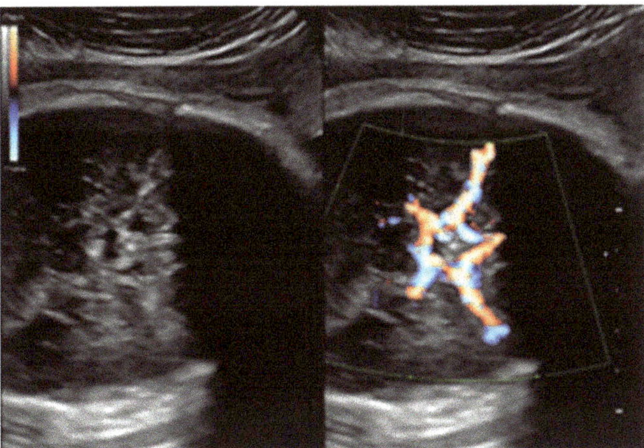

Fig. 6: At base of skull, identify circle of villus. Vertical running vessel is middle cerebral artery.

Five findings are common in all sections of head:
1. CSP
2. Lateral ventricle and choroid plexus
3. Midline intact falx
4. Posterior fossa (CM, cerebellum, and NF)
5. Intact cranium.

Face

Face malformations are not lethal usually but is more disfiguring. If you miss, that one may not pardon. 3D sonography here may be useful in better presentation of malformation to patient. We target to visualize eyeballs, lens, both nostrils, upper lip, lower lip, and chin in this sections. For tangential

TABLE 2: Malformations in transventricular and transcerebellar view.

Transventricular view	Transcerebellar view

• CP cyst (soft marker)
• Isolated borderline ventriculomegaly (soft marker)
• CSP not visible:
  – ACC
  – Holoprosencephaly
  – Anencephaly
  – Septo-optic dysplasia
• All hydrocephalus:
  – Aqueduct stenosis
  – Schizencephaly
  – Porencephaly
  – Lissencephaly
• Periventricular hemorrhage/echogenicity suggestive of fetal infection
• Tumors involving choroid
• Microcephaly
	• Obliteration of posterior fossa:
	  – Arnold–Chiari type II
	• Large CM:
	  – Mega cisterna magna
	  – Blake's pouch
	  – Partial vermian agenesis
	  – Dandy walker malformation
	  – Arachnoid cyst
	  – Rhombencephalosynapsis
	  – Joubert syndrome

(CSP: cavum septum pellucidum).

BOX 4: Findings of head.

Calvarium:
- Absent:
  - Anencephaly
  - Acrania
- Partially absent:
  - Encephalocele
- Ossification:
  - Poor—osteogenesis imperfecta
- Shape:
  - Cloverleaf—skeletal malformation
  - Lemon—Arnold–Chiari type II
  - Strawberry—Trisomy 13
  - Brachycephaly—Trisomy 21
  - Dolichocephaly—Oligo/skeletal malformation
- Lateral ventricle
- Posterior fossa
- Cavum septum pellucidum—when absent:
- Anencephaly
- Holoprosencephaly
- ACC
- Septal agenesis

section while looking at spine and head in coronal section, we have to slide transducer in ventral direction of fetus. For profile, move transducer at 90° from tangential view. For axial section, move transducer from transthalamic view caudally **(Figs. 7 and 8)**.

Three sections:
1. Tangential **(Fig. 9)**
2. Profile **(Fig. 10)**
3. Axial/transverse section **(Figs. 11 and 12)**.

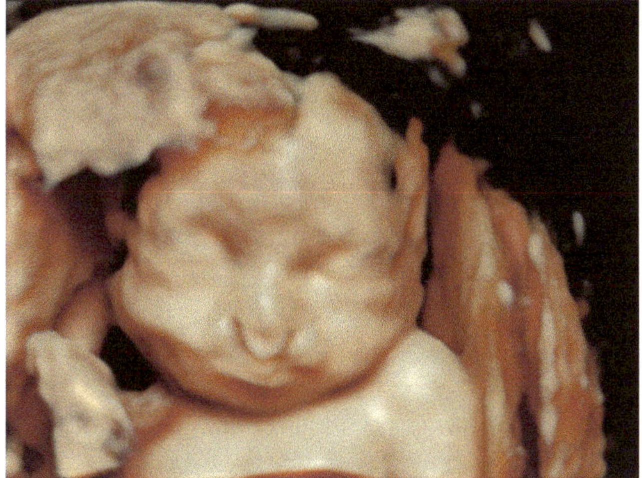

Fig. 7: Bilateral cleft lip and palate in 3D.

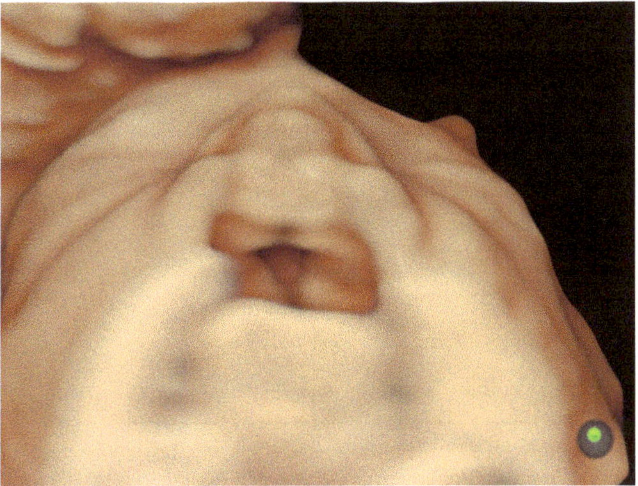

Fig. 8: Cleft palate on 3D in same patient.

NECK (FIG. 13)

Additional scan is not a part of guidelines. Any mass lesion such as thyroid enlargement, lymphangioma, teratoma, hemangioma, cord round neck, and esophageal pouch in suspicious TE fistula.

Chest

Transverse section at four-chamber view level:
- Heart:
  - Four-chamber view
  - Outflow tracts—left ventricular outflow tract (LVOT) and right ventricular outflow tract (RVOT)
  - Three-vessel view and three vessel and trachea (3VT) view

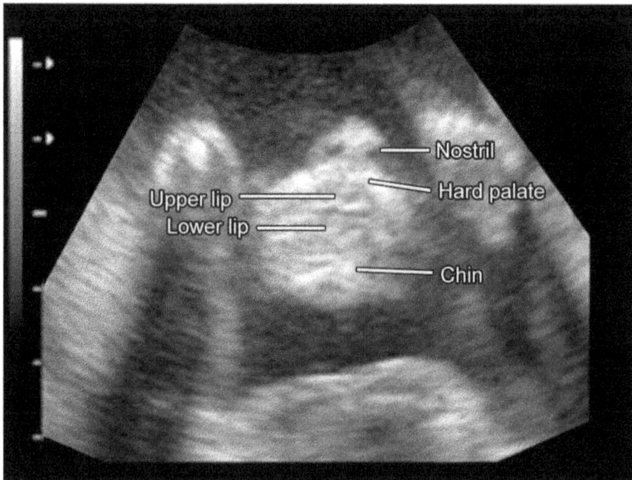

Fig. 9: Tangential view of face.

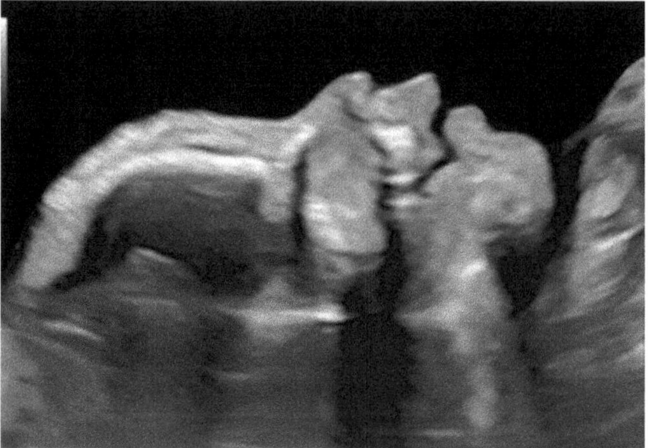

Fig. 10: Profile face: Note prefrontal edema is normal < 6 mm. Tip of nose, nasal bone, upper lip, lower lip, and chin protruding the frontal line ruling out micrognathia. Tongue is inside gum margin ruling out macroglossia.

- Lungs
- Bones—spine, ribs, and sternum.

Four-Chamber View (Fig. 14)

In this view, let us first concentrate on lungs. They look homogenously echogenic on both sides of heart visible extending from spine to wedge between heart and chest wall. Any mixed echogenicity, cystic lesion, short lung, or hyperechoic lungs are suggestive of malformation **(Fig. 15)**.

Ribs are visible usually posteriorly as to visualize heart, we have to see through intercostal space so anterior rib may not be visible, one has to see, if there is any suspicious finding. Ribs are at least two-thirds from spine to sternum. If extending short, think of short rub syndromes.

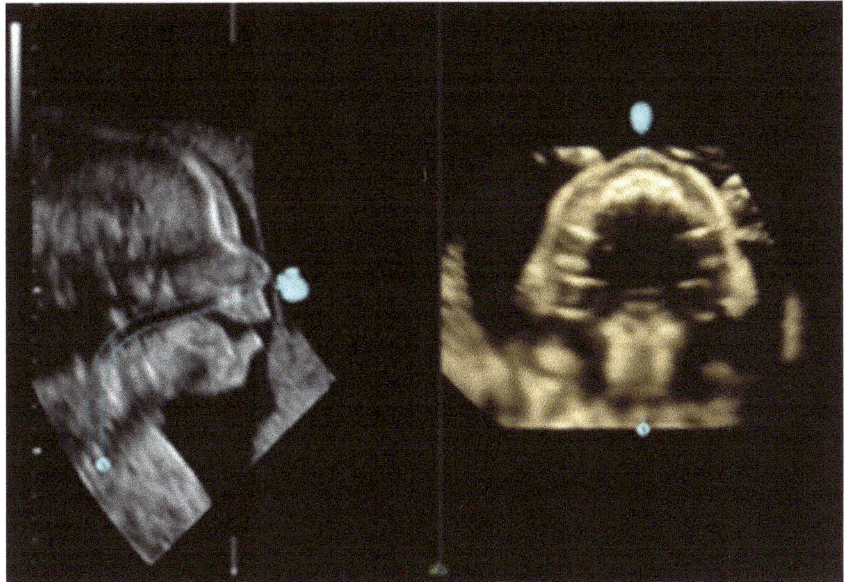

Fig. 11: With the help of 3D and Omniview, we can evaluate fetal face dynamically. Here in this image, notice hard palate.

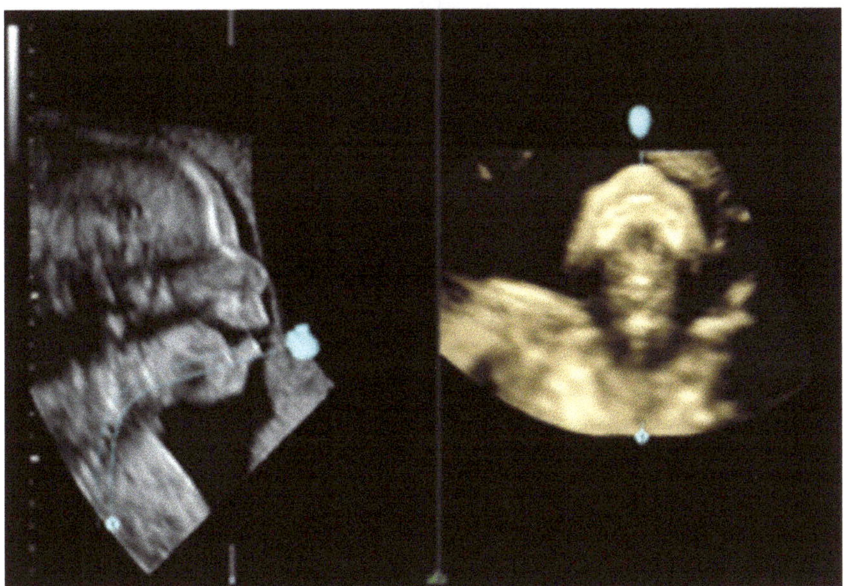

Fig. 12: With help of 3D and Omniview, we can evaluate fetal face dynamically. Here in this image, notice mandible.

Four-Chamber Heart (Figs. 16 and 17)

Position size structure and squeeze are to be seen.

Heart is centrally located with axis toward left nearly 45° ± 20 occupying less than 50% of thorax area. Toward sternal is right ventricle, which has

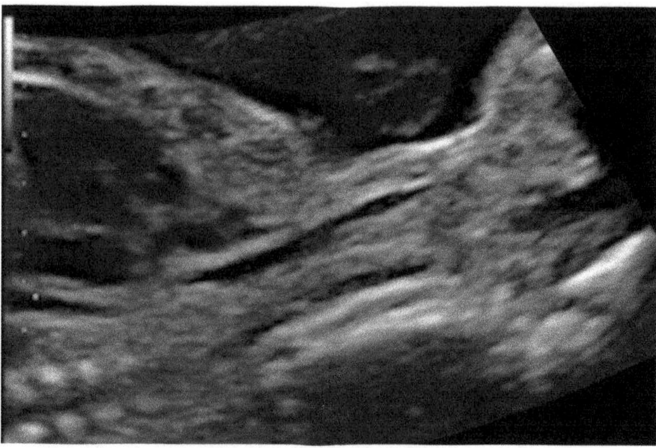

Fig. 13: Looking at neck, any mass lesion of neck cord round neck can be ruled out. Neck is not part of guideline.

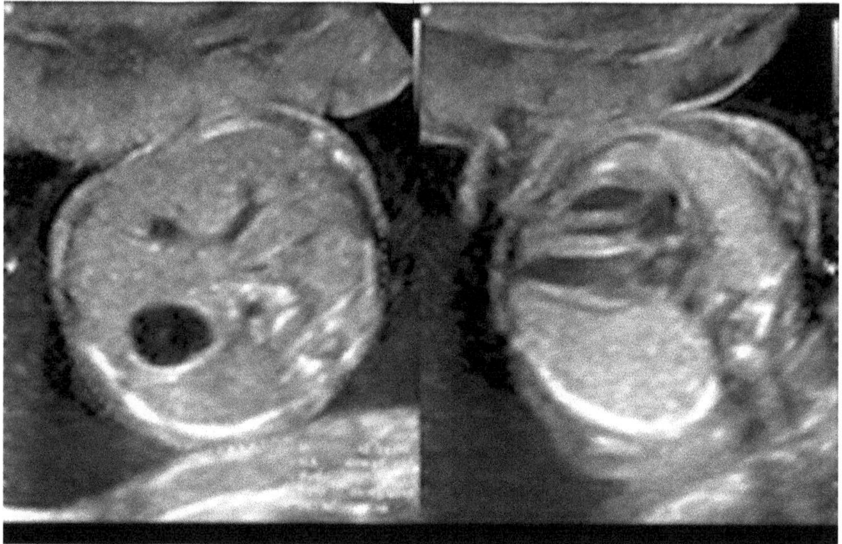

Fig. 14: On left is AC view with spine, stomach, and portal in clockwise rotation and fetus is in cephalic suggestive left-sided stomach and 4-chamber view shows heart on same side of stomach suggesting situs solitus.

moderator band at apex; AV valves are more toward apex. Left atrium is in proximity with spine, two pulmonary veins are visible entering in it, and flap of foramen ovale is visible beating in left atrium. Once these two cavities are defined, rest of two cavities can be easily labeled. Both ventricles they contract equally and simultaneously, almost of same size, inter ventricular septum is intact. Both atria are of equal size; contract and relax simultaneously with color Doppler flow from atrium to ventricle can be noted when atrium is contracting and ventricles are relaxed with AV valve open. When ventricles contract, one will identify AV valve closed and

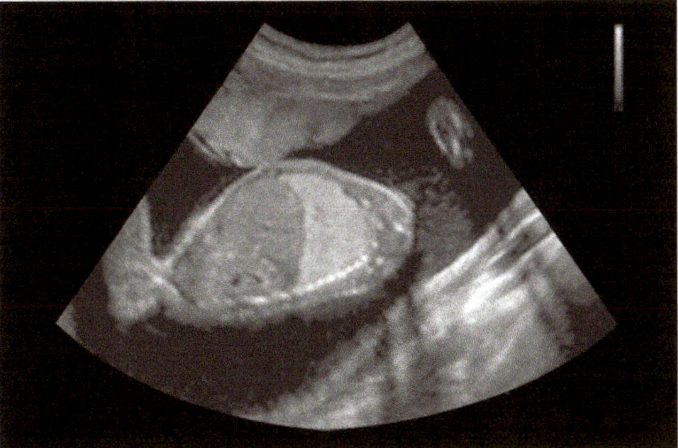

Fig. 15: Note echogenic lung separated from hypoechoic liver by upward convex diaphragm.

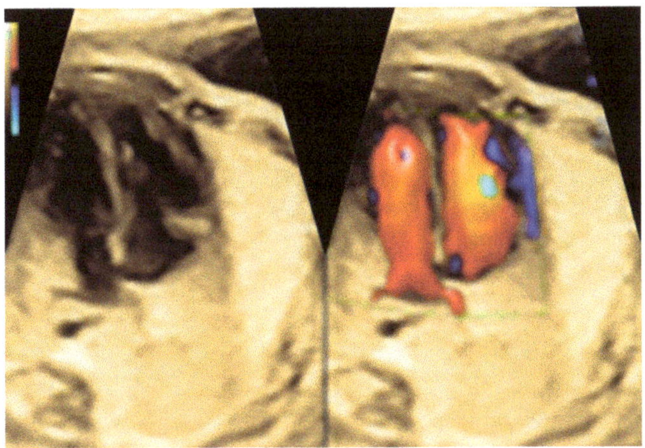

Fig. 16: Four-chamber view 2D with color. Note two pulmonary veins entering in left atrium. Flow from both atria to ventricle in red. Intact ventricular septum (IVS) and septum secundum and primum of atrial septum with foramen ovale are visible. Noted single vessel behind four chamber—aorta.

flow from ventricle to outflow tracts. Flow from right atrium to left atrium through foramen ovale can be noticed. Notice off-set at crux of heart, tricuspid valve is more toward apex, mitral is more toward base. Septum primum and secundum can be identified between two atria. Notice little fluid in pericardial space, which is <2 mm.

Outflow Tracts

*Left outflow tract (**Fig. 18**):* Just move your transducer from four-chamber view to LVOT by sliding little upward and rotating transducer to left fetal shoulder. You get left ventricle connecting to ascending aorta where anterior wall of aorta is continuous with IVS and posterior wall of aorta is continuous with

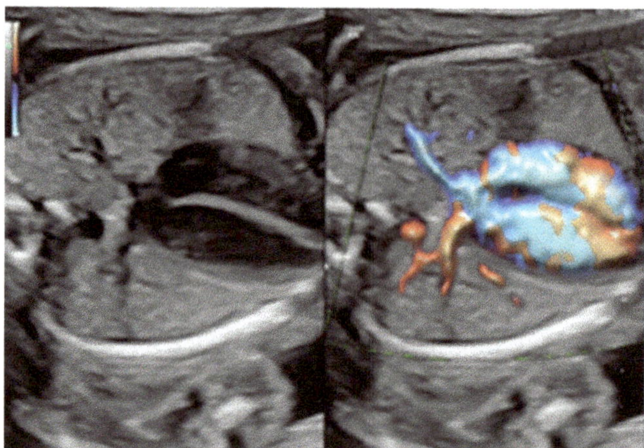

Fig. 17: Lateral 4-chamber view pulmonary entering in left atrium. Noted one pulmonary has blue color (downward direction) and other is red (upward direction flow). Aorta just anterior to spine and intact ventricular septum (IVS) noted.

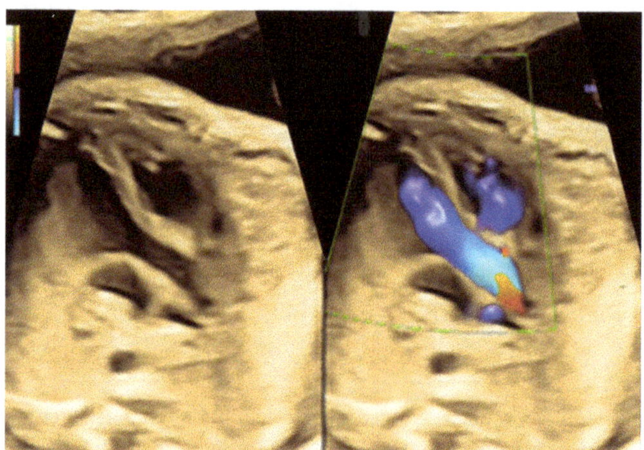

Fig. 18: Image of left outflow tract. Anterior wall of aorta in continuation with intact ventricular septum (IVS) and posterior wall of aorta with mitral valve. Note flow from ventricle to ascending aorta in blue.

flap of mitral valves. One can identify a dot in outflow tract, which is aortic valve, which is visible when valve is closed and dot disappears when valve is open. In ventricular systole on color Doppler, flow from left ventricle to aorta is visible and dot disappears; in diastole, flow stops and dot appears. Aorta is first vessel coming out of heart and it does not divide but turns posteriorly sharply to join descending aorta.

*Right outflow tract (**Fig. 19**):* To get RVOT, move transducer cephalic from LVOT view and turn transducer little toward right shoulder of fetus and you will get RVOT. This is second vessel to come out of heart and it divides into two immediately after coming out. On color Doppler in ventricular

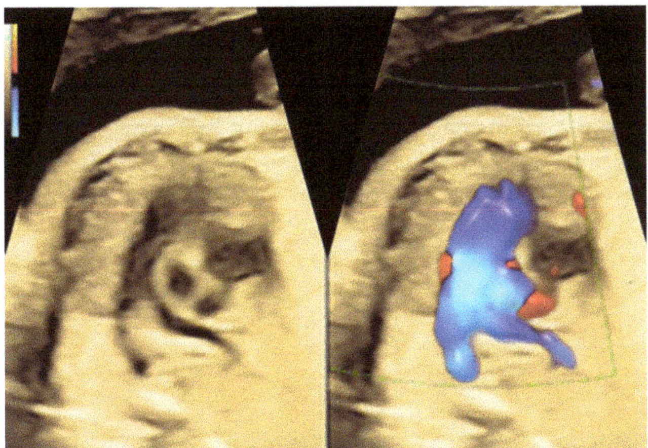

Fig. 19: Right outflow tract. Let finger walk view. Main pulmonary artery (MPA) arising from right ventricle and immediately dividing in right pulmonary and left pulmonary. Noted on right of MPS is ascending aorta. Same color in pulmonary and aorta is noted.

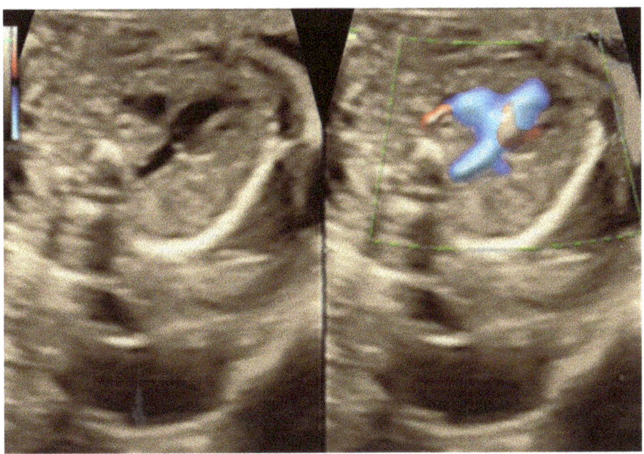

Fig. 20: Three-vessel view has three vessels as name suggest. From left main pulmonary artery (MPA), aorta, and superior vena cava (SVC). Note same color in MPA and aorta. Noted red color vessel connected to SVC is azygous vein.

systole, flow is visible in MPA and its branches whereas in diastole, it is not visible. Right branch moves rightward between ascending aorta and trachea to right lung. Left branch moves toward left lung and in this plane, it is not visible but its continuation as ductus arteriosus is visible connecting to descending aorta. This view is also called five-vessel view or let the finger move view.

Three-vessel and Three-vessel Trachea View (Fig. 20)

Move transducer little up and you will get three-vessel view and by tilting little up, you will get three-vessel trachea view. Both these views are important. Distance between all three vessels is normal and situation is almost same, when you draw a line connecting anterior border of all vessels, it is straight. Color in pulmonary and aorta is same. In 3VT view, both aortic arch and ductal arch are to left of trachea. In 3VT view, ductal arch and aortic arch form V shape where large arm of V is ductal arch and small arm is aortic arch.

Additional Views

- Hammock view **(Fig. 21)**
- Aortic arch/ductal arch view **(Fig. 22)**.

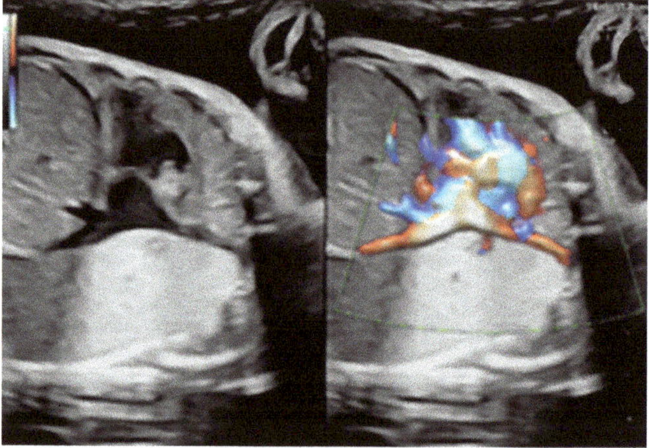

Fig. 21: Hammock view: Superior vena cava (SVC) and inferior vena cava (IVC) connecting to right atrium. Noted hepatic and ductus venosus (DV) combine before entering in right atrium.

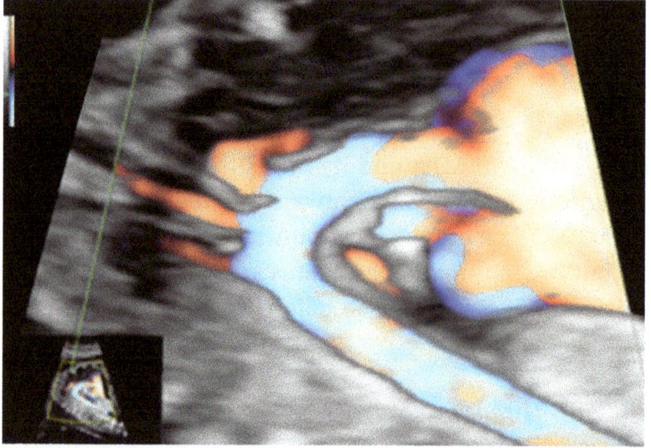

Fig. 22: In high-definition (HD) flow, aortic arch arising from middle of chest with three vessel coming out from arch. Noted walking stick shape.

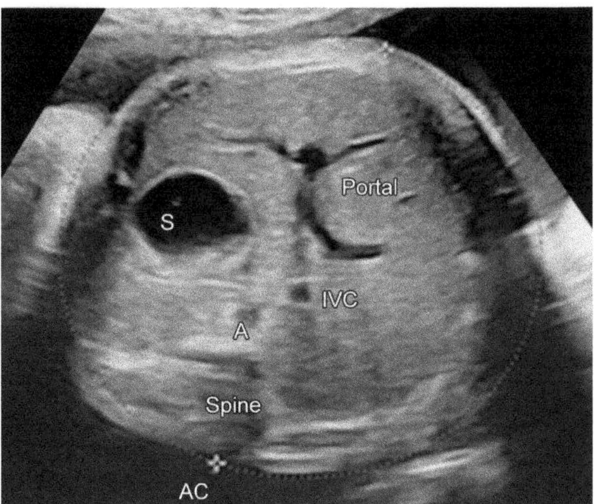

Fig. 23: Abdominal circumference (AC) view: Note spine. Orientation of spine, stomach, and portal in clockwise rotation. Fetus was cephalic presentation so stomach on left and portal turning to right. Note position of aorta—A and inferior vena cava (IVC).

Abdomen

Three sections:
1. Abdominal circumference (AC) level
2. Kidneys and cord level
3. Bladder level.

Abdominal Circumference View

Just moving caudal from four-chamber view you will get AC view. In ideal AC view, as shown in **Figure 23**, you will notice a round cut section with spine situated posteriorly. In cephalic presentation spine, stomach and portal turning to right are visible in clockwise rotation and in that case, stomach is on left side. Move up in four-chamber and you will get heart tilted to the same side as stomach and this confirms the situs solitus. Just anterior to spine and little to left notice aorta. More anterior to spine and little to right, one can see IVC and this arrangement is important to notice in normal fetus. Differing arrangement gives you diagnosis of heterotaxy. AC is to be measured at outer border including skin.

Cord and Kidney Level (Fig. 24)

As per guideline, this is second abdominal view where cord with umbilical vein and two arteries are visible entering in abdomen. At this stage, no other structure is the part of cord. At same level on both sides of spine, kidneys are visible as retroperitoneal structure and on real time in log section, one can see them moving up and down with respiration. In long coronal section, both renal arteries can be noted supplying kidneys as additional section.

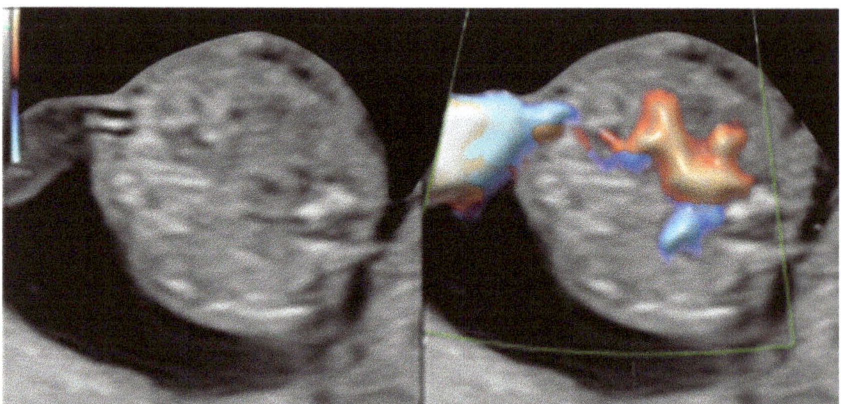

Fig. 24: Cord insertion and kidney view. At lumber region level, umbilical cord can be seen entering in abdomen. Note on back on both side of spine two kidneys.

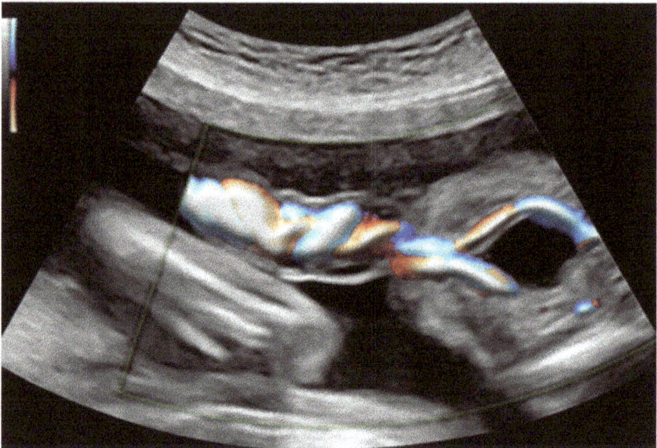

Fig. 25: Two vessel round bladder suggestive of three vessel cord.

Bladder Level (Fig. 25)

Moving down from cord level, hypoechoic rounded anechoic structure slushed to anterior abdominal wall can be noticed and on color Doppler, two vessels passing on both sides of bladder can be identified. This is a fetal urinary bladder with two umbilical arteries. Almost at same level, iliac bones with sacral promontory can be seen posteriorly suggestive of presence of sacrum **(Fig. 26)**.

Additional Section (Fig. 27)

Just below the AC view, fetal gallbladder is visible on right of portal vessel with anterior rounded bling end and on color Doppler, it is not filled with color. It is always visible in fetus after 22 week of pregnancy. At the same level on both sides of spine, slanting triple line long structure is visible—both fetal adrenals. Just below this level, large bowel as tubular structure with little echogenic

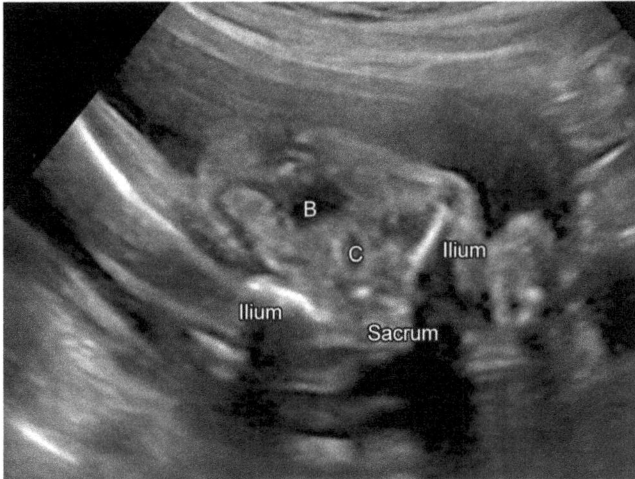

Fig. 26: Note section at iliac level. Both Ilium bone with sacrum at sacral vertebra 1 is visible noting presence of sacrum. (B: bladder; C: sigmoid colon).

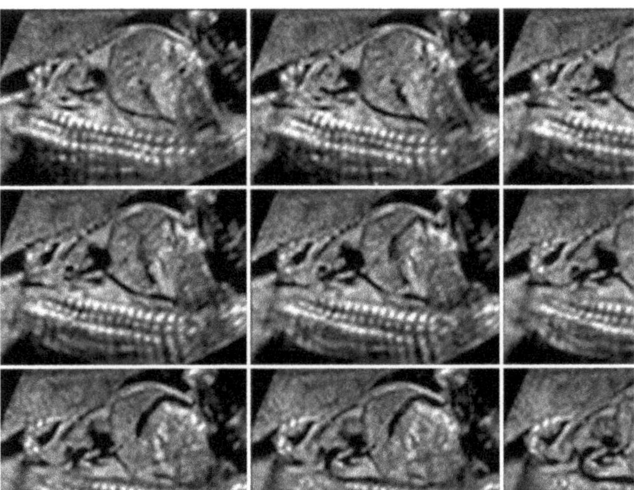

Fig. 27: In multislice view notice in sagittal section different abdominal organs and its relation.

content and after 26 weeks haustrations is visible and small bowel as little echogenic structure with hypoechoic areas is visible. Large bowel diameter is always <20 mm with no visible peristalsis and small bowel diameter is <7 mm, and measurable length is <15 mm and has peristalsis. One can record live clip in axial section as well as longitudinal section for record purpose. In mid-sagittal section, little to right note umbilical vein entering in and running underneath anterior abdominal wall than turning sharply posteriorly and enters liver as portal vessel which turns to right and before that gives left and right hepatic and continues cephalad to enter into right atrium along with IVC and hepatic forming a common conduit. In same section, one can notice intact diaphragm with heart and little more echogenic lungs compare to liver above and stomach and liver below the diaphragm. In longitudinal section parasagittal, one can see kidneys having normal renal contour with good corticomedullary differentiation. Length of kidney is between 3 and 5 vertebral length. Normal ureters are not visible.

Spine

- Longitudinal sagittal **(Fig. 28)**
- Longitudinal coronal **(Fig. 29)**
- Transverse view **(Fig. 30)**.

Fetal spine in longitudinal sagittal section has a smooth curve. Vertebral bodies are seen ventral and dorsal one side lateral ossification center with intact skin covering can be seen. Other side lateral ossification center can be seen tilting probe on other side. In coronal longitudinal section, hole in spine cannot be seen due to curve.

In transverse section, ventral body of vertebra and dorsal two lateral ossification centers with intact skin cover can be identified. When lateral ossification centers are diverging in coronal section and transverse section, think Arnold-Chiari malformation **(Fig. 31)**. In long and transverse section, skin overlying will be thin membrane and uplifted. Sacrum is to be identified as a tapering end. Look beyond tip of sacrum to rule out sacrococcygeal teratoma **(Fig. 32)**.

Limbs (Figs. 33 and 34)

All three segments of each limb with three long bones in each limb and total 12 long bones are to be identified. All long bones shall be of normal

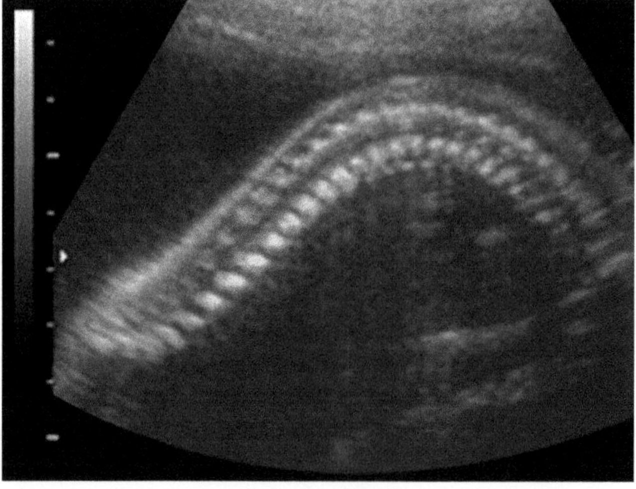

Fig. 28: Sagittal longitudinal view of spine. Vertebral bodies are ventrally and one of lateral ossification center dorsally situated with continuous skin covering. Note smooth curve.

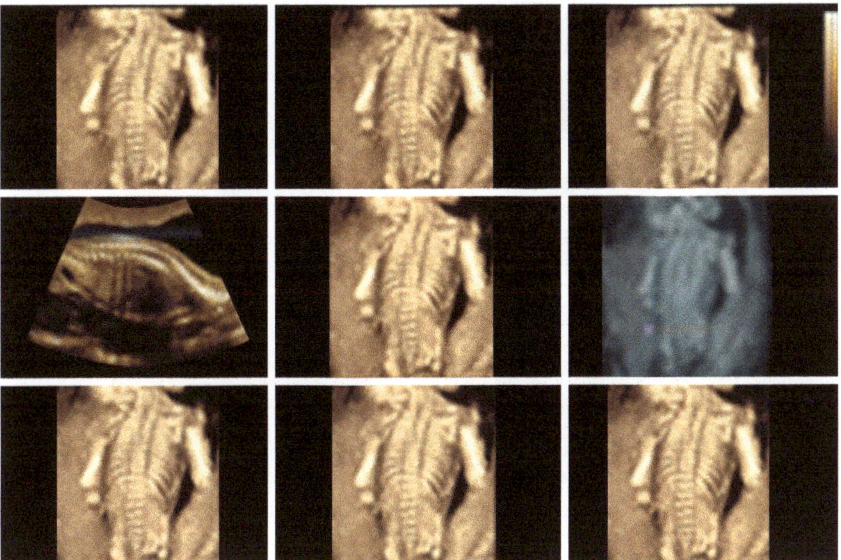

Fig. 29: Spine in 3D multislice view.

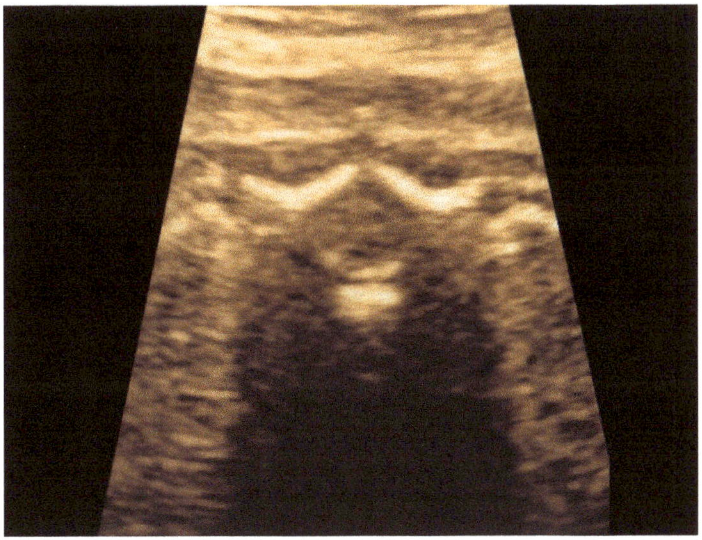

Fig. 30: Transverse spine.

shape, size, and contour with normal ossification. In long bones, as per guideline, only one femur is to be measured. Identify epiphysis on both sides and measure only diaphysis of long bone. When there is doubt for shortening of long bones, abnormal curvature, widening of end of long bones, and missing bone, one shall measure all long bones with foot also. Normal FL/foot length is >90%. Relation of foot-to-leg has to be confirmed to rule out TEV **(Fig. 35)**.

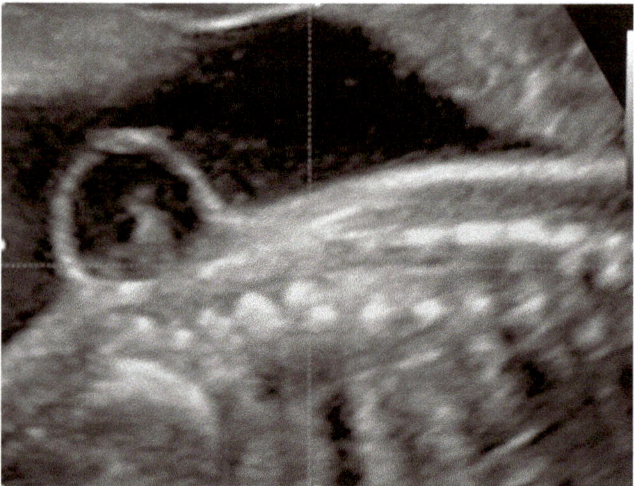

Fig. 31: Longitudinal sagittal view of spine with one lateral ossification center missing with lifter covering tissue—meningocele.

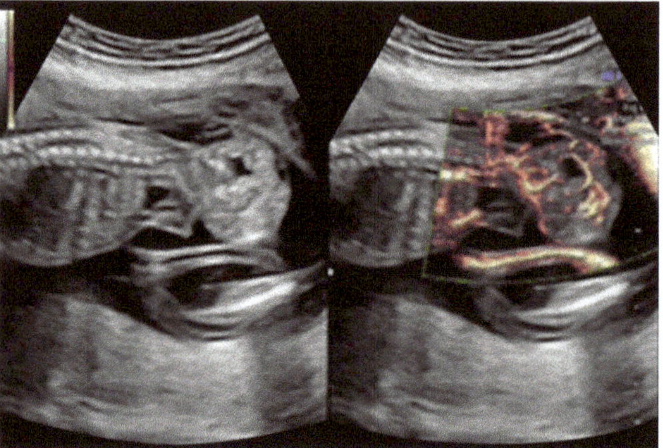

Fig. 32: Sacral spine tapering with a mixed echogenic mass beyond the tip of sacrum with high vascularity—sacrococcygeal teratoma.

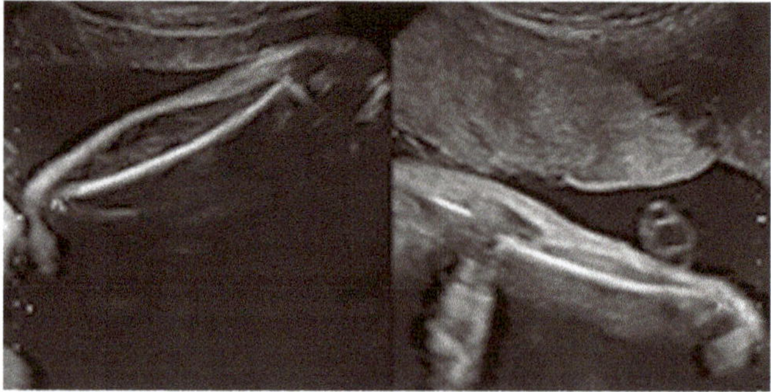

Fig. 33: Long bones to be identified with epiphysis at both end and only diaphysis to be measured.

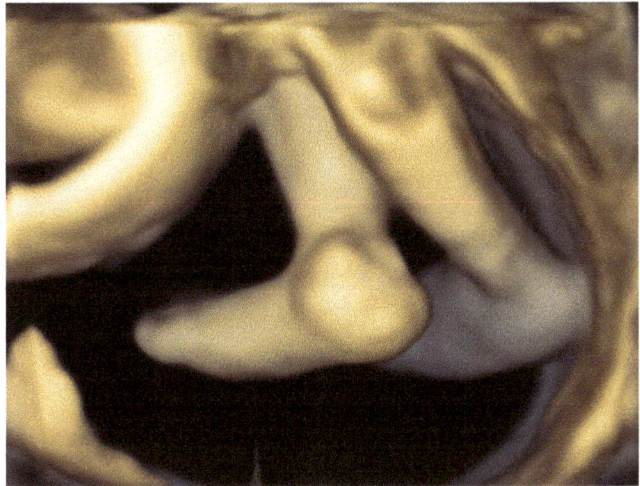

Fig. 34: Relation of foot to leg is to be identified. This is normal lower limb.

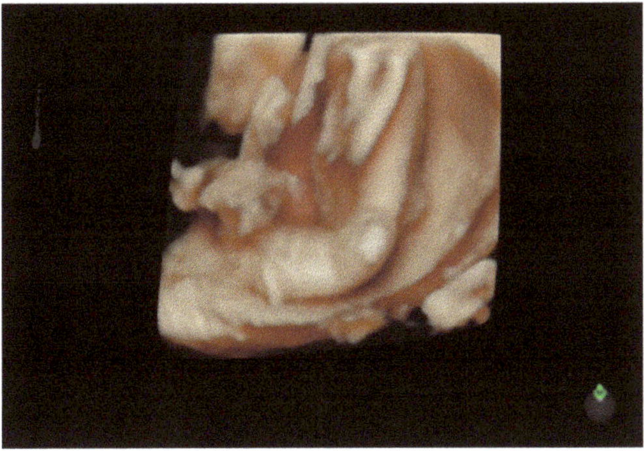

Fig. 35: Clubfoot in 3D.

Fetal Environment

Fetal placenta **(Fig. 36)** is the most important structure for fetus. It is a functional lung, kidneys and supply nourishment to fetus. So, any abnormality of placenta has direct impact on outcome of pregnancy and morbidity and mortality of fetus and neonate. Note the position of placenta, its relation, and distance from internal os. Cord insertion in placenta shall be almost in center. Placenta is little more echogenic compared to myometrium and little more hypoechoic line can be seen with on color Doppler. Retroplacental vessel separating placenta from myometrium can be identified and this rules out penetrating placenta. Normal placenta is homogenous echogenic. When one identifies in homogenous placenta, jelly-like placenta, multiple hypoechoic

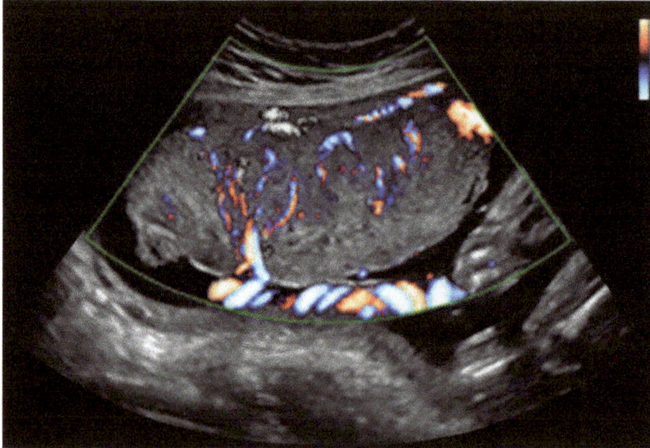

Fig. 36: Cord attachment with placenta. Myometrium can be clearly defined separate ruling out penetrating placenta.

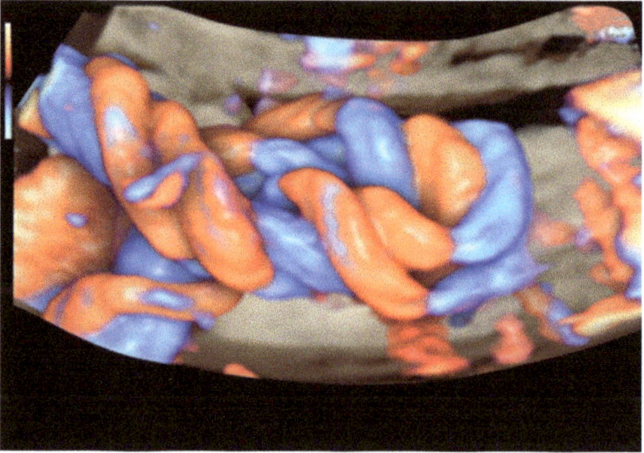

Fig. 37: Umbilical cord.

hares, bilobed or circumvallate placenta, and penetrating placenta are required to be identified precisely and reported. Any mass lesion such as lipoma and hemangioma is to be identified. Grading of placenta is of no practical value. In grade I placenta, echogenic calcified areas are noted on fetal and/or maternal surface. In grade II placenta, incomplete septa are formed from maternal to fetal surface and vice-versa. In grade III placenta, complete septa are noted.

Umbilical Cord (Fig. 37)

It is connecting pool from placenta to fetus. Note length of cord, number of vessels in cord, coiling of cord, any mass lesion, or cyst in cord. When two vessel cords are noted, scan fetus to rule out any other sonomarkers and malformations of fetus.

Amniotic Fluid (Fig. 38)

Amniotic fluid indicates health of the fetus. Oligoamnios or polyamnios indicate guarded outcome and requires fetus examination to rule out malformation and color Doppler to rule out fetal hypoxia. Amniotic fluid can be assessed by AFI. Divide gravid uterus in found equal segment by vertical and transverse line and measures largest pocket of fluid in each segment keeping probe vertical to table. Measure this pocket vertical avoiding fetal parts and cor. Sum of all four pockets gives you AFI. If it is >20 cm, suggest polyamnios and oligo is diagnosed, if it is less than 4 cm. Other more practical method is Goldman's criteria, in which if your eyeballing is suggestive of polyamnios and if largest pocket is >7 cm, it is polyamnios. If eyeballing is oligoamnios and largest pocket is <3 cm, it is oligoamnios. In multifetal pregnancy, largest pocket around each fetus is to be measured.

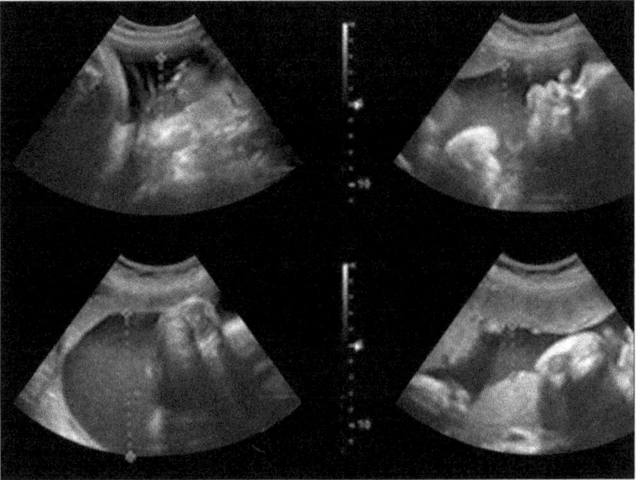

Fig. 38: Amniotic fluid index (AFI).

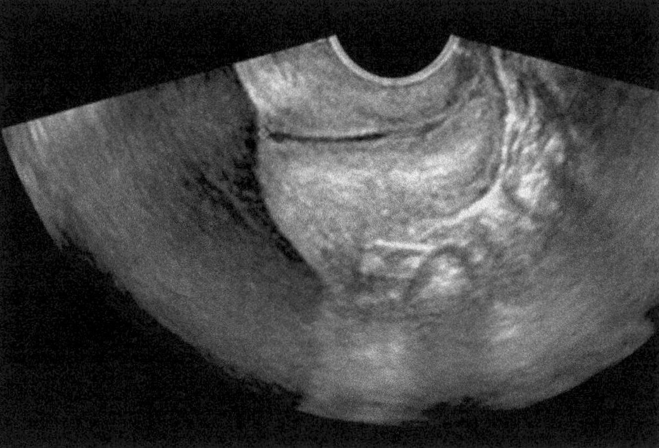

Fig. 39: Transvaginal (TV) approach is better for assessment of cervical length and ruling out incompetent os. Here is normal competent cervix.

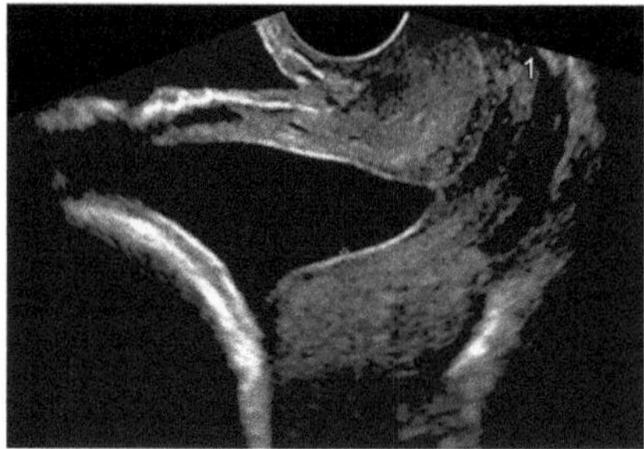

Fig. 40: By transvaginal (TV) assessment of cervix, apply pressure by abdominal hand and notice gapping internal os with short cervix suggestive of incompetent cervix. This is cervical stress test.

Cervix (Figs. 39 and 40)

Transvaginal route is preferred for measurement of cervix from internal os to external os. Cervical stress test to be carried out. While doing TV scan of cervix, apply pressures over mother's abdomen by other hand and watch gapping of internal os with shortening of cervical length.

Uterus and Adnexa

- Mass lesion or malformation may not be detectable in second and third trimester.

Genitalia [In India, as per Pre-Conception and Pre-Natal Diagnostic Techniques (PC-PNDT) act, it is not to be seen/declared].

Ultrasound in Multifetal Pregnancy

Chinmayee Ratha

INTRODUCTION

The incidence of multifetal pregnancy has increased definitely over the past decades primarily due to the advent of assisted reproduction technique (ART), although other factors contributing to lifestyle changes and even better diagnostic techniques have contributed to the same.[1] The twin birth rate increased by just under 70% between 1980 (19 per 1,000 live births) and 2006 (32 per 1,000 live births). Ultrasound has emerged as the single most important diagnostic, prognostic, and even a therapy-guiding tool for multifetal pregnancy in contemporary obstetrics.

DIAGNOSIS OF MULTIFETAL PREGNANCY

Pregnancy itself may be diagnosed by urine pregnancy tests and high levels of hormones may make us suspect multiple pregnancies, but ultrasound remains the mainstay of diagnosis of multifetal pregnancy—the number of fetuses and their amniotic/chorionic distribution **(Figs. 1 to 3)**.

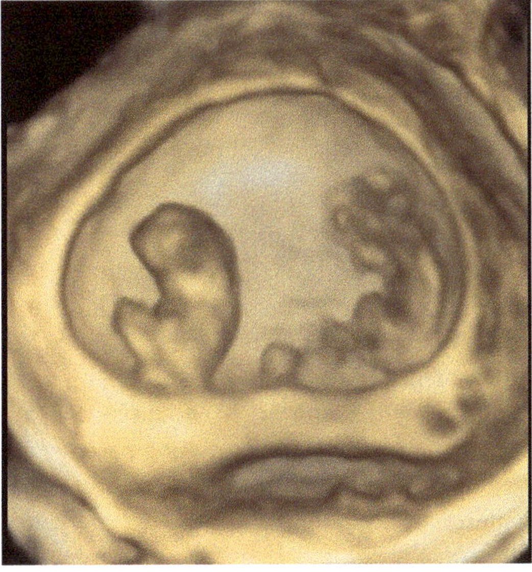

Fig. 1: Monochorionic twins.

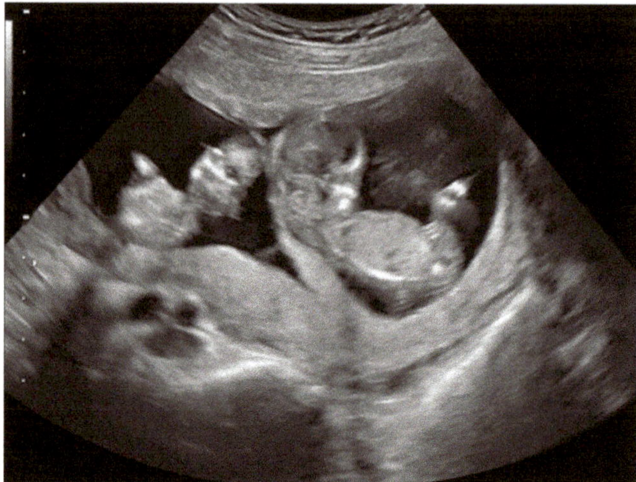

Fig. 2: Dichorionic twins.

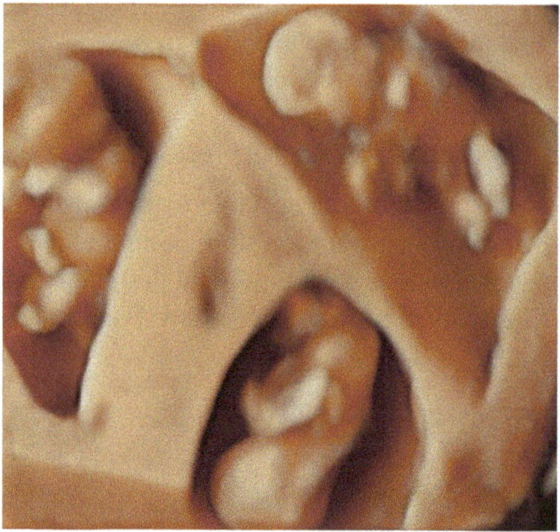

Fig. 3: Trichorionic triplets.

Establishment of Chorionicity and Amnionicity

Chorionicity is the most important determinant of the prognosis of a multifetal pregnancy. If a multiple pregnancy is "monochorionic", it means that all fetuses are connected to one placenta and hence they "share" the placental circulation. This sharing could become "unequal" and lead to problems of circulation dynamic imbalance and discordant fetal growth.

Chorionicity is therefore crucial in counseling parents about the course of a multifetal pregnancy and has to be taken into account while deciding methods of prenatal diagnosis and multifetal pregnancy reduction. The best time to determine chorionicity by ultrasonography (USG) is the first trimester of pregnancy when one can assign chorionicity with a sensitivity

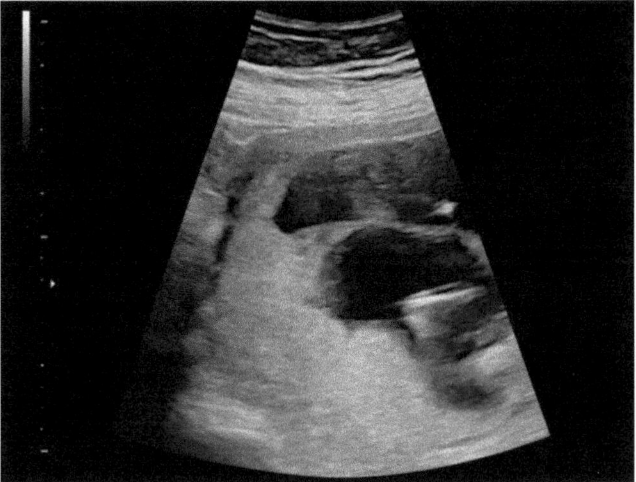

Fig. 4: Lambda sign (dichorionic).

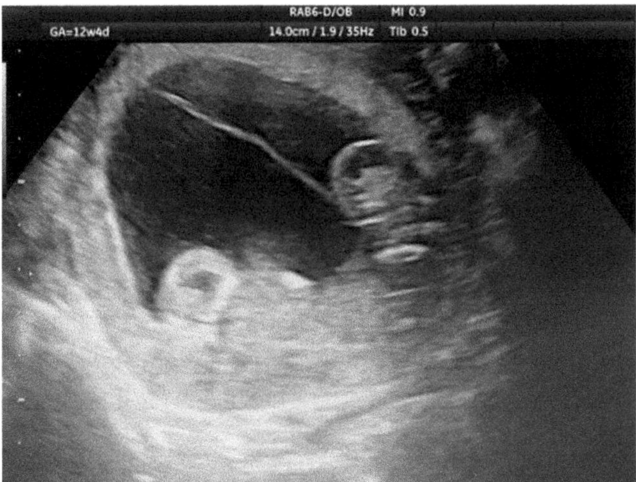

Fig. 5: "T" Sign (monochorionic).

and specificity for 100% and 99.8%, respectively.[2] If each fetus has its own placenta, ultrasound will be able to demonstrate separate placentae or the "lambda sign" or "twin peak" sign, which is the hallmark of polychorionicity **(Fig. 4)**. In contrast, the "T sign" indicates monochorionicity **(Fig. 5)**.

The International Society of Ultrasound in Obstetrics and Gynecology (ISUOG) clinical practice guidelines of 2016[3] provide the following recommendations:
- Chorionicity should be determined before 13 + 6 weeks of gestation using the membrane thickness at the site of insertion of the amniotic membrane into the placenta, identifying the T sign or lambda sign, and the number of placental masses. An ultrasound image demonstrating the chorionicity should be kept in the records for future reference (*GRADE OF RECOMMENDATION: D*).

- If it is not possible to determine chorionicity by transabdominal or transvaginal ultrasound in the routine setting, a second opinion should be sought from a tertiary referral center (*GOOD PRACTICE POINT*).
- At the time at which chorionicity is determined, amnionicity should also be determined and documented. MCMA (monochorionic monoamniotic) twin pregnancies should be referred to a tertiary center with expertise in their management (*GOOD PRACTICE POINT*).

ROLE OF ULTRASOUND IN DATING A MULTIFETAL PREGNANCY

It is an accepted fact that dating of a pregnancy should be done by early pregnancy crown-rump length (CRL), as sometimes the mother's recollection of dates may not be accurate. In twin pregnancies, there may however be discrepancy in the CRL of two fetuses and this in pregnancies conceived spontaneously, the larger of the CRLs should be used to estimate gestational age.

Similarly, in higher order multiples, the CRL of the largest fetus is considered for dating as per the current guidelines. This is an area of active research and there may be some revision of protocol, if alternate convincing evidence arises.

If the woman presents after 14 weeks of gestation, the larger head circumference should be used. Twin pregnancies conceived via in vitro fertilization should be dated using the oocyte retrieval date or the embryonic age from fertilization.[3] It is therefore important to take a detailed history of the periconception period to ascertain that the events that determine the dating of pregnancy are well documented and match the assigned gestational age calculation.

Accurate dating in early pregnancy is the most important determinant of adequate diagnosis and monitoring for fetal growth problems later in pregnancy—this fact is important in multifetal pregnancy too.

ULTRASOUND IN ANEUPLOIDY SCREENING IN MULTIFETAL PREGNANCY

Screening for aneuploidies in multifetal pregnancy is primarily based on ultrasound markers as the performance of maternal serum biochemistry is expected to be inferior as compared to singleton pregnancies due to the coexistence of multiple fetoplacental units of potentially different chromosomal composition. The role of maternal serum biochemistry is only justified in first trimester combined screening of twins with defined chorionicity. In higher order multiples, the combination of maternal age and the nutchal transluceny (NT) recorded between 11 + 0 and 13 + 6 weeks of gestation should be used as biochemical screening becomes unreliable.[1]

Twin pregnancies in the second trimester and higher order multiple pregnancies should be offered aneuploidy screening based on ultrasound parameters as the primary method. In polychorionic pregnancies, each fetus gets an individual risk for aneuploidies and there may be discordance in the NT values leading to discordant risks for both fetuses. It is important to inform women and their partners in advance of the potentially complex decisions that they will need to make on the basis of the results of combined screening, bearing in mind the increased risk of invasive testing in twins, the possible discordance between dichorionic twins for fetal aneuploidy, and the risks of selective fetal reduction.

In monochorionic twins, as they are both theoretically assumed to have similar karyotypes, the risks are allocated after taking an average of the NT of both fetuses such that both have a similar risk for aneuploidy.

Cell-free fetal DNA can be offered in multifetal pregnancy[4] after checking with the specific laboratories regarding this facility. This can act as a secondary screening method, as it may reduce the need for unnecessary invasive testing, However, if the results of cell-free DNA suggest high risk of aneuploidy, invasive testing is warranted.

In high-risk fetuses, ultrasound-guided chorionic villus sampling (CVS) and amniocentesis help in confirming the fetal chromosomal status.

ULTRASOUND-BASED SERIAL MONITORING PROTOCOL OF MULTIPLE PREGNANCIES

In dichorionic twins, both fetuses are labeled systematically based on either the position of the placentae or the cord insertion levels or the position of the membranes such that one fetus is identified as twin A and another as twin B. This labeling allows for the correct follow-up as serial growth is monitored for the same fetus without ambiguity or confusion as the pregnancy grows. If systematic labeling is not done in early pregnancy, it is difficult to ascertain proper follow-up and the allocation of first and second fetus labels may become arbitrary as fetuses move within the womb.

The current recommendations[3] of planning fetal monitoring on multiple pregnancies are essentially based on serial USG assessment of fetal growth and well-being parameters. They are demonstrated clearly on the **Flowchart 1**.

DIAGNOSIS AND MANAGEMENT OF FETAL GROWTH RESTRICTION IN TWINS

Fetal growth restriction is diagnosed when the estimated fetal weight falls below the 10th centile for gestation and may be associated with sequential Doppler changes affecting the prognosis of the fetus. In twins, the other aspect to fetal growth assessment is "intertwin discordance", which may happen if one fetus is growing much smaller than the other. If this discordance (defined

Flowchart 1: Suggested protocol for monitoring twins based on chorionicity.[3]

Dichorionic twin pregnancy

Monochorionic twin pregnancy

Dichorionic twin pregnancy

- 11–14 weeks → • Dating, labeling • Chorionicity • Screening for trisomy 21
- 20–22 weeks → • Detailed anatomy • Biometry • Amniotic fluid volume • Cervical length
- 24–26 weeks
- 28–30 weeks
- 32–34 weeks → • Assessment of fetal growth • Amniotic fluid volume • Fetal Doppler
- 36–37 weeks
- Delivery

Monochorionic twin pregnancy

- 11–14 weeks → • Dating, labeling • Chorionicity • Screening for trisomy 21
- 16 weeks
- 18 weeks → • Fetal growth, DVP • UA-PI
- 20 weeks → • Detailed anatomy • Biometry, DVP • UA-PI, MCA-PSV • Cervical length
- 22 weeks
- 24 weeks
- 26 weeks
- 28 weeks
- 30 weeks → • Fetal growth, DVP • UA-PI, MCA-PSV
- 32 weeks
- 34 weeks
- 36 weeks

(DVP: deepest vertical pocket; UA-PI: uterine artery pulsatility index; MCA-PSV: middle cerebral artery peak systolic velocity)

as the difference of weights divided by the larger weight and expressed as a percentage) is more than 25%, the condition is termed as selective intrauterine growth restriction or selective fetal growth restriction (sFGR).[3]

In dichorionic pregnancies, sFGR should be followed as in growth-restricted singletons. Fetal Doppler can be followed up 1-2 weekly, growth 2 weekly, and finally the call for delivery will depend on the gestational age as well as prognosis for survival of both fetuses. Individual cases will require senior consultant neonatologist input incase difficult decision to deliver or defer delivery have to be taken and there may be a tendency to prefer a conservative plan in the interest of the larger twin to ensure at least one intact survival in critical cases.

In monochorionic pregnancies, however, risking an intrauterine demise of a co-twin is not acceptable and hence if there arises a risk of impending fetal demise—remote to term/viability, aggressive interventions are sought for to disconnect the circulation of the twins to avoid residual neurological injury to the surviving co-twin. sFGR in monochorionic twin pregnancy occurs mainly due to unequal sharing of the placental mass and vasculature.[5]

This unequal sharing of placental vasculature in monochorionic twins can lead to other problems such as twin reversed arterial perfusion (TRAP), twin-to-twin transfusion syndrome (TTTS) and their potential complications.

ROLE OF ULTRASOUND IN PREDICTING COMPLICATIONS OF MONOCHORIONIC TWINS

Unique complications of monochorionic twins such as TRAP sequence and TTTS are now better understood and managed as our cumulative knowledge and experience have improved in these sectors because of better imaging and documentation of physiology and follow-up.

Twin reversed arterial perfusion sequence results from an acute difference in arterial pressures between the two twins early in the first trimester, which disturbs the vascular balance **(Fig. 6)**.[6] The bidirectional flow gets abolished and there develops unidirectional flow, in the reverse direction resulting in one amorphous, acardiac mass (TRAP) with a normally "pumping" twin, which is at risk of cardiac failure, if the TRAP grows very big and vascular.

Twin-to-twin transfusion syndrome affects about 15% of all monochorionic twin pregnancies and is a result of unbalanced AV anastomoses in the placenta. One twin becomes the "donor" and another "recipient" in the TTTS sequence. The donor becomes progressively hypovolemic, oliguric, and

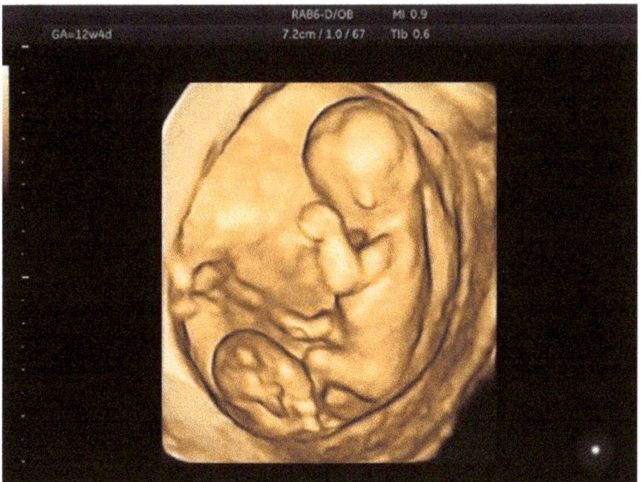

Fig. 6: Twin reversed arterial perfusion sequence with a normal co-twin.

growth restricted. The recipient becomes overperfused and at risk of cardiac failure. Both fetuses are at risk of mortality in this condition, if left untreated. TTTS is classified into five stages based on a system of staging proposed by Professor Quintero in 1999.[7] These stages are:

- *Stage I*: Discordant amniotic fluid volumes (polyamnios and oligoamnios), but urine still visible sonographically within the donor twin's bladder; 40% mortality risk
- *Stage II*: Criteria of stage I, but urine is not visible within the donor's bladder
- *Stage III*: Criteria of stage II and critically abnormal Doppler studies of the umbilical artery, ductus venosus, or umbilical vein
- *Stage IV*: Ascites or frank hydrops in either twin; (60% mortality risk)
- *Stage V*: Demise of either fetus.

As is evident, the role of ultrasound is central to the establishment of the stage of TTTS and hence in monitoring and prognosticating the condition. In cases where treatment is warranted, many ultrasound-guided procedures are used too.

All monochorionic pregnancies are advised ultrasound-guided surveillance for TTTS from 16 weeks onward every 2 weekly. Stage-1 TTTS can be managed conservatively but after stage 2, the evidence for treatment is stronger than conservative approach.[8]

Treatment of TTTS can be by fetoscopy-guided LASER ablation of placental anastomosis. In rare cases where either LASER is unavailable or not feasible, ultrasound-guided bipolar cord coagulation or radiofrequency ablation (RFA) can be done.

ROLE OF ULTRASOUND IN GUIDING THERAPY IN MULTIFETAL PREGNANCY

Ultrasound-guided therapeutic procedures have helped to improve perinatal outcomes in multifetal pregnancies. One of the most common procedures done to diagnose fetal chromosomal anomalies is ultrasound-guided amniocentesis or CVS.

Ultrasound-guided fetal reduction is done in the first trimester to reduce higher order multiple pregnancies to twin such that perinatal outcome can be optimized.[9] In some cases of critical anomalies in one co-twin, selective fetal reduction can be done under ultrasound guidance—the method of reduction would depend on the chorionicity of the pregnancy. In dichorionic pregnancies, a simple 22-g needle could be used to instill intracardiac KCl and affect an asystole for fetal reduction.

However in monochorionic twins, nonpharmacological methods are used of which needle-guided LASERs, bipolar cautery, or RFA can be done under ultrasound guidance **(Figs. 7A and B)**.

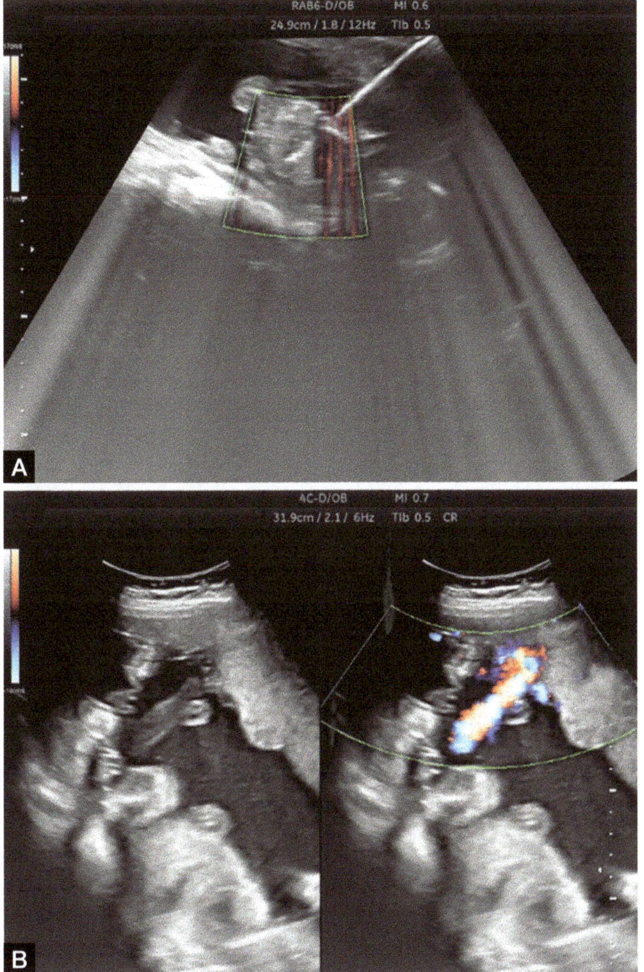

Figs. 7A and B: (A) Radiofrequency ablation (RFA) needle under ultrasonography guidance; (B) Post-RFA cessation of flow in one cord of monochorionic monoamniotic pregnancy with one anencephaly.

KEY LEARNING POINTS ABOUT ULTRASONOGRAPHY IN MULTIFETAL PREGNANCY

- An early pregnancy USG can help in diagnosing a multifetal pregnancy and dating it based on the CRL of the largest fetus.
- *Chorionicity* is the single most important determinant of prognosis in multiple pregnancies.
- Chorionicity is best established between 10 and 14 weeks and may be difficult after that.
- Aneuploidy screening in multiple pregnancies is mostly dependent on USG findings although serum biochemistry can be used in first trimester for twins with defined chorionicity.

- USG can guide CVS and amniocentesis in multiple pregnancy.
- USG is pivotal in serial growth monitoring in multiple fetuses and systematic labeling is important to avoid confusion.
- Doppler studies guide the management of growth-restricted fetuses.
- There are complications unique to monochorionic twins, which can be diagnosed, staged, and even managed with the help of USG guidance.

REFERENCES

1. National Collaborating Center for Women's and Children's Health (UK). Multiple Pregnancy. The Management of Twin and Triplet Pregnancies in the Antenatal Period. Commissioned by the National Institute for Clinical Excellence. London: RCOG Press; 2011.
2. Dias T, Arcangeli T, Bhide A, Napolitano R, Mahsud-Dornan S, Thilaganathan B. First-trimester ultrasound determination of chorionicity in twin pregnancy. Ultrasound Obstet Gynecol. 2011;38(5):530-2.
3. Khalil A, Rodgers M, Baschat A, Bhide A, Gratacos E, Hecher K, et al. ISUOG Practice Guidelines: role of ultrasound in twin pregnancy. Ultrasound Obstet Gynecol. 2016;47(2):247-63.
4. Gil MM, Quezada MS, Revello R, Akolekar R, Nicolaides KH. Analysis of cell-free DNA in maternal blood in screening for fetal aneuploidies: updated meta-analysis. Ultrasound Obstet Gynecol. 2015;45(3):249-66.
5. Lewi L, Gucciardo L, Huber A, Jani J, Mieghem TV, Doné E, et al. Clinical outcome and placental characteristics of monochorionic diamniotic twin pairs with early- and late-onset discordant growth. Am J Obstet Gynecol. 2008;199(5):511.e1-7.
6. Sueters M, Oepkes D. Diagnosis of twin-to-twin transfusion syndrome, selective fetal growth restriction, twin anemia-polycythaemia sequence, and twin reversed arterial perfusion sequence. Best practice and research. Best Pract Res Clin Obstet Gynaecol. 2014;28(2):215-26.
7. Quintero RA, Morales WJ, Allen MH, Bornick PW, Johnson PK, Kruger M. Staging of twin-twin transfusion syndrome. J Perinatol. 1999;19(8 Pt 1):550-5.
8. Quintero RA, Dickinson JE, Morales WJ, Bornick PW, Bermúdez C, Cincotta R, et al. Stage-based treatment of twin-twin transfusion syndrome. Am J Obstet Gynecol. 2003;188(5):1333-40.
9. Evans MI, Goldberg JD, Horenstein J, Wapner RJ, Ayoub MA, Stone J, et al. Selective termination for structural, chromosomal, and mendelian anomalies: international experience. Am J Obstet Gynecol. 1999;181(4):893-7.

Management of Common Problems

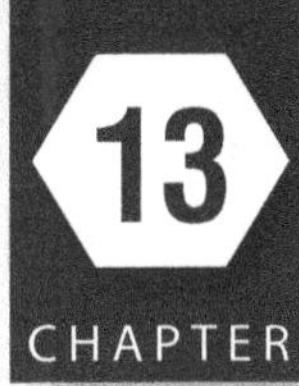

Pruritus in Pregnancy/Obstetric Cholestasis

Pratik Tambe, Preeti Deshpande

INTRODUCTION

Obstetric cholestasis or intrahepatic cholestasis of pregnancy is a multifactorial condition with intense pruritus in absence of skin rash, with abnormal liver function tests[1] with elevated serum aminotransferases and bile acid. It has an onset in 2nd/3rd trimester and there is spontaneous relief within 2–3 weeks postdelivery. Neither the skin rash nor the abnormal liver function tests have any alternate cause. Both remit following delivery.

The incidence of obstetric cholestasis is 0.5–1% in North America and England. Incidence is high in Scandinavia and South America. Incidence is as high as 9–15% in Chile and Bolivia.[2] In Scandinavia and Baltic countries, obstetric cholestasis occurs in 2%.

ETIOLOGY

The etiology of obstetric cholestasis is multifactorial. It involves genetic, hormonal, and environmental factors. Estrogen and progesterone metabolites have been demonstrated to have a role in obstetric cholestasis. The disease usually appears in 3rd trimester, when estrogen production reaches its maximum. Also, the incidence is higher in twin gestation.

Progesterone and its associated metabolites may be associated with increased plasma levels of mono- and disulfated progesterone metabolites. Impaired function of the hepatocellular bile acid transporters due to high levels of estrogen and progesterone at post-transcriptional levels has been demonstrated in vitro.[3]

Presence of the disease in ethnic groups and geographic areas points at a genetic predisposition. Mutation in hepatocellular phospholipid transporter, ABCB4 that mediates secretion of the major human phospholipid and phosphatidylcholine into the bile has been estimated to account for 15% cases.

Seasonal variation and incomplete recurrence in subsequent pregnancy may be associated with nutritional factors, which suggest that exogenous factor such as selenium deficiency may contribute.

CLINICAL PRESENTATION

Obstetric cholestasis presents in the 2nd/3rd trimester after 30 weeks of gestation and generally subsides 48 hours to 3 weeks postdelivery. It is associated with severe pruritus starting on palms and soles that is soon generalized. Very rarely, it may begin at 6-10 weeks. Pruritus is a very unpleasant symptom, which worsens at night. It can cause sleep deprivation and psychological suffering.

There is no rash at the start. Dermatographia artefacta may develop secondary to scratching. Jaundice is less common, seen in 10-15% cases. Jaundice typically develops 1-4 weeks after pruritus. Fatigue and insomnia are seen. Epigastric discomfort and malaise are common. Steatorrhea develops leading to malabsorption of fat-soluble vitamins. Vitamin K deficiency may develop leading to increased risk of postpartum hemorrhage.

Other causes of itching in pregnancy such as pruritic urticarial papules and plaques of pregnancy or prurigo of pregnancy should be ruled out. These lesions develop over the stretch marks and spread from abdomen to buttocks and the thighs. These rashes spare the umbilicus, palms, and soles.

The other skin disorders, which pose as differentials for obstetric cholestasis, include pemphigoid gestationis, which is a self-limiting condition. It is a bullous disorder seen after 20 weeks of gestation. It begins with pruritus. Papules and plaques develop around the umbilicus, which form blisters. It flares up at the time of delivery and diagnosis is by skin biopsy and immunofluorescence. Atopic eruptions in pregnancy may occur in atopic individuals.

MANAGEMENT PATHWAYS

The management pathways for pruritus in pregnancy are described in **Flowchart 1**.

DIAGNOSIS

Diagnosis is based on four points—pruritus, raised bile acid > 10 µmol/mL, spontaneous relief postdelivery in 2-3 weeks, and absence of other diseases that can cause pruritus and jaundice. In obstetric cholestasis, initially the patient develops pruritus and later on the liver function test change. Hence, the liver function tests should be done every 1-2 weeks. There may be a mild increase in up to twofold to tenfold rise in the liver transaminases including aspartate aminotransferase and alanine aminotransferase (ALT), weeks after pruritus. However, sometimes, the aminotransferase levels may rise up to 1,000 units/mL.

Bilirubin is raised only infrequently. Serum total bile acid levels may increase 10-100 times in obstetric cholestasis. Cholic acid is increased more than chenodeoxycholic acid. Bile acid levels are not routinely done. If bile acid levels are raised, it may be associated with adverse fetal outcome. Secondary

Flowchart 1: Diagnostic approach to pruritus in pregnancy.

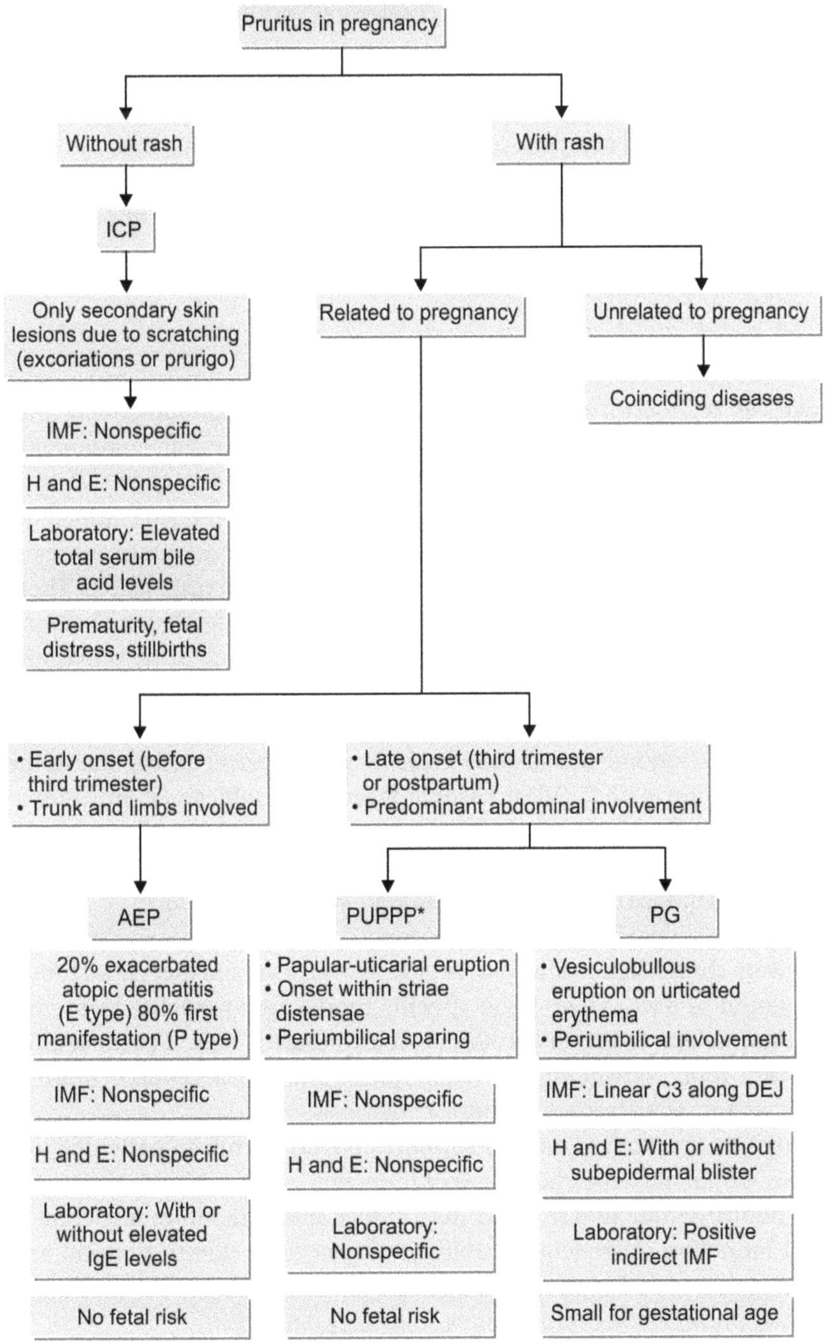

Pruritus in pregnancy

- Without rash → ICP
  - Only secondary skin lesions due to scratching (excoriations or prurigo)
    - IMF: Nonspecific
    - H and E: Nonspecific
    - Laboratory: Elevated total serum bile acid levels
    - Prematurity, fetal distress, stillbirths

- With rash
  - Related to pregnancy
    - • Early onset (before third trimester)
      • Trunk and limbs involved → **AEP**
      - 20% exacerbated atopic dermatitis (E type) 80% first manifestation (P type)
      - IMF: Nonspecific
      - H and E: Nonspecific
      - Laboratory: With or without elevated IgE levels
      - No fetal risk
    - • Late onset (third trimester or postpartum)
      • Predominant abdominal involvement
      - **PUPPP***
        - • Papular-uticarial eruption
          • Onset within striae distensae
          • Periumbilical sparing
        - IMF: Nonspecific
        - H and E: Nonspecific
        - Laboratory: Nonspecific
        - No fetal risk
      - **PG**
        - • Vesiculobullous eruption on urticated erythema
          • Periumbilical involvement
        - IMF: Linear C3 along DEJ
        - H and E: With or without subepidermal blister
        - Laboratory: Positive indirect IMF
        - Small for gestational age
  - Unrelated to pregnancy
    - Coinciding diseases

(ICP: intrahepatic cholestasis of pregnancy; AEP: atopic eruption of pregnancy; PG: pemphigoid gestationis; IMF: immunofluorescence; H and E: histopathology; DEJ: dermoepidermal junction; PUPPP: pruritic urticarial papules and plaques of pregnancy)

to vitamin K deficiency, prothrombin time may increase. Other causes of liver disorder need to be ruled out, such as viral hepatitis, preeclampsia, and acute fatty liver.

In obstetric cholestasis, the total bile acid composition shifts to hydrophobic pattern with higher lithocholic acid and unconjugated serum bile acids. Serum alkaline phosphatase may rise but it is difficult to interpret due to elevation of placental isoenzyme. Serum aminotransferases may allow better follow-up for patients with obstetric cholestasis after start of ursodeoxycholic acid than fasting total serum bile acid levels, as the latter initially increase with ursodeoxycholic acid.

PROGNOSIS

Prognosis is good for the mother. Pruritus regresses spontaneously after delivery. However, the fetus is at risk of preterm delivery, meconium, and stillbirth. Active surveillance is needed.

Although the pathophysiology of fetal risk has not yet been clarified, an elevation of maternal fetal bile acid flow and inability of the fetus to eliminate bile acids through the immature fetal liver appear to be responsible. There is excess accumulation of bile acid that is toxic in the fetal compartment. Accumulation of bile acid leads to fetal cardiotoxicity and arrhythmias and intrauterine fetal death.

There are signs of acute anoxia with serosal and pulmonary petechial bleed, but no chronic anoxia. Bile acids may cause vasoconstriction in the placenta. There is no IUGR or chronic placental insufficiency. Infusion of cholic acid in fetal lambs stimulates passage of meconium due to colonic motility. Bile acids also trigger myometrial contraction and lead to preterm delivery and induce contraction of chorionic veins of placenta.

The fetus should be delivered as soon as it is mature. However, intrauterine fetal death cannot be correlated with biochemical tests and there is no robust correlation of data. There is no specific monitoring modality to predict intrauterine fetal death. In cardiotocography, there is lack of predictability of future fetal well-being. Ultrasonography is not a reliable method for preventing fetal death in obstetric cholestasis.

There is insufficient data to support delivery or refuse early delivery (<37 weeks) in obstetric cholestasis or induction of labor aimed at reducing late stillbirth. Induction of labor may induce morbidity in mother due to failed induction. Also, fetal morbidity may increase due to preterm and respiratory distress. Hence, pharmacological treatment is needed to improve pruritus, prevent fetal complications, and delay delivery.

TREATMENT

Many pharmacological agents have been used in treatment of obstetric cholestasis. These include phenobarbital (100 mg), hydroxyzine (25–50 mg), glutathione precursor S-adenosyl methionine, cholestyramine, and dexamethasone. All these agents have shown limited clinical benefits. There is no specific therapy for maternal symptoms and neonatal outcomes.

Phenobarbitone

Phenobarbitone relieved pruritus in 50% patients but showed no reduction of enzymes.

Topical Emollients

Topical emollients relieve itching to some extent.

Antihistaminics

Antihistaminics such as chlorpheniramine may provide sedation but have no significant impact on pruritus.

Ursodeoxycholic Acid

Currently, ursodeoxycholic acid seems the most promising option among the drugs available for obstetrics cholestasis. It is a hydrophilic bile acid, which decreases liver damage in mother by cytoprotection against hepatotoxic effect of hydrophobic bile acid and improves transport and secretion of hepatobiliary bile acid. Stimulation of the hepatocellular secretions seems to be the most effective mechanism. Ursodeoxycholic acid may also have a specific effect by improving transport of bile acids across placenta.

It improves impaired hepatocellular secretion by post-transcription stimulation of the canalicular expression of key transport protein such as conjugate export pump, multidrug resistance protein 2 or bile salt pump, and BSEP. It reduces elevated levels of sulfated steroids in the serum, urine, amniotic fluid, and colostrum.

Evidence

A meta-analysis of nine randomized controlled trials (RCTs) was published in 2012.[4] The points assessed included—total resolution of pruritus, reduced pruritus, normalization of alanine transaminase, normalization of serum bile acid, and reduction of fetal complications such as preterm, respiratory distress, and need for neonatal intensive care unit (NICU). The symptoms were reviewed on day 14/day 21. The control groups included interventions such as placebo, cholestyramine, dexamethasone, S-adenosyl methionine, or no specific treatment. All the above tests and symptoms showed better improvement in ursodeoxycholic acid groups.

The dose ranges from 600 to 2,000 mg or 15 mg/kg/d in 2–3 divided doses and is effective in reducing pruritus and reducing total serum bile acid levels ALT and bilirubin levels. Ursodeoxycholic acid improved cholic acid:chenodeoxycholic acid ratio. It has no significant side effects; some patients had diarrhea, nausea, and vomiting. The meta-analysis concluded that ursodeoxycholic acid is effective in reducing pruritus and improving liver function test results and may also benefit fetal outcomes.

Ursodeoxycholic acid does not prevent intrauterine fetal death, which is a feared but rare complication. Another meta-analysis by Sophie Grand Maisen et al., which included RCTs and nonrandomized studies.[5] This suggested possible benefits of lower rates of prematurity, increase birth weight, decrease pruritus, improved LETs, and safety of ursodeoxycholic acid for use in obstetric cholestasis.

S-adenosyl Methionine

There is insufficient evidence to show whether S-adenosyl methionine is effective for control of maternal symptoms or improvement of fetal outcomes. It has to be given as an intravenous injection twice daily (800 mg/day), which is inconvenient for patients. In one trial, a combination of ursodeoxycholic acid and S-adenosyl methionine was found to be very effective.[6]

Guar Gum

It was shown to improve pruritus in a double-blind study in Finland.[7]

Dexamethasone

A randomized controlled trial comparing dexamethasone and ursodeoxycholic acid was conducted and published in 2005 by the American Association for the Study of Liver Disease.[8] Patients were randomly allocated to three groups in a double blind fashion; the first group received ursodeoxycholic acid 1 g/day as a single dose for 3 weeks, second group received dexamethasone 12 mg/day as a single dose for 1 week, and third group was given placebo for 3 weeks.

The ursodeoxycholic acid group showed reduced ALT and bile, but not bilirubin and pruritus in obstetric cholestasis. Additionally, subgroup analysis was done for changes in laboratory parameters and pruritus during treatment when serum bile acids were ≥40 µmol/L at inclusion. Fetal complication rates do not increase until bile acid levels exceed 40 µmol/L.

Subgroup analysis showed that ursodeoxycholic acid improved biochemical markers of cholestasis as well as pruritus and treatment with ursodeoxycholic acid was more effective than treatment with dexamethasone. Mean bile acid levels decrease 79% with ursodeoxycholic acid compared to 45% decrease with dexamethasone. Also, in this subgroup, alanine transaminase and bilirubin reduction were more pronounced with ursodeoxycholic acid. However, fetal complications did not reduce even in this subgroup.

It was found that the benefit of dexamethasone on pruritus and biochemical markers of cholestasis was transient. A rapid decrease in pruritus and bile acid was seen after 1 week of treatment, but was followed by an increase. On the other hand, the observation with ursodeoxycholic acid was an increase in total bile acid level in the first 2–3 days, decrease to baseline after 4–5 days treatment after which a steady decrease occurred. This RCT showed that dexamethasone was less effective than ursodeoxycholic acid.

Vitamin K

Water-soluble vitamin K needs to be supplemented. In obstetric cholestasis, bile acids are not excreted into the gastrointestinal tract and hence there is no micelle formation. There is steatorrhea and reduced absorption of fat-soluble vitamin K. This can affect coagulation factor synthesis.

CONCLUSION

Randomized controlled trials are difficult to carry out with pregnant women, particularly in a relative rare condition such as obstetric cholestasis. Though it is a benign disease for mother, it causes very distressing symptoms and may affect the fetal intrauterine milieu. Currently, investigations are unable to predict the prognosis and fetal complications accurately. There is a need for early diagnosis and effective treatment. Of all the current therapies, ursodeoxycholic acid shows promise by reducing pruritus, improving liver function, and enhancing fetal outcomes.

REFERENCES

1. Royal College of Obstetricians and Gynaecologists (2006). Obstetric Cholestasis (Green-top Guideline No. 43). [online] Available from: https://www.rcog.org.uk/en/guidelines-research-services/guidelines/gtg43/. [Last accessed June, 2020].
2. Bergman H, Melamed N, Koren G. Pruritus in pregnancy—Treatment of dermatoses unique to pregnancy. Can Fam Phys. 2013;59(12):1290-4.
3. Ozkan S, Ceylan Y, Veli O, Yildrim S. Review of a challenging clinical issue: intrahepatic cholestasis of pregnancy. World J Gastroenterol. 2015;21(23):7134-41.
4. Bacq Y, Sentilhes L, Reyes HB, Glantz A, Kondrackiene K, Binder T, et al. Efficacy of ursodeoxycholic acid in treating intrahepatic cholestasis of pregnancy: a meta-analysis. Gastroenterology. 2012;143(6);1492-501.
5. Maison SG, Durand M, Mahone M. The effects of ursodeoxycholic acid treatment of intrahepatic cholestasis of pregnancy on maternal and fetal outcomes: a meta-analysis including non-randomized studies. J Obstet Gynaecol Can. 2014;36(7):632-41.
6. Nicastri PL, Diaferia A, Tartagni M, Loizzi P, Fanelli M. A randomized placebo-controlled trial of ursodeoxycholic acid and S-adenosylmethionine in the treatment of intrahepatic cholestasis of pregnancy. Br J Obstet Gynaecol. 1998;105(11):1205-7.
7. Gylling H, Rjikonen S, Nikkilä K, Savonius H, Miettinen TA. Oral guar gum treatment of intrahepatic cholestasis and pruritus in pregnant women: effects on serum cholesterol and other non-cholesterol sterols. Eur J Clin Invest. 1998;28(5):359-63.
8. Glantaz A, Marschall HU, Lammert F, Mattsson LA. Intrahepatic cholestasis of pregnancy: a randomized controlled trial comparing dexamethasone and ursodeoxycholic acid. Hepatology. 2005;42(6):1399-405.

Vaginal Discharge in Pregnancy

Abha Rani Sinha

■ INTRODUCTION

Women during pregnancy may have vaginal discharge, which may be either physiological or pathological. Vaginal pH, glycogen content, and amount of secretion influence the quantity and type of organisms present in the vagina. Lactobacilli restrict the growth of other organisms by producing lactic acid, thus maintaining a low pH. These organisms also produce hydrogen peroxide, which is toxic to anaerobes. The normal vaginal bacterial population assists in inhibiting the growth of pathologic vaginal organisms. If the normal vaginal ecosystem is altered, there is a greater chance of proliferation of pathogenic organisms. Factors that alter vaginal environment include feminine hygiene products, contraceptives, vaginal medications, antibiotics, sexually transmitted diseases (STDs), sexual intercourse, and stress. The challenge to the clinician is to differentiate and recognize the abnormal vaginal discharge and provide specific treatment.

Common causes of abnormal vaginal discharge in pregnancy:
- Candida vulvovaginitis
- Anaerobic bacterial infection and bacterial vaginosis (BV)
- *Trichomonas vaginitis*
- Mixed infection or STD

■ VULVOVAGINAL CANDIDIASIS

Higher estrogen levels and higher glycogen content in vaginal secretions during pregnancy increase a woman's risk of developing vulvovaginal candidiasis (VVC). *Candida albicans* infection occurs in the vast majority (80–90%) of diagnosed VVC cases, while infection with other species, such as *Candida glabrata* or *Candida tropicalis,* occurs less frequently. With adequate pharmacotherapy and avoidance of contributing factors (e.g., douching and wearing tight pants), VVC and associated symptoms resolve in a short period of time. Predisposing factors to VVC include pregnancy, diabetes mellitus, immunosuppressive therapy, antibiotics, oral contraceptives, immunodeficient conditions, and tight fitting and nylon undergarments. Heat and moisture favor the growth of *Candida* species. The VVC can be sexually transmitted, and several studies reported an association between candidiasis and orogenital sex.

Classification of Vulvovaginal Candidiasis

Uncomplicated Vulvovaginal Candidiasis

- Sporadic or infrequent vulvovaginal candidiasis
- Mild-to-moderate vulvovaginal candidiasis
- Likely to be *Candida albicans*
- Nonimmunocompromised women

Complicated Vulvovaginal Candidiasis

- Recurrent vulvovaginal candidiasis
- Severe vulvovaginal candidiasis
- Nonalbicans candidiasis
- Women with diabetes, immunocompromising conditions [e.g., HIV (human immunodeficiency virus) infection], debilitation, or immunosuppressive therapy (e.g., corticosteroids)

Symptoms and Signs

Most patients with VVC complain of vaginal discharge, dyspareunia, vulval pruritus, and burning. Patients commonly complain of pruritus and burning after intercourse or upon urination. Erythema and edema of the labia majora and minora and rashes on the perineum and thighs may be seen on physical examination, and a whitish, thick, and curd-like vaginal discharge is usually present.

Diagnosis

The diagnosis is made on both clinical examination and laboratory by identification of *Candida* by positive wet-mount test or potassium hydroxide (KOH) preparation. In the wet-mount test, the spores and *Candida* are seen when vaginal discharge or scrapings from vulval lesions are mixed with normal saline and viewed under high-power magnifications. The presence of yeast blastospores or pseudohyphae can be detected in approximately 30–50% of patients with symptoms. The addition of 10% KOH to the solution lyses white blood cells, red blood cells, and vaginal epithelial cells, making the alkali-resistant branching budding hyphae of *Candida* easier to see. Positive results from these two tests in combination with a normal vaginal pH are helpful in confirming the diagnosis. Most studies demonstrate that most of vaginal isolates are *Candida albicans*. Therefore, fungal cultures have not been used by most clinicians as part of the initial evaluation.

Treatment

There are several treatment options for *Candida* infection, such as antifungals and antiseptics, with corticosteroids as a useful addition for pruritus and erythema.

Antifungal agents commercially available for the treatment of VVC include imidazole antifungals (e.g., butoconazole, clotrimazole, and miconazole), triazole antifungals (e.g., fluconazole and terconazole), and polyene antifungals (e.g., nystatin). These agents are available in oral and topical formulations. The topical formulations of imidazole and triazole antifungals are collectively known as azole antifungals. Azole antifungals are considered the therapy of choice during pregnancy owing to the safety data collected from animals as well as humans. Prospective and observational studies involving the use of topical antifungals did not reveal an increased risk of major malformations when mothers were exposed any time during pregnancy. Systemic absorption of these topical medications is minimal, posing little risk of transfer to the unborn baby. Azole therapy should be recommended for 7 days instead of a shorter duration because of improved treatment success.

Low-potency topical corticosteroids can be prescribed to alleviate acute symptoms such as itching and redness. A meta-analysis conducted by Park-Wyllie et al., combining five prospective human studies, found that for mothers who were exposed to oral corticosteroids, there was a nonsignificant increased odds ratio for total major malformations. There was a small but statistically significant increased risk of cleft palate compared with controls (odds ratio: 3.35; 95% confidence interval: 1.97–5.69). For topical corticosteroids, approximately 3% of the dose applied onto the skin is systemically absorbed. Two population-based studies found no increased risk of major malformations in the babies of mothers who used topical corticosteroids during pregnancy.

ANAEROBIC BACTERIAL INFECTION AND BACTERIAL VAGINOSIS

Vaginal flora of a normal asymptomatic reproductive-aged woman includes multiple aerobic or facultative species as well as obligate anaerobic species. Of these, anaerobes are predominant and outnumber aerobic species. These anaerobes include gram-negative organisms such as *Prevotella, Bacteroides, Fusobacterium* species, and *Veillonella* species and gram-positive bacilli such as *Propionibacterium* species, *Eubacterium* species, and *Bifidobacterium* species. These anaerobic bacteria cause nonspecific vaginitis.

Bacterial vaginosis is characterized by a shift from normal vaginal population of lactobacilli to anaerobes such as *Gardnerella vaginalis, Prevotella, Bacteroides,* and *Mobiluncus* species and other bacteria such as *Mycoplasma* and *Ureaplasma* species. It is one of the most frequent conditions encountered in reproductive health clinics throughout the world. The condition had been previously called *Haemophilus vaginalis* vaginitis, nonspecific vaginitis, and *Gardnerella vaginalis* vaginitis.

Bacterial vaginosis has been strongly associated with poor pregnancy outcomes such as preterm delivery and low-birth weight infants, and several studies have now established the associations between BV, HIV, and puerperal sepsis.

Bacterial vaginosis usually occurs in sexually active patients. Some of the other risk factors include multiple sexual partners, low socioeconomic status, lesbians, presence of intrauterine device, and prior STD.

Symptoms and Signs

Bacterial vaginosis is characterized by a malodorous, profuse, thin, homogeneous yellow, white, or gray discharge that is adherent to the anterior and lateral vaginal walls. Typically, the patient may complain of a fishy odor during or shortly after coitus and also during menses. The alkaline nature of blood or semen (pH > 7) brings about a transient increase in the vaginal pH, and this causes the release of amines, which the patient perceives as fishy odor. Vulvitis and pruritus are very minimal or totally absent. Nearly half of patients with BV have no symptoms.

Obstetric complications include premature rupture of fetal membranes, late miscarriage, and postpartum endometritis; whereas, pelvic inflammatory disease (PID), posthysterectomy cuff infection, and postabortal sepsis are some of the gynecological complications.

Diagnosis

Diagnosis of BV can be based on the Amsel's clinical criteria or Gram stain.

A Gram stain (considered the gold standard laboratory method for diagnosing BV) is used to determine the relative concentration of lactobacilli (i.e., long Gram-positive rods), Gram-negative and Gram-variable rods and cocci (i.e., *Gardnerella vaginalis*, *Prevotella*, *Porphyromonas*, and peptostreptococci), and curved Gram-negative rods (i.e., *Mobiluncus*) characteristic of BV.

In Amsel's criteria, three of the following are required to diagnose BV:
- Homogeneous, thin, and white discharge that smoothly coats the vaginal walls
- Clue cells (e.g., vaginal epithelial cells studded with adherent coccobacilli) on microscopic examination
- pH of vaginal fluid > 4.5
- A fishy odor of vaginal discharge before or after addition of 10% KOH (i.e., the whiff test)

The Nugent's method relies on the identification of categories of vaginal microflora based on quantitative assessment of a vaginal gram-stained smear. The Nugent's method has been extensively validated in industrialized countries where assessment of vaginal microflora is an important step in understanding the pattern of flora association with BV. Culture is the least accurate in making a diagnosis of BV, as there is overgrowth of many vaginal organisms in this condition. Though virtually, all patients with BV have *Gardnerella vaginalis* isolated on culture, it must also be noted that the organism can also be cultured in 40–50% of women with normal flora.

Treatment

Treatment is recommended for all symptomatic pregnant women. Studies have revealed that treatment with oral metronidazole 500 mg twice daily to be equally effective as metronidazole gel, with cure rates of 70% using Amsel's criteria to define cure. Multiple studies and meta-analyses have failed to demonstrate an association between metronidazole use during pregnancy and teratogenic or mutagenic effects in newborns. Symptomatic pregnant women can be treated with either of the oral or vaginal regimens recommended for nonpregnant women. Although adverse pregnancy outcomes, including premature rupture of membranes, preterm labor, preterm birth, intra-amniotic infection, and postpartum endometritis have been associated with symptomatic BV in some observational studies, treatment of BV in pregnant women can reduce the signs and symptoms of vaginal infection. A meta-analysis has concluded that no antibiotic regimen prevented preterm birth (early or late) in women with BV (symptomatic or asymptomatic). However, in one study, oral BV therapy reduced the risk for late miscarriage, and in two additional studies, such therapy decreased adverse outcomes in the neonate. Treatment of asymptomatic BV among pregnant women who are at high risk for preterm delivery (i.e., those with a previous preterm birth) has been evaluated by several studies, which have yielded mixed results. Seven trials have evaluated treatment of pregnant women with asymptomatic BV at high risk for preterm delivery—one showed harm, two showed no benefit, and four demonstrated benefit.

■ TRICHOMONIASIS

Trichomoniasis is the most common STD worldwide. It was originally thought to be innocuous but has now been found to be associated with preterm labor, premature rupture of membranes, increased perinatal loss, and PID.

Trichomonas vaginitis is caused by the *Trichomonas* organism, which is a small, flagellated, motile, and anaerobic protozoan. The particular trichomonad responsible for vaginitis is *Trichomonas vaginalis*, which is the type found in the vagina *Trichomonas vaginalis* is usually transmitted sexually. Males are usually asymptomatic, but they can easily infect treated female.

The vaginal discharge of trichomoniasis is malodorous, frothy and profuse, thin creamy or slightly greenish, and may cause itching. The classic yellow–green discharge is found in 20–50% of patients more often, the discharge is gray or white. The patient may also complain of dyspareunia, postcoital bleeding, pruritus vulvae, frequency of micturition, and dysuria. On speculum examination, apart from the discharge, a cervical erosion may be seen, and in severe cases, multiple, small punctuate hemorrhages and swollen papillae may be found on the cervix ("strawberry" cervix) and vagina.

Diagnosis

The most common method for *Trichomonas vaginalis* diagnosis is microscopic evaluation of wet preparations of genital secretions because of convenience and relatively low cost. The sensitivity of wet mount is low (51–65%) in vaginal specimens. Clinicians using wet mounts should attempt to evaluate slides immediately because sensitivity declines as evaluation is delayed, decreasing by up to 20% within 1 hour after collection.

When highly sensitive [e.g., nucleic acid amplification test (NAAT)] testing on specimens is not feasible, a testing algorithm (e.g., wet mount first, followed by NAAT if negative) can improve diagnostic sensitivity in persons with an initial negative result by wet mount. Although *Trichomonas vaginalis* may be an incidental finding on a Pap test, neither conventional nor liquid-based Pap tests are considered diagnostic tests for trichomoniasis, because false negatives and false positives can occur.

Culture was considered the gold standard method for diagnosing *Trichomonas vaginalis* infection before molecular detection methods became available. Culture has a sensitivity of 75–96% and a specificity of up to 100%. In women, vaginal secretions are the preferred specimen type for culture, as urine culture is less sensitive. The benefit of routine screening for *Trichomonas vaginalis* in asymptomatic pregnant women has not been established. However, screening at the first prenatal visit and prompt treatment, as appropriate, are recommended for pregnant women with HIV infection, because *Trichomonas vaginalis* infection is a risk factor for vertical transmission of HIV. Pregnant women with HIV who are treated for *Trichomonas vaginalis* infection should be retested 3 months after treatment.

Treatment

Treatment reduces symptoms and signs of *Trichomonas vaginalis* infection and might reduce transmission. Likelihood of adverse outcomes in women with HIV also is reduced with *Trichomonas vaginalis* therapy.

The recommended regimen in pregnant women is metronidazole 2 g orally in a single dose. Symptomatic pregnant women, regardless of pregnancy stage, should be tested and considered for treatment. Treatment of *Trichomonas vaginalis* infection can relieve symptoms of vaginal discharge in pregnant women and reduce sexual transmission to partners. Although perinatal transmission of trichomoniasis is uncommon, treatment also might prevent respiratory or genital infection of the newborn.

Although metronidazole crosses the placenta, data suggest that it poses a low risk to pregnant women. No evidence of teratogenicity or mutagenic effects in infants has been found in multiple cross-sectional and cohort studies of pregnant women. Women can be treated with 2-g metronidazole in a single dose at any stage of pregnancy. Tinidazole should be avoided in pregnant women, and breastfeeding should be deferred for 72 hours following a single 2-g dose of tinidazole. Clinicians should counsel symptomatic pregnant women with trichomoniasis regarding the potential risks for and benefits of treatment and about the importance of partner treatment and condom use in the prevention of sexual transmission.

Metronidazole is secreted in breast milk. With maternal oral therapy, breastfed infants receive metronidazole in doses that are lower than those used to treat infections in infants, although the active metabolite adds to the total infant exposure. Plasma levels of the drug and metabolite are measurable, but remain less than maternal plasma levels. Although several reported case series found no evidence of adverse effects in infants exposed to metronidazole in breast milk, some clinicians advise deferring breastfeeding for 12–24 hours following maternal treatment with a single 2-g dose of metronidazole. Maternal treatment with metronidazole (400 mg three times daily for 7 days) produced a lower concentration in breast milk and was considered compatible with breastfeeding over longer periods of time.

GONORRHEA AND CHLAMYDIAL INFECTION

Chlamydia and gonorrhea can both cause vaginal discharge in pregnancy and a major cause of morbidity among women in developing countries. Both infections have been associated with adverse pregnancy outcomes. *Chlamydia* is characteristically asymptomatic. About one-third of patients may have symptoms including mucopurulent vaginal discharge. Most women with gonorrhea are asymptomatic. When symptoms occur, they are localized to the lower genitourinary tract and include vaginal discharge, urinary frequency or dysuria, and rectal discomfort.

Diagnosis (Chlamydia)

The NAAT is the preferred test for chlamydia because of its high sensitivity and specificity and its use on specimens obtained noninvasively. It can be performed using cervical or urine specimens. Nonamplified nonculture tests, such as the DNA probe test, remain an option when the NAAT is not available or is too expensive. Repeat testing three weeks after completion of therapy is recommended for pregnant women.

Diagnosis (Gonorrhea)

Screening can be performed with a culture on Thayer–Martin media, which is recommended in a population with a low prevalence of infection. Nucleic acid hybridization tests of cervical specimens and NAATs of cervical specimens or urine are also used, with NAATs being the most sensitive and specific. Culture is the most widely available test and has the advantage of providing antimicrobial susceptibility. A repeat test is recommended in the third trimester for those at continued risk.

Treatment

Azithromycin has been shown to be safe in pregnant women and is recommended as the treatment of choice for chlamydia during pregnancy.

A Cochrane review of treatment for gonorrhea in pregnancy concluded that ceftriaxone 125 mg intramuscularly and spectinomycin 2 g intramuscularly have similar cure rates to oral amoxicillin plus probenecid. One randomized trial found cefixime 400 mg orally to be as effective as ceftriaxone 125 mg intramuscularly for the treatment of gonorrhea in pregnancy. The CDC (Centers for Disease Control and Prevention) recommends either of these as the treatment of choice for gonorrhea.

■ SUGGESTED READING

1. Baron EJ, Cassell GH, Duffy LB, Eschenbach JR, Greenwood SM, Harvey NE, et al. Laboratory diagnosis of female genital tract infections. In: Baron EJ (Ed). Cumulative Techniques and Procedures in Clinical Microbiology (Cumitech) 17A. Washington, DC: ASM Press; 1993. pp. 1-28.
2. Brocklehurst P, Gordon A, Heatley E, Milan SJ. Antibiotics for treating bacterial vaginosis in pregnancy. Cochrane Database Syst Rev. 2013;(1):CD000262.
3. Brocklehurst P. Antibiotics for gonorrhoea in pregnancy. Cochrane Database Syst Rev. 2002;(2):CD000098.
4. Burtin P, Taddio A, Ariburnu O, Koren G. Safety of metronidazole in pregnancy: a meta-analysis. Am J Obstet Gynecol. 1995;172(2 Pt 1):525-9.
5. Carey JC, Klebanoff MA, Hauth JC, Hillier SL, Thom EA, Ernest JM, et al. Metronidazole to prevent preterm delivery in pregnant women with asymptomatic bacterial vaginosis. National Institute of Child Health and Human Development Network of Maternal-Fetal Medicine Units. N Engl J Med. 2000;342:534-40.
6. Cook RL, Hutchison SL, Ostergaard L, Braithwaite RS, Ness RB. Systematic review: noninvasive testing for *Chlamydia trachomatis* and *Neisseria gonorrhea*. Ann Intern Med. 2005;142:914-25.
7. Cotch MF, Pastorek JG 2nd, Nugent RP, Hillier SL, Gibbs RS, Martin DH, et al. *Trichomonas vaginalis* associated with low birth weight and preterm delivery. Sex Transm Dis. 1997;24:353-60.
8. Czeizel AE, Rockenbauer M. Population-based case-control study of teratogenic potential of corticosteroids. Teratology. 1997;56(5):335-40.
9. Doering PL, Santiago TM. Drugs for treatment of vulvovaginal candidiasis: comparative efficacy of agents and regimens. DICP. 1990;24(11):1078-83.
10. Golightly P, Kearney L. Metronidazole—is it safe to use with breastfeeding? United Kingdom National Health Service, UKMI; 2012.
11. Gumbo FZ, Duri K, Kandawasvika GQ, Kurewa NE, Mapingure MP, Munjoma MW, et al. Risk factors of HIV vertical transmission in a cohort of women under a PMTCT program at three peri-urban clinics in a resource-poor setting. J Perinatol. 2010;30:717-23.
12. Kigozi GG, Brahmbhatt H, Wabwire-Mangen F, Wawer MJ, Serwadda D, Sewankambo N, et al. Treatment of *Trichomonas* in pregnancy and adverse outcomes

of pregnancy: a subanalysis of a randomized trial in Rakai, Uganda. Am J Obstet Gynecol. 2003;189:1398-400.

13. King CT, Rogers PD, Cleary JD, Chapman SW. Antifungal therapy during pregnancy. Clin Infect Dis. 1998;27(5):1151-60.

14. Kingston MA, Bansal D, Carlin EM. 'Shelf life' of *Trichomonas vaginalis*. Int J STD AIDS. 2003;14:28-9.

15. Lamont RF, Nhan-Chang CL, Sobel JD, Workowski K, Conde-Agudelo A, Romero R. Treatment of abnormal vaginal flora in early pregnancy with clindamycin for the prevention of spontaneous preterm birth: a systematic review and metaanalysis. Am J Obstet Gynecol. 2011;205:177-90.

16. Lawing LF, Hedges SR, Schwebke JR. Detection of trichomonosis in vaginal and urine specimens from women by culture and PCR. J Clin Microbiol. 2000;38:3585-8.

17. Lee BE, Feinberg M, Abraham JJ, Murthy AR. Congenital malformations in an infant born to a woman treated with fluconazole. Pediatr Infect Dis J. 1992;11(12):1062-4.

18. McDonald HM, O'Loughlin JA, Vigneswaran R, Jolley PT, Harvey JA, Bof A, et al. Impact of metronidazole therapy on preterm birth in women with bacterial vaginosis flora (*Gardnerella vaginalis*): a randomised, placebo controlled trial. Br J Obstet Gynaecol. 1997;104:1391-7.

19. Mohamed OA, Cohen CR, Kungu D, Kuyoh M, Onyango J, Bwayo J, et al. Urine proves a poor specimen for culture of *Trichomonas vaginalis* in women. Sex Transm Infect. 2001;77:78-9.

20. Monif GR, Baker DA. *Candida albicans*. In: Monif GR, Baker DA (Eds). Infectious Diseases in Obstetrics and Gynecology, 5th edition. New York, NY: Parthenon Press; 2003. pp. 405-21.

21. Nørgaard M, Pedersen L, Gislum M, Erichsen R, Søgaard KK, Schonheyder HC, et al. Maternal use of fluconazole and risk of congenital malformations: a Danish population-based cohort study. J Antimicrob Chemother. 2008;62(1):172-6.

22. Obiero J, Mwethera PG, Wiysonge CS. Topical microbicides for prevention of sexually transmitted infections. Cochrane Database Syst Rev. 2012;(6):CD007961.

23. Odendaal HJ, Popov I, Schoeman J, Smith M, Grové D. Preterm labour—is bacterial vaginosis involved? S Afr Med J. 2002;92(3):231-4.

24. Olshen E, Shrier LA. Diagnostic tests for chlamydial and gonorrheal infections. Semin Pediatr Infect Dis. 2005;16:192-8.

25. Oren D, Nulman I, Makhija M, Ito S, Koren G. Using corticosteroids during pregnancy. Are topical, inhaled, or systemic agents associated with risk? Can Fam Physician. 2004;50:1083-5.

26. Passmore CM, McElnay JC, Rainey EA, D'Arcy PF. Metronidazole excretion in human milk and its effect on the suckling neonate. Br J Clin Pharmacol. 1988;26:45-51.

27. Piper JM, Mitchel EF, Ray WA. Prenatal use of metronidazole and birth defects—no association. Obstet Gynecol. 1993;82:348-52.

28. Pursley TJ, Blomquist IK, Abraham J, Andersen HF, Bartley JA. Fluconazole-induced congenital anomalies in three infants. Clin Infect Dis. 1996;22(2):336-40.

29. Ramus RM, Sheffield JS, Mayfield JA, Wendel GD Jr. A randomized trial that compared oral cefixime and intramuscular ceftriaxone for the treatment of gonorrhea in pregnancy. Am J Obstet Gynecol. 2001;185:629-32.

30. Stoner KA, Rabe LK, Meyn LA, Hillier SL. Survival of *Trichomonas vaginalis* in wet preparation and on wet mount. Sex Transm Infect. 2013;89:485-8.

31. Ugwumadu A, Manyonda I, Reid F, Hay P. Effect of early oral clindamycin on late miscarriage and preterm delivery in asymptomatic women with abnormal vaginal flora and bacterial vaginosis: a randomised controlled trial. Lancet. 2003;361: 983-8.

32. Ugwumadu A, Reid F, Hay P, Manyonda I. Natural history of bacterial vaginosis and intermediate flora in pregnancy and effect of oral clindamycin. Obstet Gynecol. 2004;104:114-9.

33. Vermeulen GM, Bruinse HW. Prophylactic administration of clindamycin 2% vaginal cream to reduce the incidence of spontaneous preterm birth in women with an increased recurrence risk: a randomised placebo-controlled double-blind trial. Br J Obstet Gynaecol. 1999;106:652-7.

34. Workowski KA, Berman SM; Centers for Disease Control and Prevention. Sexually transmitted diseases treatment guidelines, 2006 [Published correction appears in MMWR Recomm Rep 2006;55:997]. MMWR Recomm Rep. 2006;55(RR-11):1-94. [online] Available from: http://www.cdc.gov/mmwr/PDF/rr/rr5511.pdf. [Last accessed July, 2020].

35. Young GL, Jewell D. Topical treatment for vaginal candidiasis (thrush) in pregnancy. Cochrane Database Syst Rev. 2001;4:CD000225.

36. Yudin MH, Landers DV, Meyn L, Hillier SL. Clinical and cervical cytokine response to treatment with oral or vaginal metronidazole for bacterial vaginosis during pregnancy: a randomized trial. Obstet Gynecol. 2003;102(3):527-34.

Pain in Early Pregnancy

Fessy Louis T, Parvathy T

INTRODUCTION

Complications arise more frequently during the first trimester than at any other stage of pregnancy. These are mostly present with bleeding, pain, or both. These cause considerable anxiety for the woman and her partner. In the vast majority of cases, no intervention alters the outcome. The main aim of clinical management is a prompt and accurate diagnosis **(Box 1)**. If the pregnancy is appropriately developed and viable, reassurance can be given, if not, appropriate intervention may be done.

RATIONAL APPROACH TO "ABDOMINAL PAIN" IN PREGNANCY

Abdominal pain or discomfort is a common symptom during significant intra-abdominal pathology. Anatomical changes during pregnancy such as rapid expansion and enlargement of the pregnant uterus and the consequent stretching of supporting ligaments and muscles as well as the pressure exerted by the gravid uterus on other intra-abdominal structures and the layers of the anterior abdominal wall may result in such "physiological" pain or discomfort. However, it is essential to differentiate such a "physiological"

BOX 1: Differential diagnosis of first trimester pain.

Pregnancy related:
- Miscarriage (threatened, inevitable, incomplete, complete, missed, or septic)
- Ectopic pregnancy
- Hydatidiform mole
- Cervical pregnancy

Coincidental to the pregnancy—gynecologic:
- Ruptured corpus luteum of pregnancy
- Ovarian cyst accident
- Torsion or degeneration of pedunculated fibroid
- Bleeding from cervical malignancy

Coincidental to the pregnancy:
- Appendicitis
- Renal colic
- Cholecystitis
- Pelvic inflammatory disease
- Endometriosis

pain or discomfort from a "pathological" pain that results from inflammatory, neoplastic, or traumatic causes. It is essential to "look beyond" the uterus and the genital tract while analyzing the cause of abdominal pain. Failure to do so may increase maternal and fetal morbidity and mortality as may such pathological causes may be potentially life threatening. Requirement of stronger analgesics to control pain and/or worsening pain or clinical condition should alert the clinician to explore rare causes and to seek multidisciplinary input early.

EFFECT OF PREGNANCY ON THE DIAGNOSIS OF UNDERLYING PATHOLOGY

Pregnancy is associated with anatomical, physiological, and biochemical changes that may alter classical symptoms and signs that would be normally associated with various clinical conditions. However, it is not always possible to elicit all the signs during pregnancy as the expansion of gravid uterus may displace intra-abdominal organs from their normal anatomical site and also may displace the bowel and omentum cranially. This may lead to the loss of protective effect by the "abdominal policeman" (omentum) to localize and limit the infection. A classic example of such "masking" of infection is acute appendicitis during pregnancy. As the pregnancy advances, uterus may displace the appendix cranially, which is usually wedged within the right hypochondrium (under the liver). As a consequence, the classical tenderness around the "McBurney's point" may be absent in late pregnancy and a woman with acute appendicitis may present with pain in the upper abdomen. Moreover, usual signs of peritonitis (tenderness, guarding, rigidity, and rebound tenderness) may not be elicited, as the large gravid uterus lies underneath the parietal peritoneum of the anterior abdominal wall. This may prevent the parietal peritoneum to be "irritated" by the inflamed intra-abdominal organ. As mentioned earlier, the gravid uterus can also obstruct and inhibit the movement of the omentum to an area of inflammation, thereby preventing this "policeman" of the abdomen from localizing the infection. This may not only distort the "expected" clinical signs, but also facilitate spread of infection into "general" peritoneal cavity, leading to a generalized peritonitis and rapid deterioration of the patient's condition. Increased plasma volume observed during pregnancy coupled with changes in the plasma proteins, increased renal clearance, and altered hepatic metabolism may pose difficulties with interpretation of biochemical markers of pathological conditions. Physiological leukocytosis and raised alkaline phosphatase that are associated with normal pregnancy may also contribute to diagnostic difficulty.

Lastly, the presence of a fetus may modify or delay investigations and treatment that would be normally instituted in a nonpregnant state. Clinicians may delay imaging techniques such as abdominal X-ray, magnetic resonance imaging (MRI), or computerized tomography (CT scan) to avoid exposing the fetus to irradiation or due to technical difficulties. Although there is a fear of teratogenesis in the first trimester and a possible link to childhood cancers, with late fetal exposure to ionizing radiation, exposures of less than 0.05 Gy have not been associated with pregnancy loss or fetal malformations.

PAIN ABDOMEN IN EARLY PREGNANCY

The gravid uterus becomes an abdominal organ by approximately 12 weeks. The most common causes of pain include threatened or incomplete miscarriage, round ligament strain, rupture of corpus luteum cyst, ectopic pregnancy, septic miscarriage with peritonitis, and acute urinary retention due to retroverted gravid uterus or an impacted ovarian cyst in the pelvis.

Miscarriage

Threatened, incomplete, inevitable, and septic miscarriages can present with abdominal pain. Contraction of the myometrium producing transient ischemia is the most likely cause of pain in threatened abortion. The fetal membrane separation produced by the blood may release local prostaglandins and inflammatory mediators, which may aggravate pain. Patients having threatened abortion will be presenting with abdominal pain and bleeding per vaginam. On clinical examination, the cervical os will be closed and minimal bleeding through os which may be blood stained or brownish discharge. Examination reveals the uterine size corresponding to period of amenorrhea. Ultrasound examination will show an intrauterine pregnancy corresponding to period of amenorrhea and it helps in confirming the viability. Counseling, reassurance, and support are the cornerstone of management. Mild analgesics like paracetamol can be prescribed, if abdominal pain is persisting.

In incomplete and inevitable miscarriage, dilatation of the cervical canal by the products of conception may cause acute abdominopelvic discomfort and pain often compounded by the contractions of the gravid uterus, as it tries to expel its content from a failed pregnancy. On examination, the internal os is dilated and the products of conception may be felt through the os. Removal of these with a sponge forceps may relieve acute colicky pain. In case of incomplete abortion, ultrasound examination shows retained products of conception in uterus. The management options include expectant, medical and surgical mode, and depend on the clinical presentation, size of the retained products, presence of bleeding and compliance for follow-up.

Septic miscarriages are common in those countries where termination of pregnancy is illegal; criminal abortion contributes a lot to maternal morbidity and mortality. While in developed countries, infection of retained products of conception following an incomplete miscarriage or failed evacuation of retained products is the common cause of sepsis. The infection can spread through the fallopian tube into peritoneal cavity and can cause peritonitis, first pelvic and then can even become general resulting in acute abdomen. The infection can spread rarely to myometrial vessels resulting in septicemia and rapid deterioration of clinical condition. General examination may reveal pallor, pyrexia, and a rapid thready pulse, suggestive of shock. On abdominal examination, tenderness, guarding, rigidity, and rebound tenderness may be elicited. Blood investigations may reveal leukocytosis and neutrophilia. Blood cultures and ultrasound examination may help in diagnosis. Treatment involves a multidisciplinary approach with broad-spectrum antibiotics and maintenance of intravascular volume, renal, and cardiac functions.

Ectopic Pregnancy

Ectopic pregnancy and corpus luteal cyst rupture can present with pain abdomen and usually as acute abdomen due to irritation of the parietal peritoneum by hemoperitoneum. History of acute abdominal pain, fainting attacks, bleeding per vaginam after a period of amenorrhea with past history of pelvic inflammatory disease or ectopic pregnancy should arouse a suspicion of ectopic pregnancy. On clinical examination, they may have unilateral iliac fossa tenderness, presence of free fluid, cervical excitation test positive, and adnexal tenderness. Transvaginal ultrasound scan and serum beta-hCG measurement may help in diagnosis. On ultrasound (USG), there might be an empty uterine cavity despite a serum beta-hCG of more than 1,500 IU/L or more than 6,000 IU/L with transvaginal sonography (TVS) and transabdominal sonography (TAS) respectively. USG might also demonstrate presence of adnexal mass, free fluid in pelvis with absent doubling of serum beta-hCG in 48 hours may point toward the diagnosis of ectopic pregnancy. Based on the clinical condition, presenting symptoms, serum beta-hCG level, and TVS finding, we can decide on the management. The management options include expectant, medical, and surgical management. Presence of abdominal pain or other symptoms will preclude expectant management or medical treatment with methotrexate. In such a case, laparoscopic treatment is the requisite and can go for salpingectomy, salpingostomy, or milking depending on the clinical condition. If the patient is hemodynamically unstable with significant amount of hemoperitoneum, an exploratory laparotomy is warranted.

Rupture of Corpus Luteal Cyst

The presentation of corpus luteal cyst almost mimics an ectopic pregnancy acute presentation, when an intrauterine pregnancy cannot be demonstrated. The presence of hemoperitoneum often necessitates the need for a laparoscopy especially to rule out an ectopic pregnancy. In most cases, conservative treatment is all that required. Sometimes, diathermic cauterization to the bleeding area of the corpus luteum may be required to arrest bleeding. If this is associated with ongoing pregnancy, progesterone support is essential in the postoperative period.

Heterotopic Pregnancy

Occasionally, a patient can present with an acute abdomen with hemoperitoneum with documented intrauterine pregnancy on transvaginal scan. The differential diagnosis in such a case includes ruptured corpus luteal cyst or ovarian cyst or a heterotopic pregnancy. The term heterotopic pregnancy refers to the coexisting intra- and extrauterine pregnancies. The incidence of heterotopic pregnancy is rare in general population accounting for about 1 in 22,000 pregnancies. But, its incidence is higher in women undergoing assisted reproduction about 1 in 100. Often a diagnostic laparoscopy is warranted in such a case. Sometimes, women may rarely present with ectopic pregnancy in a uterine scar.

Other Causes

Abdominal pain due to acute urinary retention can occur as a sequela to retroverted gravid uterus or an impacted pelvic mass such as an ovarian cyst or fibroid. The diagnosis in such a case can be made from the history and confirmed by ultrasound scan. The treatment includes indwelling catheter for continuous bladder drainage, which may relieve abdominal pain. The retroverted gravid uterus correction can usually occur after 12 weeks of gestation, when it becomes an abdominal organ.

An impacted ovarian cyst or fibroid also can present with pain abdomen due to urinary retention due to compression of urethra and the bladder neck thereby causing mechanical obstruction. If suspicion of malignancy on USG including bilateral cysts, capsular involvement, presence of thick septa (>3 mm), solid areas and papillary projections, and increased Doppler blood flow, then MRI or even laparotomy may be required. The benign urinary cysts large enough to cause urinary obstruction may be removed during second trimester. The posterior wall fibroid may compress the bladder neck leading to urinary retention. The condition usually resolves after 12 weeks when the uterus becomes an abdominal organ.

SUGGESTED READING

1. American College of Obstetricians and Gynecologists. Guidelines for Diagnostic Imaging During Pregnancy. ACOG Committee Opinion 158. Washington, DC: ACOG; 1995.
2. Chandraharan E, Arulkumaran S. Painful uterine contractions. In: Arulkumaran S (Ed). Emergencies in Obstetrics & Gynaecology. Oxford: Oxford University Press; 2006.
3. Confidential Enquiries into Maternal and Child Health (CEMACH). (2007). Saving Mothers' Lives (2003–2005). [online] Available from: https://www.publichealth. hscni.net/sites/default/files/Saving%20Mothers%27%20Lives%202003-05%20.pdf. [Last accessed June, 2020].
4. Dellinger RP, Carlet JM, Masur H, Gerlach H, Calandra T, Cohen J, et al. Surviving Sepsis Campaign guidelines for management of severe sepsis and septic shock. Crit Care Med. 2004;32(3):858-73.
5. Pedrosa I, Levine D, Eyvazzadeh AD, Siewert B, Ngo L, Rofsky NM. MR imaging evaluation of acute appendicitis in pregnancy. Radiology. 2006;238(3):891-9.
6. Royal College of Obstetricians and Gynecologists (RCOG). (2006). Management of Early pregnancy Loss. Green Top Guideline No.25. [online] Available from: https://www.rcog.org.uk/en/guidelines-research-services/guidelines/gtg25/. [Last accessed June, 2020].

Fever in Pregnancy

Alpesh Gandhi, Janki Munjal Pandya

INTRODUCTION

Pregnancy is a physiological state, wherein the immunity of mother gets lowered and increases vulnerability towards pathogens. Fever, as it is known, is a sign of tipping off of balance in homeostasis of body. Fever in pregnancy can bring in a lot of medical problems for mother as well as for fetus. An elevated temperature, which may be associated with other symptoms, can be due to various infectious or noninfectious reasons. Infections can be subdivided into viral, bacterial, parasitic and fungal, which can be transmitted vertically to fetus in utero/intrapartum/postpartum.

ETIOLOGY

Various reasons can reset thermoregulatory center to a higher temperature by pyrogenic polypeptides, which include interleukin-1-alpha and beta, tumor necrosis factor alpha, and beta and interferon alpha.

Pyrexia can be due to pathogens or can be due to noninfectious reasons.

Infectious diseases causing pyrexia in pregnancy:

- *Urinary tract infections (UTI)*: Pregnancy causes a lot of changes in renal system, including decreased bladder and ureteral tone, vesicoureteral reflux, and decreased local immunity against pathogens. These factors collectively contribute toward increased propensity toward developing UTI.
- *Respiratory tract infections*: Majorly, upper respiratory tract infections in form of common cold/flu are encountered, lower respiratory ones being rare in absence of risk factors. Tuberculosis, being rampant in developing countries, can be hazardous in already immunocompromised pregnant state.
- *Vector-borne diseases*: Malaria and dengue.
- *Gastrointestinal disease*: Appendicitis, typhoid fever, hepatitis, parasitic intestinal infestations, and cholecystitis.
- *Blood-borne and sexually transmitted diseases (STDs)*: Bacterial vaginosis, gonorrhea, trichomoniasis, candidiasis, HIV, hepatitis, syphilis, abscesses, and septicemia.

Various pathogens responsible for pyrexia are *Mycobacterium tuberculosis, Salmonella typhi, Staphylococcus, Neisseria gonorrhoeae,*

Plasmodia, Chlamydia, hepatitis viruses, HIV, influenza, herpes, varicella, dengue, rubella, and *Cytomegalovirus (CMV)*. Socioeconomic status, poor hygiene, high-risk behavior, and epidemic/endemic disease in premises are additional factors increasing pregnant woman's vulnerability toward getting infections. Center for Disease Control has recommended screening for STDs in first trimester, as well as in third trimester in case of high-risk pregnant woman.

Noninfectious reasons:
- Autoimmune diseases
- Connective tissue diseases
- Neoplasm.

CLINICAL PRESENTATION

Pregnant patient is labeled with having fever when body temperature rise above 99°F. Accompanying symptoms may help in establishing diagnosis, and proper management, curtailing further maternal and fetal damage. Various conditions are enlisted below, which can be associated with characteristic presentation:
- *Fever with abdominal pain*: Viral diarrhea and typhoid fever
- *Fever with rigors*: Malaria and urinary tract infections
- *Fever with rash*: Chikungunya, dengue, typhoid, and measles
- *Fever with altered neurological symptoms*: Cerebral malaria and meningitis
- *Persistent fever*: Typhoid, malaria, tuberculosis, and HIV.

CLINICAL IMPLICATIONS

Pyrexia affects mother as well as fetus according to the duration of fever and stage of fetal growth. Raised maternal body temperature interferes within fetal protein metabolism. Heat shock proteins are expressed increasingly leading to raised cellular resistance to thermal impact. This, in turn, inhibits cellular proliferation, causing impairment if fetal development. When maternal body temperature rises significantly during embryonic stage, chances of miscarriage are increased. Animal studies have found fever to be teratogenic, and in humans, fever during embryonic stage may lead to congenital anomalies.[1] Three times increase in neural tube defects, congenital cardiac anomalies, and facial defects has been noted in pregnancies having pyrexia during first trimester.[2,3]

Fever during mid and last trimester may lead to premature labor, intrauterine growth restriction (IUGR), intrauterine fetal death (IUFD), and stillbirth. Chronic vulvovaginitis causes micropores in amniotic membranes and ruptures them in long run. Infections such as malaria cause micro-obstructions/clogging by parasites and may lead to IUGR/IUFD/SB. Out of all preterm deliveries, almost one quarter is due to infection or inflammation during pregnancy, causing pyrexia. A study linked fever during pregnancy with twofold increase in chances of child having autism and developmental delays.[4]

Timely administration of antipyretic medications has been found to be effective against such catastrophes.[5,6]

Usage of acetaminophen during pregnancy has been linked to increased chances of ADHD-like behaviors in children.[7]

CLINICAL EVALUATION

A proper history taking in form of origin, duration, and progress of fever and associated symptoms, along with specific history of travelling, needs to be done. General examination in form of vitals, signs of pallor, rash, icterus, edema, lymphadenopathy, and built and nourishment is mandatory. Systemic examination according to system involved, followed by obstetric examination for proper progress of pregnancy and fetal status, is to be done. These steps of systemic evaluation will guide the clinician toward a set of diagnosis, which can be pinpointed to one in particular with the help of investigations, in form of specific ones for specific diseases and ultrasonography for fetal condition.

Characteristic skin rash may indicate various diagnoses. Chickenpox manifests as centrifugal rash, starting from trunk, in form of macules, papules, vesicles, pustules, and scabs. Measles manifests as centripetal rash, starting from face, in form of maculopapular, along with Koplik spots on buccal mucosa and conjunctivitis. Painful vesicular eruptions are seen in herpes simplex, orofacial in HSV-1 and genital in HSV-2 type. Secondary syphilis may present with roseolar rash, with mucus patches in pharynx. Widespread transient maculopapular rash may be seen with viral fever.

Systemic evaluation for neurological symptoms such as headache, altered behavior, and convulsions may reveal signs of raised intracranial pressure and signs of meningitis. Abdominal examination will help in diagnosing enlarged liver and spleen, though the locations may vary due to enlarged uterus.

Investigations in form of common blood investigations such as complete blood count, urine routine micro, renal and liver function tests, blood sugar, and ultrasonography of abdomen and fetus are to be carried out. Specific investigations according to probable diagnosis would give confirmation, helping further management.

Fetal ultrasonography for condition of fetus, amount of amniotic fluid, and placental grading is done. Middle cerebral artery peak systolic velocity is a useful tool for diagnosing fetal anemia. Congenital anomalies need to be ruled out in cases of early pregnancy infections.

PREVENTIVE MEASURES

Screening for some of the infectious diseases such as HIV, hepatitis B, and syphilis can be done prior to planning for pregnancy. During antenatal visit, screening for HIV, hepatitis B, syphilis, and in at risk pregnancies, screening for gonorrhea and hepatitis C is recommended. The preventive steps in form of avoiding high-risk behavior, proper dietary advices, adequate rest and exercise, and avoiding alcohol and drugs are important for better pregnancy outcome. Awareness for symptoms such as burning micturition, common cold-cough, discharge per vaginam, and abdominal pain is important so as to treat the conditions at an earlier step.

URINARY TRACT INFECTION

Asymptomatic bacteriuria is common during pregnancy due to urinary stasis and reduced bladder and ureteric tones.[8] Symptomatic urinary tract infections can lead to pyelonephritis, anemia, sepsis, renal failure, hypertension in mother and prematurity, IUGR, and perinatal deaths in fetus. Various organisms such as *Escherichia coli* (80–90%), *Proteus*, and *Klebsiella* are commonly implicated. Other pathogens involved are *Staphylococcus*, Group B streptococcus (GBS), and *Enterobacter* species. Atypical pathogen such as chlamydia may cause sterile pyuria. GBS bacteriuria may lead to PPROM and preterm labor. Intrapartum infection of GBS may lead to neonatal pneumonia, meningitis, sepsis, and even death.

Asymptomatic bacteriuria, if left untreated, can lead to cystitis and pyelonephritis in mother and prematurity and LBW in neonate. Acute pyelonephritis presents with fever, flank pain, nausea, vomiting, frequency, urgency, and dysuria.

Urine routine micro and culture are preferred during first antenatal visit.[9] In suspected cases of UTI, urine studies in from of culture and routine micro are to be done, along with CBC, renal function tests, and ultrasonography of abdomen—pelvis and fetus. Nitrofurantoin is the drug of choice, as it is safe during pregnancy and highly effective. Culture can be repeated after 1–2 weeks to conclude completion of therapy. Fosfomycin single dose has been found to be effective and safe for treatment in pregnant women. In case of acute pyelonephritis, hydration and intravenous antibiotics (beta lactams) are preferred. Ceftriaxone 1–2 g every 24 hours for 10 days or antibiotics can be chosen on basis of culture report. Recurrent UTI should be properly evaluated for finding its cause, and can be treated with nitrofurantoin effectively in absence of surgical cause.

Surgical causes such as bladder stones, diverticula, and trauma can be treated surgically, but surgery should be preferred during 2nd trimester, because of increased risk of miscarriage during 1st trimester and increased risk of preterm labor during 3rd trimester.

RESPIRATORY INFECTIONS

- *Upper respiratory tract infections*: It may present with rhinitis, sinusitis, pharyngitis, and laryngitis. The causative organisms can be bacterial such as Group A and C *Streptococci, N. gonorrhoeae,* and atypical bacteremia; or it can be of viral origin such as rhinovirus, Adenovirus, *Coxsackievirus,* and influenza virus. Culture helps in diagnosing pathogen. Influenza is a self-limiting condition in nonpregnant state; but in pregnancy, it may complicate to the level of pneumonia if not properly dealt with. Pregnancy increases propensity of developing severe disease by fourfold to fivefold, risk being highest in third trimester.

Influenza may lead to higher chances of adverse outcomes in form of miscarriage, preterm birth, or nonreassuring fetal heart patterns. It may have teratogenic effect when occurs during first trimester, but larger trials are required to conclude.

Vaccine against influenza has been recommended during 2nd and 3rd trimesters in all women by WHO. The antibodies developed will be transmitted to fetus, protecting him/her.

In mild infections, symptomatic treatment in form of decongestants, antipyretics, and anti-inflammatory medicines is done. In case of severe infection, penicillin group of drugs are preferred.

- Lower respiratory tract infections.
- *Swine flu:* It is caused by H1N1 strain of influenza virus, RNA virus of orthomyxoviridae family. Officially declared as pandemic by WHO, this disease presents with fever, cough, sore throat, headache, malaise, diarrhea, and vomiting. Pregnant women typically present with breathlessness along with constitutional symptoms, and may lead to acute respiratory distress syndrome rapidly, leading to increased chances of maternal mortality. Culture from throat swabs of throat secretions for virus detection, rapid diagnostic tests, direct immunofluorescence assay, and detection of virus-specific antibodies are modalities. CDC has recommended reverse transcriptase polymerase chain reaction (PCR) to be the method of choice, which is known to yield the results within 4 hours. Oseltamivir 75 mg BD for 5 days is recommended. Prophylactic dose is 75 mg OD for 10 days. Dose and duration can be increased in advanced stage of disease.
- *Pneumonia:* Depending upon the origin, maternal and fetal morbidity and mortality vary. Earlier the gestational age at the time of disease, milder are the symptoms. Bacterial pneumonia would present as fever, cough, dyspnea, and chills. In addition to pregnancy, as a risk factor, anemia, smoking, and use of steroids and tocolytic agents increase vulnerability toward contracting pneumonia. Pathogens involved are *Streptococcus pneumoniae, Haemophilus influenzae, Mycoplasma pneumoniae,* and *Staphylococcus aureus.* Fungal pneumonia is rare during pregnancy, which is self-limited and mild. Viral and fungal pneumonia are rare. Aspiration pneumonitis may occur due to elevated diaphragm and reduced gastric motility. Maternal complications in form of bacteremia, empyema, anemia, and even death can occur. Pneumonia in HIV is

seen in majority of patients due to opportunistic infections. A thorough investigation in from of CBC, blood culture, sputum examination for gram, AFB stain and culture, and chest X-ray will help in arriving on diagnosis. Supportive therapy in form of IV fluids, nasal oxygen, nebulization, ionotropic support, and in hypoxic patients, ventilator support is done. Beta-lactams and macrolides (ceftriaxone/penicillin/coamoxiclav/azithromycine/clindamycin/clarithromycin) for bacterial, acyclovir (800 mg 5 times a day) for viral, and cotrimoxazole for fungal pneumonia are drugs of choice.

- *Tuberculosis*: Evening rise of temperature is noticed in case of tuberculosis. Low-grade fever of 100°F is noted in evening.

  Fetus can get affected in utero, leading to miscarriage, severe IUGR, premature delivery, and stillbirth.

  Sputum culture for AFB and chest X-ray are modalities to confirm the diagnosis. Drugs of choice are rifampicin, isoniazid, pyrazinamide, and ethambutol. Streptomycin can cause damage to 8th cranial nerve, thus its use has to be calculated with risk–benefit keeping in mind. The pregnant woman needs to be treated according to the category she falls in. Categories for management of tuberculosis in India are revised. Category 1 is new patients, which include new sputum smear positive, new sputum smear negative, new extrapulmonary, and new others. They are treated with 2 months of intensive phase in form of H3R3Z3E3, followed by 4 months of continuation phase in from of H3R3. Category 2 includes smear-positive relapse, smear-positive failure, smear-positive treatment after default, and others. They are treated with 2 months of intensive phase H3R3Z3E3 or 1 month of intensive phase H3R3Z3E3, followed by 5 months of H3R3E3.

- *Chickenpox*: Characteristic skin rashes start from trunk and spread centrifugally, usually 1–2 days after the onset of fever. Chickenpox during pregnancy increases chances of pneumonia and maternal mortality. Primary varicella infection during pregnancy is a medical emergency, increasing maternal as well fetal compromise, pneumonia and congestive cardiac failure being major causes of maternal morbidity and mortality. Spontaneous miscarriage is reported in around 5% of cases when varicella zoster infection is acquired during first trimester. It leads to congenital varicella syndrome in fetus, characterized by chorioretinitis, microphthalmia, cataract, microcephaly, mental retardation, limb hypoplasia, cutaneous scars, and low birth weight (LBW) babies. Varicella infection in the window of 5 days before and 2 days after delivery will lead to neonatal varicella infection, manifesting as pneumonia and cutaneous lesions. It has mortality rate of almost 30%.

  Acute response in form of IgM can be seen from around 3–10 days, and IgM stays till 6 months after the exposure. IgG antibodies appear after 3 weeks and may persist for years. Culture and PCR from lesions can be confirmative.

Acyclovir 800 mg 5 times a day for 7 days is an effective and safe therapy during pregnancy. The maximum infectivity is when the skin vesicles start rupturing and the fluid starts oozing out, wherein the affected patient needs isolation. Lesions take 5 days to get crusted from appearance of rash.

If there is maternal infection in last 4 weeks of pregnancy, planned delivery should be deferred at least till 7 days after onset of rash, in absence of maternal and/or fetal compromise. If cesarean section is required for any maternal/fetal indication, epidural/spinal anesthesia should be given by needle traversing through skin part, which is not affected. Breastfeeding is not contraindicated.

Passive immunity in form of Ig and antiviral therapy will prevent serious congenital infection.

- *Parvovirus infection*: *Parvovirus B$_{19}$* (DNA virus) is transmitted through respiratory secretions and hand to mouth. It is also known as fifth disease or erythema infectiosum. Adults infected may not manifest typical cutaneous changes (slapped cheek appearance), but they may develop arthralgia. There is low risk to fetus when pregnant woman contracts the disease. The infection is thought to cause fetal anemia, by destroying precursors of erythroid series. It may manifest as miscarriage, hydrops fetalis, myocarditis, and IUFD. Transplacental transfer may lead to fetal loss in around 10% of the cases when infection occurs before 20 weeks of gestation.

  Parvovirus can be diagnosed with serological testing. Correction of fetal anemia can be attempted by intrauterine transfusion through fetal abdomen or through umbilical vessels, the latter being preferred method, as it leads to better absorption and associated with higher survival rate than the former route.

- *Rubella*: Congenital rubella syndrome (CRS) has become extremely rare for last few decades. Serological testing of pregnant female is advised, and if IgG antibody is found, there are no chances of maternal or fetal morbidity. Pregnancy should be deferred at least till 3 months after vaccination. CRS occurs when pregnant woman acquires infection in first 16 weeks of gestation. Characteristics of CRS are—IUGR, microcephaly, cataract, cardiac defects (patent ductus arteriosus and pulmonary arterial hypoplasia), neurological disease, hepatosplenomegaly, and blueberry muffin appearance (due to extramedullary hematopoiesis).

  Serum IgM peaks around a week after onset and persists till 6 weeks. IgG start appearing 2-3 weeks from the onset of illness.

- *Measles*: It can cause miscarriage, premature labor, and LBW babies.

HEPATITIS

Acute viral hepatitis causes maternal as well as fetal morbidity and mortality depending upon type of virus, load of virus, and stage of gestation. Hepatitis E has been found to be associated with adverse maternal and fetal outcome, with risk amounting to maternal mortality, especially when disease presents during third trimester. Hepatitis A can be transmitted perinatally and very rarely transplacentally. Hepatitis B is transmitted mainly during second stage of labor. Fetus may not suffer from clinical problems, but may stay as a carrier of hepatitis B. Breastfeeding is not contraindicated when mother suffers from hepatitis A, E, and C.

Enzyme-linked immunosorbent assay (ELISA) test can be useful for detection of HBsAg, HBeAg, anti-HBC, anti-HAV, and anti-HEV antibodies. Measuring viral loads for hepatitis B and C is also important.

Hepatitis E has grave maternal as well as fetal outcomes. As pregnancy is considered immunocompromised state, viral load increases rapidly, leading to acute hepatic failure, cerebral complications, and disseminated intravascular coagulation in the last stage.[10] It has manifestations in from of fever, loss of appetite, nausea, vomiting, abdominal pain, and jaundice. Virus-specific antibodies and detection of virus RNA by reverse transcriptase are diagnostic modalities. The disease may complicate pregnancy by causing maternal hypertension, pre-eclampsia, renal complications, premature labor, and hepatic failure leading to encephalopathy. Early detection and symptomatic and supportive treatment in form of treatment of jaundice and fluid management will be the right approach.

Hepatitis B has an incubation period of 45–160 days. Risk of transmission is very low in early pregnancy; it is maximum during intrapartum period. Transmission rate of hepatitis B, in case of cesarean section, has not been significantly low than those who delivered vaginally.[11] Neonates who receive vaccine and immunoglobulin still remain at risk of getting infection depending on maternal viral load.[12] If the fetus has received HpB Ig and HpB vaccine, breastfeeding carries no additional risk even in hepatitis B infection. Treatment is usually supportive, and lamivudine (100 mg/day) may be necessary only when there is acute hepatic failure. If antiviral therapy was started to reduce maternal-child transmission, it can be discontinued after 4–10 weeks of delivery.

Hepatitis A is transmitted via fecal-oral route, and is usually self-limited. Bilirubin and liver enzymes are elevated. It presents with nausea and vomiting and leads to preterm labor. Fetus is rarely affected, except during intrapartum phase. Anti-HAV IgG antibodies get transferred via placenta to fetus giving protection even in neonatal phase. Pregnant woman who may be at risk of HAV infection can be vaccinated with inactivated or recombinant vaccine during pregnancy. Neonate can be administered Ig within 48 hours of birth, if mother gets infected during third trimester.

MALARIA

Characteristic feature is fever of tertian or quotidian pattern. Fever may occur daily or every other day in paroxysm. Cold stage is usually followed by hot stage, lasting for around 6–10 hours.

In low transmission area, the implications are more severe in with regards to maternal and fetal morbidity, increasing chances of fetal mortality as well.

Malaria can complicate pregnancy by causing and/or aggravating associated conditions, which can lead to severe maternal anemia, jaundice, acute respiratory distress syndrome, fluid and electrolyte disturbances, and, in the most dreaded scenario, can cause circulatory collapse. Maternal anemia may predispose to infections alike urinary tract infection and respiratory infections. Pulmonary edema due to fluid overload immediately after delivery is a grave complication.

Peripheral blood smear is the gold standard investigation. Thick smear is used for low-density parasite load, and thin is used for differentiation of plasmodia species. Quantitative buffy coat layer, rapid malaria Ag detection techniques, fluorescent staining, malaria PCR, and stick test are other diagnostic modalities.

Treatment

During first trimester, chloroquine, quinine, and clindamycin are safe. During 2nd and 3rd trimesters, artemisinin therapy is safe. Avoid primaquine in pregnancy.

National vector-borne disease control program recommends quinine 10 mg/kg thrice a day for 7 days for *P. falciparum* malaria, for 1st trimester and artemisinin-based combination therapy (ACT) in 2nd and 3rd trimesters. ACT can be implemented with artemether (80 mg) and lumefantrine (480 mg) BD for 3 days. Severe and complicated malaria needs artesunate 2.4 mg/kg loading dose IV or IM followed by 1.2 mg/kg at 12 and 24 hours, and daily for 7 days.

DENGUE

Classical dengue fever manifests as fever with rigors, headache, retro-orbital pain, and myalgia. It is also known as break bone fever, the temperature may rise up to 105–106°F, associated with thrombocytopenia, leukopenia, and resolves after 5–6 days. Classical fever may complicate pregnancy further by progressing toward dengue shock syndrome and dengue hemorrhagic fever. The former characterized by tachycardia with shallow pulse, hypotension, cold extremities, and the later manifests as acute fever for 2–6 days, hemorrhagic manifestations, thrombocytopenia, pleural effusion, ascites, and hypoalbuminemia.

Dengue increases chances of preterm birth and LBW babies.

Polymerase chain reaction from blood confirms the diagnosis within 1–5 days. Serum NS1 Ag within 2–7 days has high sensitivity and specificity. Cell culture for virus isolation and detection of virus-specific antibodies are other modalities.

Treatment

Early detection and timely management are the keys for reducing maternal and perinatal morbidity and mortality. Symptomatic management and fluid management along with transfusion of blood and blood products accordingly may require.

■ TYPHOID FEVER

Stepladder pattern of fever is unique to enteric fever, which is increasing temperatures, not coming back to baseline. The fever is of high grade, associated with headache, poor appetite, weakness and fatigue, and rose-colored skin rash.

Enteric infection in mother gets transplacentally transmitted leading to miscarriage, IUFD, and neonatal infections.

Antibody detection by serum Widal test and culture from stool, urine, blood, and bone marrow confirm the diagnosis. Ceftriaxone 2–4 g/day for 7 days or azithromycin 500 mg daily for 7 days is the treatment of choice.

■ HERPES

The HSV-1 majorly causes orofacial lesions and HSV-2 causes genital lesions, the latter accounting for 70% of herpes simplex infection cases. Approximately, in 90% cases, neonate gets affected during passage from birth canal. In around 10% cases, congenital infection may occur. Neonate can acquire infection in postpartum phase, from infected puerpera or caregiver. Presence of antibody against any of the types gives protection against the other type as well. Intrauterine infection is associated with IUGR, preterm labor, and miscarriage.

Herpes simplex virus infection can lead to localized orofacial disease, meningitis, or may involve multiple organs in fetus. Type-specific antibodies for HSV-1 and -2 will confirm diagnosis. PCR and culture are the modalities used. In suspected neonatal involvement, HSV PCR can be applied on spinal fluid of neonate. Culture can be taken from lesions from skin, urine, stool, blood, and rectum.

Herpes simplex virus infection can further be subdivided into primary, nonprimary, recurrent, and asymptomatic shedding:

- *Primary infection*: Around 75% of patients remain asymptomatic. Lesions appear around 2–14 days after exposure, and can last up to 20 days. Antibody response starts after 3–4 weeks of exposure, and stays for lifetime, but is not protective against recurrence. Symptoms can be in form of vulval itching, vaginal discharge, dysuria, tender vesicles, and ulcers. Fever, nausea, malaise, and myalgia may occur.
- *Nonprimary*: Heterogeneous antibody is present at the time of exposure and appearance of symptoms. Viral shedding lasts only for 7 days.

- *Recurrent*: Women may be asymptomatic. Localized pain, vulval itching, and vaginal discharge are the symptoms in some of the women encountering recurrence.
- *Asymptomatic viral shedding*: It is episodic, lasting for a day or two.

Cesarean section is the preferred method of delivering baby so as to protect neonate from intrapartum exposure.

Treatment

- Acyclovir 200 mg 5 times a day, for 7 days, and for recurrent infections, 400 mg TDS for 5 days. Acyclovir gets concentrated in amniotic fluid during pregnancy and can also get secreted in breast milk. Acyclovir effectively reduces dysuria, pain, and viral shedding.
- *Valacyclovir*: 1,000 mg BD for 7 days for first episode. 500 mg BD for 3 days for recurrent episode. It has increased bioavailability than acyclovir.
- *Famciclovir*: 250 mg TDS for 7 days. For recurrence, 1,000 mg BD for a day. It has higher intracellular concentration as compared with acyclovir.

When primary herpes in 1st and 2nd trimesters, treatment course, f/b daily suppressive therapy from 36th week till delivery (CS). Primary infection in 3rd trimester requires daily suppressive therapy till delivery (CS). Recurrent infection needs daily suppressive antiviral at or beyond 36 weeks till termination.

Preventive Measures

Avoid tight fitting clothes that might hold in heat and moisture. Use Barrier contraception during intercourse. Usage of warm water only and no soap to clean outside vagina (wipe front to back). Complete treatment of male partner is mandatory.

HUMAN IMMUNODEFICIENCY VIRUS

The HIV is a major threat to mother and fetus, the later getting affected mainly at the time of delivery and breastfeeding. Intrauterine vertical transmission is also a possibility. Infected neonate may suffer from recurrent infections, chronic diarrhea, and failure to thrive.

CYTOMEGALOVIRUS

Cytomegalovirus can be transmitted via body fluids, through sexual contact, or blood transfusion. Fetus can be affected by transplacental transmission, and neonate is at risk of getting infected via breast milk. CMV vertical transmission can occur at any stage during pregnancy, risk being highest during third trimester. Earlier the disease, more severe will be its form. Majority pregnant women affected with CMV are asymptomatic, but vertical transmission can affect fetus leading to congenital CMV infection, manifesting in form of IUGR and congenital defects like microcephaly, hydrocephalus, sensorineural hearing loss, optic atrophy, delayed development.

Cytomegalovirus can be diagnosed by using urine or serum for PCR. Rapid culture from urine is also highly sensitive and specific. Fourfold or more of increase in IgG within 2 weeks suggests recent infection with CMV.

Congenital CMV can be diagnosed by using amniotic fluid for PCR, with highest specificity and sensitivity.

SYPHILIS

Fetus can get affected during primary, secondary, and latent phase of syphilis. Primary syphilis may be asymptomatic, manifesting as chancre, and lymphadenopathy. Secondary stage reveals nonpruritic rash, arthritis, optic neuritis, keratitis, and meningitis. Fetus can get affected in utero leading to miscarriage, stillbirth, and premature birth. The earlier the stage of disease, the higher the risk of morbidity. Untreated primary or secondary syphilis during pregnancy lead to fetal infection rate of almost 100%. It can cause SB, late abortion, neonatal disease, death, or latent infection. Latent phase does not have any symptoms, and is still transmissible to fetus. All pregnant women should be screened for syphilis. Nontreponemal Ab test results (RPR and VDRL) are often false positive in pregnant women, therefore, positive results should be confirmed with specific antitreponemal Ab tests such as micro-hemagglutination assay-T pallidum (MHA TP) and fluorescent treponemal Ab absorption test (FTA-ABS). Antitreponemal Ab test findings are not indicators of current infection, because results may remain positive for life. Once diagnosed, consider other STDs, especially HIV. 1st, 2nd, and early latent syphilis patients are to be treated with 2.4 million units of benzathine penicillin G single dose. Late latent stage of syphilis needs to be treated with three doses of benzathine penicillin at the interval of 1 week. Penicillin being the only drug for syphilis during pregnancy; patients having sensitivity toward it must be desensitized.

VULVOVAGINITIS AND CHORIOAMNIONITIS

Chorioamnionitis may lead to miscarriage, preterm labor, prelabor rupture of membranes (PROM), preterm prelabor rupture of membranes (PPROM) or fetal complications in form of IUGR, cerebral ischemia, neurodevelop-mental delays, cerebral palsy, and chronic pulmonary disease in neonate. In severe form, neonate can develop neonatal sepsis, septic shock, and multiorgan failure.

Evaluation is done by history of extent, nature, location, duration of symptoms, followed by physical examination. Mid-vaginal pH is raised in bacterial vaginosis and trichomoniasis. Whiff test is positive with bacterial vaginosis and trichomoniasis. Saline smear helps in detecting Clue cells indicating bacterial vaginosis, hanging drop for motile trichomonads, and

10% KOH treated smear for hyphae and spores of Candida. Strawberry cervix and vagina are characteristically seen with trichomoniasis:

- *Bacterial vaginosis*: Polymicrobial from abnormal condition of vagina marked by reduced or absent H_2O_2 producing lactobacilli, which encourages overgrowth of facultative aerobes and anaerobes. Organisms identified are *G. vaginalis, M. hominis, M. urealyticum*, bacteroides, and other species. Predisposing factors are level of sexual activity, frequency of intercourse, and attention to personal hygiene (50% are asymptomatic). Cardinal symptom is malodorous discharge during menses or after intercourse when high pH of semen or blood increases volatility of odor producing amines. Vulval itching, strong fishy white/gray unpleasant odor, and dysuria. Preterm labor caused by it is usually unresponsive to tocolytic therapy. Oral and local metronidazole is preferred agent, and clindamycin should be avoided in second half of pregnancy to avoid preterm labor.
- *Vulvovaginal candidiasis*: Colonization by Candida is significantly higher in pregnancy than in nonpregnant state, but these pregnant women were more asymptomatic than nonpregnant ones. External dysuria causing burning at vulval outlet during micturition and dyspareunia occurs. Physical examination reveals labial swelling, erythema, presence of scratch marks. Thick curdy or crusted discharge at introitus, scraping of discharge often reveals ulcers. Culture of vaginal discharge on Sabouraud's or Nickerson's media may be required to establish diagnosis. Counseling, correction of predisposing factors, antifungals (oral and/or topical). Avoid fluconazole during pregnancy.
- *Vaginal trichomoniasis*: Metronidazole/tinidazole/secnidazole can be used, but avoid these drugs during 1st trimester, if benefit does not outweigh the risk.
- *Chlamydia*: Chlamydia is the most common bacterial STD, around 75% of patients being asymptomatic. Chlamydial cervicitis should be considered in presence of yellow or green vaginal discharge, greater than 10 polymorphs per HPF, and bleeding or edema of the cervix. CDC-accepted screening methods are nucleic acid amplification test (NAAT) on urine or endocervical swab. Unamplified nucleic acid hybridization test, an enzyme immunoassay, or direct fluorescent Ab test on endocervical swab are other modalities. Cervical swab is taken for gram stain, culture and serology, and PCR. *Treatment*—azithromycin (first line, 1 g single dose), amoxicillin (alternative, 500 mg TDS for 7 days), erythromycin (2nd line coz of compliance limiting GI adverse effects).
- *Gonorrhea*: This is second only to chlamydia in cases of bacterial STDs. 50% patients are asymptomatic. Pregnancy is a predisposing factor to disseminated gonococcal infection, which classically presents as an arthritis-dermatitis syndrome. Pregnant woman with gonorrhea can transmit infection to her infant at the time of delivery, causing

life-threatening infections. Newborns exposed during vaginal delivery can develop acute conjunctivitis (ophthalmia neonatorum), sepsis, arthritis, and/or meningitis. Recommended screening method is endocervical culture. Alternatives are NAAT and nucleic acid hybridization test. Treatment—single dose IM ceftriaxone (250 mg) and oral azithromycin (1 g).

- *Vulvovaginitis due to Group B Streptococcus*: This is the most common cause of life-threatening infections in newborn. Intrapartum transmission is the most common. GBS causes cystitis, amnionitis, endometritis, SB, endocarditis, or meningitis. UTI and pelvic abscess may occur during postpartum. Newborn may suffer from bacteremia, meningitis, and pneumonia. Surviving babies may suffer from visual of hearing loss, developmental delays, and neurological sequelae. Penicillin or ampicillin is started during labor, until delivery.

NONINFECTIVE FEVER

- *Neoplasm*:
  - *Lymphoma*: Hodgkin's lymphoma during pregnancy may present with fever with unknown origin, fatigue, weight loss, and painless lymph nodes. Diagnosis is confirmed by CBC, ESR, lymph node biopsy, and immunophenotyping. MRI and ultrasonography will help in establishing primary and metastasis. Radiation therapy and chemotherapy may be deferred till delivery, but in necessary cases, at times, it is given even during pregnancy after explanation of risks to fetus.
  - *Leukemia*: As leukemia is acutely detrimental to maternal health, diagnosis of it during initial phase of pregnancy usually warrants termination of pregnancy. Chemotherapy during pregnancy will lead to various fetal morbidities depending upon the stage of gestation and dose of chemotherapy.
- *Connective tissue disorders*: Hereditary connective disorders may complicate in form of uterine rupture, vaginal/cervical tears, postpartum hemorrhage, and aortic dissection.
- Autoimmune diseases may create fertility problems, and during pregnancy, there will be risks of teratogenesis, if the patient is kept on chemotherapeutic agents.

REFERENCES

1. Czeizel AE, Puho EH, Acs N, Bánhidy F. Delineation of a multiple congenital abnormality syndrome in the offspring of pregnant women affected with high fever-related disorders: a population-based study. Congenit Anom (Kyoto). 2008;48(4): 158-66.
2. Dreier JW. Systemic review and meta-analyses: fever in pregnancy and health impact in the offspring. Pediatrics. 2014;133(3):e674-88.

3. Wang M1, Wang ZP, Gong R, Zhao ZT. Maternal flu or fever, medications use in the first trimester and the risk for neural tube defects: a hospital-based case control study in China. Childs Nerv Syst. 2014;30(4):665-71.

4. Zebro O, Losif AM, Walker C, Ozonoff S, Hansen RL, Hertz-Picciotto I. Is maternal influenza or fever during pregnancy associated with autism or developmental delays? Results from the Childhood Autism Risks from Genetics and Environment Study. J Autism Dev Disord. 2013;43:25-33.

5. Suarez L, Felkner M, Hendricks K. The effect of fever, febrile illnesses, and heat exposures on the risk of neural tube defects in a Texas-Mexico border population. Birth Defects Res A ClinM ol Teratol. 2004;70(10):815-9.

6. Czeizel AE, Puho EH, Acs N, Bánhidy F. High fever related maternal diseases as possible causes of multiple congenital abnormalities: a population-based case-control study. Birth Defects Res A Clin Mol Teratol. 2007;79(7):544-51.

7. Liew Z, Ritz B, Rebordosa C, Oslen J. Acetaminophen use during pregnancy, behavioral problems, and hyperkinetic disorders. JAMA Pediatr. 2014;168(4):313-20.

8. Dafnis E, Sabatini S. The effect pregnancy on renal function: physiology and pathophysiology. Am J Med Sci. 1992;303(3):184-215.

9. American College of Obstetricians and Gynecologists, Washington, DC. Antimicrobial Therapy for Obstetric Patients. ACOG Educational Bulletin No. 245. Int J Gynaecol Obstet. 1998;245:8-10.

10. Kar P, Jilani N, Husain SA, Bhudev C. Does hepatitis E viral load and genotypes influence the final outcome of acute liver failure during pregnancy? Am J Gastroenterol. 2008;103:2495.

11. Yang J, Zeng XM, Men YL, Zhao LS. Elective cesarean section versus vaginal delivery for preventing mother to child transmission of hepatitis B virus: a systemic review. Virol J. 2008;5:100.

12. Chen HL, Lin LH, Hu FC, Lee JT, Lin WT, Yang YJ, et al. Effects of maternal screening and universal immunization to prevent mother to infant transmission of HBV. Gastroenterology. 2012;142:773.

Clinical Approach to First Trimester Bleeding in Pregnancy

Neha Agarwal, Saroj Singh

INTRODUCTION

Vaginal bleeding is a common occurrence during early pregnancy. 20–40% of pregnant women experience bleeding during the first trimester of pregnancy.[1] This bleeding is usually of maternal origin.

Vaginal bleeding in early pregnancy is associated with a 1.6-fold increased risk of adverse outcomes, including preterm labor (PTL), preterm premature rupture of membranes (PPROM), and intrauterine growth restriction.[2] As bleeding persists or recurs later in pregnancy, the risk of associated morbidities grows.[3] Although 50% of the women who suffer from vaginal bleeding during early pregnancy go on to have a normal pregnancy,[2] vaginal bleeding in the second half of pregnancy is linked to perinatal mortality, disorders of the amniotic fluid, premature rupture of membranes (PROM), preterm deliveries, low birth weight, and low neonatal Apgar scores.[4]

CAUSES OF BLEEDING IN EARLY PREGNANCY

The major causes of vaginal bleeding in early pregnancy are miscarriage (10–20% of clinical pregnancies) and ectopic pregnancy (1–2%).[5] Bleeding occurring very early in pregnancy may be due to endometrial implantation. Gestational trophoblastic disease (GTD) should be considered, especially if serum beta-human chorionic gonadotropin (β-hCG) is abnormally raised. It is vital to establish the site of the pregnancy, as failure to correctly diagnose an ectopic can have potentially life-threatening consequences. **Box 1** shows the causes of first trimester bleeding.

It is not difficult to diagnose vaginal bleeding in a pregnant patient; what is important is recognizing life-threatening situations needing urgent treatment (ectopic pregnancy, a miscarriage with heavy vaginal bleeding and infected abortion with septic shock).

CLINICAL ASSESSMENT

The initial assessment of a woman with vaginal bleeding in early pregnancy must first consider hemodynamic stability and the degree of pain or bleeding. It should be recognized that young women may suffer significant blood loss before any signs of hemodynamic instability are evident.[6] The most likely diagnoses of a hemodynamically unstable patient with early pregnancy

---

BOX 1: Causes of bleeding in first trimester.

Obstetric causes:
- Implantation bleeding
- Miscarriage
- Ectopic pregnancy
- Molar pregnancy
- Subchorionic hemorrhage
- Idiopathic bleeding in a viable pregnancy

Gynecological causes (cervix, vagina, or vulva):
- Infection (*Chlamydia*, etc.)
- Trauma and laceration of skin
- Malignancy
- Ruptured varicose veins
- Cervical abnormalities (polyp, ectropion, etc.)

Surrounding structures (bladder or anus):
- Hemorrhoids
- UTI and schistosomiasis
- Trauma, infection, or malignancy

(UTI: urinary tract infection)

---

bleeding are a ruptured ectopic pregnancy, an incomplete miscarriage with "cervical shock" (parasympathetic stimulation caused by products in the cervical is leading to hypotension and bradycardia), or massive hemorrhage secondary to miscarriage or molar pregnancy.[6]

A speculum examination must be performed and any products of conception (POC) protruding from the cervical os should be removed. These patients may require urgent surgical management like suction curettage, laparoscopy, or laparotomy. In a hemodynamically stable patient, a more detailed assessment can be done. The initial evaluation, as a rule, should include a detailed history and gynecological examination. Imaging by ultrasonography (US) is an integral part of the initial assessment.

HISTORY

The history should include:
- Last menstrual period, regularity of menstrual cycles, confirmation of pregnancy, likely gestational age
- Characterization and quantification of bleeding to assess the severity—onset of bleeding, frequency of occurrence, fresh (red), or old (darker, brown) bleeding. If bleeding is less than that a woman perceives as a normal menstruation, it probably needs no urgent treatment. Although an ectopic pregnancy can present with little loss of blood.
- *Precipitating factor:* Bleeding after intercourse or defecation could indicate a cervical origin—infection or malignancies, or even hemorrhoids.
- *Accompanying symptoms:*
  - *Abdominal cramps and pain:* Acute, continuous, localized, or general
  - Nausea and fainting, shoulder tip pain—a sign of hypotension due to intra-abdominal bleeding in ectopic pregnancy

- Syncope, chest pain, and shortness of breath may point toward anemia from significant blood loss.
- Passage of products points toward an incomplete abortion.
- Fever can be due to recent unsterile procedure or of septic abortion. It could also be a symptom of an infection which may cause miscarriage, e.g., malaria.[7]
- *Dysuria*: Sometimes, a urinary tract infection (UTI) presents with fresh blood in the toilet. Painless macrohematuria occurs in urinary schistosomiasis.
- Vaginal discharge could point toward sexually transmitted infection (STI) such as gonorrhea and *Chlamydia*.
- *Detailed medical and obstetric history*: Poorly controlled diabetes and thyroid disease are associated with an increased risk of miscarriage.[8] Any prior intervention that may not have been aseptic or has been incomplete. Any previous surgery—an ectopic pregnancy due to pelvic inflammatory disease (PID) can reoccur.
- History of bleeding and coagulation disorders
- Use of medications, especially anticoagulation therapy
- Some drugs [e.g., diuretics, antiepileptic drugs, nonsteroidal anti-inflammatory drugs (NSAIDs), misoprostol, retinoids, and cytostatic drugs], toxins (lead, mercury, formaldehyde, ethylene oxide, and benzene), and large doses of radiation also increase the risk of miscarriage.[9]
- If the bleeding started before pregnancy, she might have cervical or vaginal lesions.
- History of trauma or sexual assault

EXAMINATION

The physical examination should include:
- *Vital signs*: Blood pressure, temperature, pulse, and respiratory rate
- *Abdominal examination* for tenderness, distension, guarding, or rigidity:
  - The fundus is palpable above the pubic symphysis when the uterus reaches the size of 12-week gestation. It may be palpable earlier in a multiple pregnancy, GTD, and pelvic or uterine masses such as fibroids or ovarian cysts.
- *Inspection of the perineum* for amount of bleeding, signs of trauma, or lesions
- *Speculum examination* to:
  - Inspect vagina, cervix, and uterus to localize the origin of bleeding
  - Assess the amount of bleeding
  - Check the cervix for dilatation of the os, cervical polyps, ulcers, or other lesions
  - Tissue present in the open cervical os must always be removed and sent for histopathological examination to confirm retained POC.
- *Bimanual examination* for assessment of uterine size, shape, position, and consistency; examination of the adnexae for masses or tenderness and

cervical motion tenderness. Be careful in a suspected ectopic pregnancy; it can rupture with too much manipulation.

- If the cervical os is open, it may be an incomplete or an inevitable miscarriage. If the os is closed, it may indicate a threatened miscarriage, complete miscarriage, missed abortion, or ectopic pregnancy.

Investigations

A combination of ultrasound assessment and measurement of serum β-hCG is required to determine the location and viability of an early pregnancy when the woman presents with bleeding.

Serum hCG levels rise exponentially up to 6–7 weeks of gestation, increasing by at least 66% every 48 hours.[10]

Repeat measurements after 48–72 hours showing a falling β-hCG is consistent with a nonviable pregnancy, but does not indicate whether it is a failed intrauterine pregnancy (IUP), or an involuting ectopic.

Plateaued or very slow to rise levels of β-hCG (<50% in 48 hours) are suggestive of an ectopic or nonviable intrauterine pregnancy.[8] However, it should be noted that an apparently appropriately rising β-hCG is found in 21% of ectopic pregnancies.[3]

Ultrasonography is the cornerstone of evaluating early pregnancy bleeding. On transvaginal ultrasound (TVS), a gestational sac will usually be visible from 4 weeks and 3 days after the last menstrual period,[11] assuming the dates are correct and menstrual cycle is regular.

A nonviable pregnancy is diagnosed on ultrasound, if there is:

- No live fetus visible in a gestational sac where the mean sac diameter (MSD) is >25 mm, or
- A visible fetal pole with a crown rump length (CRL) of >7 mm, with no fetal heart activity after a period of observation of at least 30 seconds.[11]

Before making a diagnosis, do a review scan after 7 days.

If an intrauterine gestational sac is not visible, the adnexa should be carefully evaluated for evidence of an ectopic pregnancy. An adnexal mass is the most common ultrasound finding in ectopic pregnancies, present in >88% of cases.[12] In case of a ruptured ectopic pregnancy, free fluid (blood) will be seen in pouch of Douglas.

The discriminatory zone is the serum β-hCG level above which a gestational sac should be visualized on TVS. Usually, this is set at 1,500 or 2,000 IU/L, although a number of variables, including skill of the sonologist and quality of the ultrasound, can alter the level.[7]

Other Tests

- Maternal blood group and antibody status to determine the need for RhD immunoglobulin administration.
- Hemoglobin and cross-matching in case of severe bleeding or suspected ectopic pregnancy.

- Erythrocyte sedimentation rate (ESR) or leukocytes in case of infection.
- Urine pregnancy test (UPT) to confirm pregnancy, if in doubt.
- Midstream urine analysis for leukocytes, blood to look for UTI
- Culdocentesis can assess the presence of blood or pus in the pouch of Douglas, if an ultrasound is not feasible.[4]

PREGNANCY OF UNKNOWN LOCATION

If a woman with a positive UPT has no signs on a TVS of an intra- or extrauterine pregnancy, and no obvious retained POC are seen, this is defined as a pregnancy of unknown location (PUL). Under these circumstances, the possible scenarios are:[11]

- Complete miscarriage
- Early intrauterine pregnancy
- Ectopic pregnancy
- A spontaneously resolving intrauterine or tubal pregnancy.

When interpreting the scan result of a woman with a PUL, serum β-hCG levels at zero and 48 hours are helpful in diagnosis of the ectopic location.[11]

Until the location is determined, a woman with a PUL could be having an ectopic pregnancy. It is, therefore, important to reassess the woman, if symptoms change. Clinical symptoms may necessitate admission to hospital while further investigations are being done.

MISCARRIAGE

By definition, miscarriage refers to the loss of a pregnancy before the fetus has reached a viable gestational age (WHO defines as <20 weeks or <500 g). Unfortunately, the cut-off point for a viable gestational age varies worldwide. Survival of preterm neonates from 20 to 22 weeks of gestational age onwards has increased because of medical advancements, especially in developed countries. In our country, the age of viability is still taken as 28 weeks.

Several terms are used to describe clinical scenarios around the process of miscarriage. These are defined in **Table 1**.[13]

TABLE 1: Definitions of subcategories of miscarriage.[13]

Miscarriage	Pregnancy loss before 20 weeks' gestation or fetal weight <500 g
Threatened	Uterine bleeding prior to 20 weeks' gestation without any cervical dilatation
Inevitable	Passage of POC of a nonviable IUP occurring or expected to occur imminently
Incomplete	Some retention of POC of a nonviable IUP
Missed	Ultrasound diagnosis of a nonviable IUP in the absence of vaginal bleeding
Septic	Miscarriage complicated by infection of the uterus and its appendages
Recurrent	Three or more consecutive miscarriages
Complete	Full expulsion of POC of an IUP

(IUP: intrauterine pregnancy; POC: products of conception)

Miscarriage is the main reason for vaginal bleeding early in pregnancy. 10–20% of clinically recognized pregnancies result in spontaneous miscarriage.[14] Ectopic pregnancies do not occur as commonly as miscarriage, but are definitely more prevalent in areas where PID is highly endemic.

Miscarriage can be a life-threatening condition when it results in massive hemorrhage (even more dangerous in the presence of anemia) or septicemia as the result of unsafe, induced abortion.

Threatened miscarriage is treated expectantly. 50% of these pregnancies continue to be viable. There is a 2.6 times increased risk of miscarriage later in the same pregnancy in cases of early threatened miscarriage, and 17% of women go on to have further complications in pregnancy (such as preterm labor or intrauterine growth restriction).[12] Cochrane review suggest that progestogens are probably effective in the treatment of threatened miscarriage but may have little or no effect in the rate of preterm birth. The evidence on congenital abnormalities is uncertain, because the quality of the evidence for this outcome was based on only two small trials with very few events and was found to be of very low quality.[15]

A *complete miscarriage* requires evaluation of any ongoing bleeding, with confirmation that the cervical os is closed, and, if necessary, a TVS to rule out retained POC.

For *inevitable, incomplete, and missed miscarriages*, management options include expectant, medical, and surgical treatments. Depending on the method chosen, follow-up will be required to ensure complete evacuation of the uterus.

- *Expectant management* involves allowing the natural process of expulsion of uterine POC to occur without intervention. The woman must be informed regarding the expected length of the process, symptoms of pain, and bleeding that she is likely to experience, and how to seek emergency medical assistance. For incomplete miscarriages, 60% of women experience complete expulsion of products in the ensuing 2 weeks and 90% by 6–8 weeks.[16] Missed miscarriages generally take longer to expel.

  Ongoing review should occur at 1–2 weeks, and if pain and bleeding have ceased, a repeat serum hCG should be performed at 3 weeks. If this is positive, further assessment with serial hCG measurements, to ensure these fall to negative levels, or an ultrasound scan may be required to assess for retained POC.

  If no bleeding or pain occurs within 7–14 days of the initial consultation, repeat the ultrasound and further discuss all treatment options as appropriate.

- *Medical management* involves the use of misoprostol (a prostaglandin E1 analog), which has been shown to be highly effective for medical evacuation of the uterus given either vaginally or orally.[17]

- *Surgical evacuation* or manual vacuum aspiration (MVA) is the treatment of choice for women with hemorrhage or sepsis. A woman may choose a surgical evacuation in order to avoid pain, bleeding, and prolongation of the process. Medical management is contraindicated in some cases, such as for a woman on anticoagulant therapy. Complications of surgical evacuation include anesthetic risks, hemorrhage, perforation, retained POC, and endometritis.

The MIST trial,[18] a large, randomized controlled trial, compared expectant, medical, and surgical management options for the treatment of miscarriage. It showed comparable efficacy and no significant difference in infection rates (2–3%). The trial reported that unplanned hospital admissions were significantly increased in the expectant (49%) and medical (18%) groups, compared with the surgical group (8%). Surgical management was required in 44% of the expectant group and 13% of those given medication; 5% of the surgical group required a further surgical procedure.

Septic abortion: An infected miscarriage can either be due to prior incomplete spontaneous miscarriage, which has not evacuated completely, or due to an unsterile procedure like MVA.

It is characterized by fever, uterine tenderness, and foul smelling discharge. The patient may develop septic shock. Septic shock has a mortality rate of approximately 25–50%, even with proper treatment in high-care facilities.[19]

Signs of disseminated sepsis are—high fever and prostration, tachycardia, tachypnea or respiratory distress and hypotension.[20] Infecting organisms are usually vaginal or bowel bacteria. There is abdominal guarding and rebound tenderness in case of peritonitis. This can be due to uterine perforation or infection, tubo-ovarian abscess, or bowel perforation.

Immediately start fluid resuscitation and a combination of broad-spectrum injectable antibiotics.

If no signs of septic shock are present, it is probably wiser to perform the MVA after 12–24 h of intravenous antibiotic treatment. When performing an MVA, look carefully for signs of perforation and for foreign bodies in the vagina or uterus. An infected uterus is easily perforated on evacuation.

ECTOPIC PREGNANCY

Ninety-five percent of ectopic pregnancies are situated in the fallopian tube.[21] Other, rarer sites include the cervical, ovarian, abdominal, or a cesarean scar pregnancy. Rarely, an ectopic pregnancy and an intrauterine pregnancy may coexist (heterotopic pregnancy).

Management options for tubal ectopic pregnancy include surgery (salpingectomy or salpingostomy), medical management with methotrexate, and possibly expectant management in a limited population of carefully selected cases.

Surgery is needed for a hemodynamically unstable patient, evidence of rupture of ectopic, after failed medical management, and if contraindications to methotrexate exist (including the possibility of noncompliance with follow-up).

Laparoscopic surgery should be performed whenever possible.[22] A salpingectomy is usually performed unless the contralateral tube is damaged. A salpingostomy may result in a need for further treatment (4–15%)[23] with methotrexate or a salpingectomy, if follow-up hCG levels do not fall appropriately. In women who have had a salpingostomy, hCG levels should be measured weekly until negative due to the risk of persistent ectopic pregnancy. In case of a salpingectomy, histological confirmation of a tubal pregnancy is usually all that is required.

About one-third of women with ectopic pregnancy are suitable for medical management with methotrexate. These women should be hemodynamically stable, be able to comply with treatment and follow-up, ideally have an hCG < 5,000 IU/L (the greatest predictor of success)[7,24] and an adnexal mass <3.5 cm with no fetal cardiac activity. Initial treatment is with a single intramuscular dose of methotrexate (50 mg/m^2), with 14% of women requiring a further dose. Success rate is up to 85%, which is similar to salpingostomy.[16] Up to 15% of women may require surgical intervention.

Ongoing fertility in the 2–3 years following surgical or medical treatment for ectopic pregnancy appears to be similar between methotrexate, salpingotomy, and salpingectomy groups.[24]

MOLAR PREGNANCY (HYDATIDIFORM MOLE, GESTATIONAL TROPHOBLASTIC DISEASE)

A molar pregnancy is an abnormal form of pregnancy where the chorionic villi around the fetus degenerate and form clusters of fluid-filled sacs or vesicles.

The classic features of molar pregnancy are irregular painless vaginal bleeding, hyperemesis gravidarum, excessive uterine enlargement, and passage of vesicles. hCG levels can vary and range from excessively high in early pregnancy (>100,000 IU/mL) to normal and slowly rising in case of a partial molar pregnancy. Conclusive diagnosis can only be made by histopathology, which shows hydropic swelling of the chorionic villi and hyperplasia of the trophoblastic cells.

Treatment

Suction evacuation is the method of choice of evacuation for complete and partial molar pregnancies except when the size of the fetal parts deters the use of suction curettage and then medical evacuation can be used.[25]

Anti-D prophylaxis is required following evacuation of a molar pregnancy.

It is safe to prepare the cervix immediately prior to evacuation. There can be excessive vaginal bleeding while evacuating molar pregnancy and a senior surgeon should directly supervise the surgical evacuation.

The use of oxytocin infusion prior to completion of the evacuation is not recommended.[25]

If the woman is experiencing significant hemorrhage prior to evacuation, surgical evacuation should be expedited and the need for oxytocin infusion weighed up against the risk of tumor embolization.

A urinary pregnancy test should be performed 3 weeks after medical management of failed pregnancy and if POC are not sent for histological examination.[25]

As persistent trophoblastic neoplasia may develop after any pregnancy, it is recommended that POC, obtained after all repeat evacuations, should also undergo histological examination.

Follow-up after GTD is highly individualized. If hCG has returned to normal within 56 days of the pregnancy event then follow-up will be for 6 months from the date of uterine evacuation. If not, then follow-up will be for 6 months from normalization of the hCG level.[25]

OTHER INCIDENTAL CONDITIONS CAUSING VAGINAL BLEEDING

- *Cervical malignancies*: In developing countries, cervical carcinoma is the most common malignancy in women. The malignancy usually presents itself at 30–50 years of age.[26] As a result, it is not unusual to encounter a cervical carcinoma in pregnancy in low-resourced settings. Unfortunately, medical professionals are usually not aware that a cervical malignancy might be a possibility when encountering (recurrent, minimal) vaginal bleeding in pregnancy. The key to a proper diagnosis is speculum examination and digital vaginal examination. Bleeding can occur spontaneously, but classically, due to direct contact of the cervix, i.e., vaginal bleeding after intercourse, inserting tampons or passage of hard stools. Bleeding due to cervical erosions is usually self-limiting and not severe (as in miscarriage or ectopic pregnancy). On bimanual examination, a solid painless mass or irregularity is palpated.
- *Infections causing vaginal bleeding*: *Chlamydia, Gonorrhea,* urogenital schistosomiasis, and urogenital tuberculosis.
- *Urinary tract infection*: A lower UTI (or cystitis) can cause hematuria, which can easily be mistaken for vaginal bleeding. Cystitis is quite common condition in pregnancy due to increased urinary stasis. Oral antibiotics are needed.
- An upper UTI (or pyelonephritis) is a more serious condition, which calls for intravenous antibiotics.
- *Cervical polyps*: In general, they bleed after intercourse, but also spontaneously. Most polyps do not bleed profusely. Diagnosis is made on speculum examination. The stem of the polyp is usually avascular. The majority (99%) of cervical polyps are benign.
- Their management depends on the symptoms. Most of the time, conservative approach is preferred, especially for small pedunculated

polyps. On the other hand, if symptoms occur with intermittent vaginal bleeding, vaginal discharge, change in the appearance aspect of the polyp such as ulceration with additional cervicitis, polypectomy can be done under antibiotic cover.

- *Cervical ectropion*: In pregnancy, the endocervical epithelium everts and becomes the exterior part of the cervix. This ectropion will bleed easily on contact. On speculum examination, there is a very specific shallow, vascular, red area.

  Symptoms are more common in pregnant women due to hormonal changes and high estrogen levels.

  Besides reassurance, no specific treatment is required during pregnancy and symptoms will resolve by themselves. These usually disappear by themselves within 3–6 months following delivery.

- *Vaginal or perigenital lacerations* can be a result of trauma or STIs or a skin infection like fungal infection or eczema.

- *Subchorionic or idiopathic bleeding*: This can only be diagnosed when other more serious causes have been excluded and no specific cause can be found. In some cases, the blood originates from the subchorionic area. In theory, due to growth of the uterus and its components in pregnancy, small lacerations occur below the chorionic layer and the uterine wall, which presents as fresh vaginal bleeding. Treatment is reassurance, but no specific treatment. Sometimes subchorionic hematomas may lead to bothersome uterine contractions or even miscarriage. In 10% of cases the bleeding reoccurs.[27]

- *Hemorrhoids* are also easily diagnosed. Sometimes anal bleeding is mistaken for vaginal bleeding. They usually disappear after pregnancy and conservative treatment is the first option—painkiller (local) and laxatives may be added, if hard stools are present as well.

BLEEDING IN LATE PREGNANCY

Common causes of bleeding in late pregnancy are placenta previa, abruption, ruptured vasa previa, uterine scar disruption, cervical polyp, bloody show, cervicitis or cervical ectropion, vaginal trauma, and cervical cancer. The first four conditions are life-threatening and should be promptly diagnosed and managed.

CONCLUSION

Early pregnancy bleeding can cause great anxiety and distress for a woman, her partner, and family, especially where a diagnosis of a nonviable pregnancy is made. It is important that the situation is dealt with both safety and sensitively and that the woman and her family are well supported throughout this time.

KEY POINTS

- Twenty to forty percent of pregnant women experience bleeding during the first trimester of pregnancy.
- Always rule out ectopic pregnancy when encountering a patient with vaginal bleeding early in pregnancy.
- Proper patient history, adequate physical examination, and ultrasound are the cornerstone to diagnose and manage early pregnancy bleeding.
- For inevitable, incomplete, and missed miscarriages, management options include expectant, medical, and surgical treatments.
- Septic shock presents with high fever, tachycardia, tachypnea, and hypotension. Removal of infected focus is necessary.
- Management options for tubal ectopic pregnancy include surgery (salpingectomy or salpingostomy), medical management with methotrexate, and possibly expectant management in a limited population of carefully selected cases.
- Suction evacuation is the method of choice of evacuation for complete and partial molar pregnancies.
- The incidental causes of bleeding in the first trimester should only be diagnosed, if more serious conditions of miscarriage, ectopic pregnancy, infections, and malignancies have been ruled out first.

REFERENCES

1. Queensland Clinical Guidelines. Maternity and neonatal clinical guideline. Early pregnancy loss. Brisbane: Queensland Health; 2011.
2. Snell BJ. Assessment and management of bleeding in the first trimester of pregnancy. J Midwifery Womens Health. 2009;54(6):483-91.
3. Hossain R, Harris T, Lohsoonthorn V, Williams MA. Risk of preterm delivery in relation to vaginal bleeding in early pregnancy. Eur J Obstet Gynecol Reprod Biol. 2007;135(2):158-63.
4. Koifman A, Levy A, Zaulan Y, Harlev A, Mazor M, Wiznitzer A, et al. The clinical significance of bleeding during the second trimester of pregnancy. Arch Gynecol Obstet. 2008;278(1):47-51.
5. King Edward Memorial Hospital. Clinical guidelines – Ectopic pregnancy. Subiaco, WA: Department of Health; 2014.
6. Breeze C. Early pregnancy bleeding. The Royal Australian College of General Practitioners 2016. AFP2016;45(5):283-6.
7. National Institute for Health and Clinical Excellence. NICE Guidelines 154: Ectopic pregnancy and miscarriage. London: NICE; 2015.
8. UpToDate. Approach to the evaluation of early pregnancy bleeding. Alphen aan den Rijn, South Holland: Wolters Kluwer; 2016.
9. Duff P, Edwards RK, Davis JD, Rhoton-Vlasak A. Obstetrics & Gynaecology: Just the Facts. New York: McGraw-Hill; 2004.
10. Barnhart KT, Sammel MD, Rinaudo PF, Zhou L, Hummel AC, Guo W. Symptomatic patients with an early viable intrauterine pregnancy: hCG curves redefined. Obstet Gynecol. 2004;104(1):50-5.
11. Australasian Society for Ultrasound in Medicine. Guidelines for the performance of first trimester ultrasound. Sydney: ASUM; 2014.

12. Dogra V, Paspulati RM, Bhatt S. First trimester bleeding evaluation. Ultrasound Q. 2005;21(2):69-85.

13. American College of Obstetricians and Gynecologists. ACOG Practice Bulletin No. 200 Summary: Early Pregnancy Loss. Obstet Gynecol 2018;132(5):1311-3.

14. Alberman E. Spontaneous abortion: epidemiology. In: Stabile S, Grudzinkas G, Chard T (Eds). Spontaneous Abortion: Diagnosis and Treatment. London: Springer Verlag; 1992. pp. 9-20.

15. Wahabi HA, Fayed AA, Esmaeil SA, Bahkali K. Progestogen for treating threatened miscarriage. Cochrane Database Syst Rev. 2018;(8):CD005943.

16. Nanda K, Lopez LM, Grimes DA, Peloggia A, Nanda G. Expectant care versus surgical treatment for miscarriage. Cochrane Database Syst Rev. 2012;(3):CD003518.

17. Neilson JP, Gyte GM, Hickey M, Vazquez C, Dou L. Medical treatments for incomplete miscarriage (less than 24 weeks). Cochrane Database Syst Rev. 2010;(1):CD007223.

18. Trinder J, Brocklehurst P, Porter R, Read M, Vyas S, Smith L. Management of miscarriage: Expectant, medical, or surgical? Results of randomised controlled trial (miscarriage treatment (MIST) trial). BMJ. 2006;332(7552):1235-40.

19. Kumar V, Abbas AK, Fausto N, Mitchell RN. Robbins Basic Pathology, 8th edition. Philadelphia: Saunders; 2007. pp. 102-3.

20. Stubblefield PG, Averbach SH, Grimes DA. (2008; Updated 2012). Septic abortion: prevention and management. [online] Available from: https://www.glowm. com/section_view/heading/septic-abortion-prevention-and-management/ item/437#:~:text=PRIMARY%20PREVENTION%20OF%20SEPTIC%20 ABORTION,occurrence%20of%20disease%20or%20injury.&text=Primary %20prevention%20of%20septic%20abortion%20includes%20access%20to %20effective%20and,appropriate%20medical%20management%20of%20 abortion. [Last accessed June, 2020].

21. Farquar CM. Ectopic pregnancy. Lancet. 2005;366(9485):583-91.

22. Hajenius PJ, Mol F, Mol BW, Bossuyt PM, Ankum WM, van der Veen F. Interventions for tubal ectopic pregnancy. Cochrane Database Syst Rev. 2007;(1):CD000324.

23. Fernandez H, Capmas P, Lucot JP, Resch B, Panel P, Bouyer J, et al. Fertility after ectopic pregnancy: The DEMETER randomized trial. Hum Reprod. 2013;28(5):1247-53.

24. Menon S, Colins J, Barnhart KT. Establishing a human chorionic gonadotropin cutoff to guide methotrexate treatment of ectopic pregnancy: A systematic review. Fertil Steril. 2007;87(3):481-4.

25. Royal College of Obstetricians and Gynaecologists. (2010). The management of gestational trophoblastic diseases. RCOG Green-top Guideline No. 6of 12 38 ©. [online] Available from: https://www.rcog.org.uk/globalassets/documents/ guidelines/gtg_38.pdf. [Last accessed June, 2020].

26. Onwudiegwu U, Bako A, Oyewumi A. Cervical cancer—a neglected health tragedy. J Obstet Gynaecol. 1999;19(1): 61-4.

27. Jager B. Chapter 2: Vaginal Bleeding in the First Trimester of Pregnancy. In: Dadelszen PV (Ed). Gynecology for Less-Resourced Locations. London: Sapiens Publishing; 2012. pp. 21-34.

5

SECTION

What Next—Time to Act

- **Management of Rh-negative Pregnancy**
  Mandakini Pradhan

- **What Next: Time to Act Hepatitis B Positive in Any Partner**
  Shelly Agarwal

- **HIV-positive Discordant Couple**
  Madhuri Chandra

- **Interpretation of TORCH Test**
  Charmila Ayyavoo

- **After Glucose Intolerance: What Next?**
  Susheela Rani

Management of Rh-negative Pregnancy

Mandakini Pradhan

INTRODUCTION

Blood group is usually described as ABO+ or ABO–, signifying the presence (+) or absence (–) of the RhD antigen on the surface of the red blood cell. The prevalence of Rh-negative blood group in different populations varies ranging from 1% in Native Americans to 30% in Spanish Basque. In India, it has been reported to be 3–5%. Development of antibodies to RhD antigens is usually referred to as Rh alloimmunization. It is usually due to fetomaternal hemorrhage (FMH) with transplacental passage of Rh-positive fetal erythrocytes into the maternal circulation. Rarely, it is due to transfusion of Rh-positive blood or blood products such as platelet unknowingly or knowingly in emergency life-saving situations. As little as 0.1 mL of fetal blood can generate an immune response in maternal blood, an amount that routinely passes into maternal circulation. Antigens are expressed on fetal red blood cell (RBC) by 38 days of gestation and hence first trimester events can cause alloimmunization, including ectopic pregnancy, spontaneous or therapeutic abortion, molar pregnancy, and threatened abortion. Invasive procedures such as amniocentesis, chorionic villous sampling, cordocentesis or external cephalic version, and maternal trauma can also lead to FMH and alloimmunization. FMH is most likely to occur at delivery. Cesarean delivery, multifetal delivery, abruption, bleeding placenta previa, or manual removal of placenta may increase the quantity of FMH.

MANAGEMENT OF Rh-NEGATIVE PREGNANCY

Management of Rh-negative pregnancy is described in **Flowchart 1**.

PREVENTION (BOX 1)

- Without any prophylaxis, 17% women developed antibodies following delivery of Rh-positive fetus and 10% of them are affected by hemolytic diseases of fetus or newborn.
- With use of preventive measures, only 0.1% of pregnancies in Rh-negative women are complicated by anti-RhD antibody production. Preventive measure is by use of polyclonal anti-D, i.e., pooled sterile human IgG antibodies to RhD antigens. It prevents alloimmunization by clearing

Flowchart 1: Management of Rh-negative pregnancy.

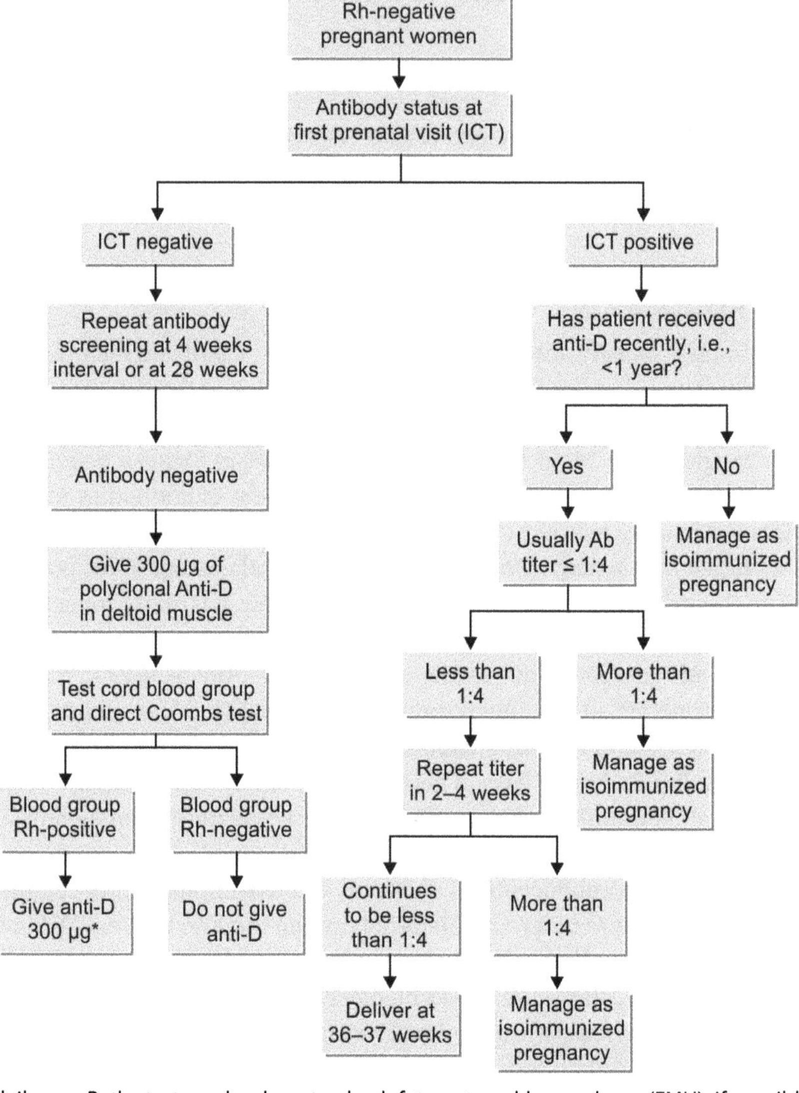

*Kleihauer–Betke test can be done to check fetomaternal hemorrhage (FMH), if possible. Dose of anti-D is decided depending on the FMH.
(ICT: indirect Coombs test)

RhD-positive RBCs from maternal circulation, downregulating the maternal B-cell-mediated immune response and possibly obscuring antigen sites on fetal RBCs.

- The standard dose of polyclonal anti-D is 300 µg IM given in the deltoid muscle (not to be given in the buttock) and that can neutralize 30 mL of fetal Rh-positive RBCs. Additional dosing of anti-D especially in multiple pregnancy, severe abruption placentae leading to fetal death is guided by quantification of FMH with Kleihauer–Betke test.

> **BOX 1:** Indication of anti-D administration in Rh-negative unsensitized women.
>
> - First trimester spontaneous and elective abortion (medical or surgical)
> - Threatened abortion
> - Ectopic pregnancy
> - Molar pregnancy
> - Bleeding during pregnancy
> - Fetal death
> - Antenatal procedures such as amniocentesis, CVS, and cordocentesis
> - External cephalic version
> - Abdominal trauma
> - Routine prophylaxis at 28 weeks
> - Birth of Rh-positive infant
>
> (CVS: chorionic villus sampling)

- Most societies world over recommend to give anti-D at 28 weeks and again postpartum after neonatal Rh-positive status is confirmed. Smaller dose of 50 µg IM is recommended for first trimester event. If not available, then giving 300 µg is safer than not giving anything.
- The half-life of anti-D is 24 days but can be detected in maternal circulation for up to 12 weeks and maximum up to 1 year. Indirect Coombs test (ICT) done within one year of receiving anti-D may indicate presence of antibody in low titer and should not be interpreted as alloimmunization.

■ MANAGEMENT OF Rh-ISOIMMUNIZED PREGNANCY

Management of Rh-isoimmunized pregnancy is described in **Flowchart 2**.

■ DETECTION OF FETAL ANEMIA

Measurement of peak systolic velocity (PSV) of middle cerebral artery (MCA), if properly measured, can detect moderate-to-severe fetal anemia with 87–90% sensitivity. A MCA PSV of more than 1.5 MoM for that gestation indicates fetal anemia requiring intrauterine transfusion and hence referral to a center with this facility.

Appearance of fetal hydrops is the result of decompensated fetal heart and late detection of fetal anemia. Moreover, success of intrauterine transfusion (IUT) is as high as 90–95% in non-hydropic fetus but 60–70% in hydropic fetus. Hence, the importance of early detection of fetal anemia by serial MCA PSV measurement in women who have ICT titers more than the critical titer (more than 1:8 for author's laboratory).

■ CONCLUSION

Rh-negative is as common as 5% in India. There is an urgent need for the use of both antenatal (at 28 weeks) and postnatal prophylaxis (Rh-positive infant even if it is malformed) to prevent alloimmunization. Early detection of alloimmunization should be done by doing ICT. Serial measurement of

Flowchart 2: Management of Rh-isoimmunized pregnancy.

ICT titer more than the critical titer, i.e., laboratory specific; Usually 1:8 or 1:16 titer

Previous obstetric history
Start fetal monitoring 10 weeks before the previous affection, i.e., fetal hydrops, fetal death, fetal transfusion or delivery, and severe hemolytic disease of newborn

Fetal monitoring: By MCA PSV

MCA PSV more than 1.5 MoM for that gestation

MCA PSV less than 1.5 MoM

Intrauterine transfusion (send the patient to appropriate center)

Monitor every 1–2 weekly

More than 1.5 MoM

Continues to be less than 1.5 MoM

Indicates moderate-to-severe fetal anemia and needs intrauterine fetal transfusion

Deliver at 34–36 weeks

Note: If technology is available then genotype of Rh-positive partner can be done. If genotype is +/+, then fetal blood group is definitely Rh-positive and hence fetal blood group determination is not helpful. If genotype is ±, then fetal blood group determination can be done by isolating fetal DNA from maternal circulation or by polymerase chain reaction (PCR) technique of fetal tissue such as CVS/amniotic fluid. If fetus is Rh-negative, then further monitoring is not necessary.

(ICT: indirect Coombs test; MCA: middle cerebral artery; PSV: peak systolic velocity; MoM: multiples of median)

MCA PSV is recommended for those who are ICT positive in high titer and referral to centers with intrauterine transfusion facility, if it is more than 1.5 MoM for that gestation.

Treatment is possible by IUT, but we should aim for prevention.

What Next: Time to Act Hepatitis B Positive in Any Partner

Shelly Agarwal

INTRODUCTION

Hepatitis B is a major health problem of global concern, which results in a potentially life-threatening liver infection. The disease is caused by hepatitis B virus (HBV), which can cause chronic liver infection and thereby increase the risk of death from cirrhosis and liver cancer.

In July 2018, WHO estimated that 257 million people are living with hepatitis B virus infection (also defined as hepatitis B surface antigen positive). Highest prevalence is observed in the WHO Western Pacific Region and the WHO African Region, where 6.2% and 6.1% of adult population are infected.[1] As far as Indian statistics is concerned, India falls in the intermediate endemicity zone (prevalence of 2–7%, with an average of 4%), with disease burden of about 50 million carriers, second largest in the world.[2]

HEPATITIS B VIRUS

The HBV DNA contains three principal antigens:
1. *Hepatitis B surface antigen (HBsAg)*: It is present on the surface of the virus and circulates freely in the serum.
2. *Hepatitis B core antigen (HBcAg)*: It is present only in hepatocytes and does not circulate in the serum.
3. *Hepatitis B e antigen (HBeAg)*: Its presence is indicative of active viral replication and hence high infectivity.[3]

Transmission

The hepatitis B can survive outside the body for at least 7 days. During this time, the virus can still cause infection, if it enters the body of a person who is not immunized. The incubation period usually ranges between 30 and 80 days, with an average of about 75 days.

Transmission can be a horizontal transmission (exposure to infected blood or parenteral, mucosal, and sexual exposure) or a vertical mother-to-child transmission. Important to note is that the development of chronic infection is most common in infants who are infected from their mothers or acquire infection before 5 years of age. In fact, 80–90% of infants infected during 1st year of life develop chronic infections and only less than 5% of otherwise healthy persons who are infected, as adults will develop chronic infections.[1] *Therefore, universal screening for hepatitis B is advocated for all pregnant women, regardless of previous testing or vaccination.*[4]

In mother to child transmission, fetus usually does not get infected during the antenatal period. HBV, because of its size, is not able to cross the placenta and therefore does not infect the fetus antenatally unless there is breach in fetal–maternal barrier. However, infected women transmit HBV to infants during delivery and, hence, perinatal transmission is a major threat to the newborn.[5]

Course of the Disease during Pregnancy

A pregnant lady suffering from acute viral hepatitis usually presents with flu-like symptoms such as nausea, vomiting, malaise, and abdominal pain and are at a lower risk of having various obstetric complications when compared with other potential hepatic complications such as HELLP (hemolysis, elevated liver enzymes, and low platelet count) and acute fatty liver of pregnancy. In fact, majority (90–95%) patients will clear the infection and have complete recovery.

Those women with chronic infection also generally do well during pregnancy and studies show no significant difference in viral loads during pregnancy. However, mothers with chronic hepatitis B should receive appropriate treatment during pregnancy and should be monitored in postpartum period for hepatic flares.

Understanding Different Serological Markers (Table 1)

When infection occurs, HBsAg can be detected in serum. Most of the patients are able to clear this infection as a part of normal immune response to infection, with subsequent formation of hepatitis B surface antibody (anti-HBs). But in some cases, HBsAg persists, resulting in chronic infection. Hence, its (HBsAg) presence indicates either acute or chronic infection and that the women is potentially infectious.

Hepatitis B surface antibody appears once recovery occurs from acute infection and it indicates immunity from HBV infection. It also develops in a person who is vaccinated against hepatitis B.

Hepatitis B core antibody (anti-HBc): Anti-HBc antibodies can be IgM and IgG. IgM anti-HBc appears during the acute phase and usually disappears by 6 months of acquiring infection. So, its presence indicates a recent infection. IgG anti-HBc appears in convalescence state and thereafter generally remains detectable for the entire lifetime.[6]

The HBeAg is a marker of active replication and its presence is indicative of infectivity and disease severity.[6,7]

The HBV DNA indicates the viral load or HBV virus particles.

TABLE 1: Interpretation of different serological markers of hepatitis B.[8]

HBsAg	Negative	Susceptible
Anti-HBc	Negative	
Anti-HBs	Negative	
HBsAg	Negative	Immune due to natural infection
Anti-HBc	Positive	
Anti-HBs	Positive	
HBsAg	Negative	Immune due to hepatitis B vaccination
Anti-HBc	Negative	
Anti-HBs	Positive	
HBsAg	Positive	Acutely infected
Anti-HBc	Positive	
IgM anti-HBc	Positive	
Anti-HBs	Negative	
HBsAg	Positive	Chronically infected
Anti-HBc	Positive	
IgM anti-HBc	Negative	
Anti-HBs	Negative	
HBsAg	Negative	Interpretation unclear; four possibilities:
Anti-HBc	Positive	1 Resolved infection (most common)
Anti-HBs	Negative	2 False-positive anti-HBc, thus susceptible
		3 "Low level" chronic infection
		4 Resolving acute infection

(HBc: hepatitis B core antibody; HBsAg: hepatitis B surface antigen)

How to manage, if only male partner is affected?

Postexposure prophylaxis for susceptible pregnant women depends upon:

- HBsAg status of the source
- Vaccination and anti-HBs response status of the pregnant woman
- *If a pregnant lady, susceptible to HBV infection, is exposed to a person who has acute hepatitis B infection and sexual contact has occurred within 14 days,* then the lady requires *hepatitis B immunoglobulin (HBIg)*, 0.06 mL/kg, intramuscular and a complete course of HBV vaccine.
- If a pregnant lady is unvaccinated and is exposed to an HBsAg-positive person (sex or needle sharing contact), then also she requires postexposure prophylaxis with HBIg and complete course of hepatitis B vaccine.
- However, if the pregnant lady is previously vaccinated and is exposed to HBsAg, she requires only a booster dose of hepatitis B vaccine.[9]

Hepatitis B vaccine is given in three doses of 1 mL in adults, intramuscularly, at 0, 1, and 6 months. Anti-HBs titer >10 IU/L after 2/3 months is considered protective.[3]

How to manage, if female partner is affected?

Recommendations for screening and vaccination during pregnancy (Flowchart 1):

- Universal screening for hepatitis B is advocated for all pregnant women, regardless of previous testing or vaccination.[4]

Flowchart 1: Screening and referral algorithm for hepatitis B virus (HBV) infection among pregnant women.

HBsAg −

HBsAg (hepatitis B surface antigen)

HBsAg +

- Report HBsAg positive pregnant women to perinatal hepatitis B prevention program
- Identify all household and sexual contacts and recommend screening by primary care provider

Assess if at high risk* for acquiring HBV infection

No

Yes

No further action needed

- Consider vaccination during pregnancy or postpartum
- Repeat HBsAg testing when admitted for delivery

Order additional tests:
- HBeAg (hepatitis B e-antigen)
- HBV DNA concentration
- ALT (alanine aminotransferase)

HBeAg No

HBeAg + or HBV DNA >20,000 IU/mL or ALT ≥19 IU/L

Yes

Refer for care postpartum

Refer to specialist immediately during pregnancy

*High risk for HBV infection includes: Household or sexual contacts of HBsAg-positive persons; injection drug use; more than one sex partner during the past six months; evaluation or treatment for sexually transmitted disease; HIV infection, chronic liver disease, or end-stage renal disease; and international travel to regions with HBsAg prevalence of >2%

U.S. Department of Health and Human Services
Centers for Disease Control and Prevention

The American College of Obstetricians and Gynecologists
WOMEN'S HEALTH CARE PHYSICIANS

Source: Adapted with permission from the Hepatits B Foundation Original publication: Apuzzio J, Block J, Cullison S, et al. Chronic Hepatitis B in pregnancy: A workshop consensus statement on screening, evaluation, and management, part 2. The female patient. 2012;37(5):30–34.

- *All HBsAg-positive women should have household contacts, other children, and other sexual partners screened.[4] Those who are nonimmune or not already infected should be vaccinated* (grade A evidence).

Antenatal management: During the antenatal period, all HBsAg-positive women should have the following tests:

- Complete blood count (CBC), baseline liver function tests, and prothrombin time
- HBeAg/Anti-HBe status to indicate severity of infection
- Total anti-HBc/IgM anti-HBc to diagnose acute or chronic infections
- *HBV DNA level*: All HBsAg-positive women should be tested of HBV DNA, but this can be deferred until third trimester, especially if initial liver function test (LFT) results are normal or results prior to pregnancy are unavailable.[10]

Women with high viral load in the third trimester (28–32 weeks) with HBV DNA > 200,000 IU/mL or >106 copies/mL or 6 log copies/mL *should be offered antiviral therapy to reduce the viral load prior to delivery and to decrease the risk of mother to child transmission.*[8] Similarly, those women with chronic HBV infection should also receive antiviral therapy in the third trimester.

World Health Organization recommends the use of oral treatment—tenofovir or entecavir, because these are most potent drugs to suppress hepatitis B virus. They rarely lead to drug resistance as compared with other drugs, are simple to take (1 pill a day), and have fewer side-effects and so require only limited monitoring. Of these, however, *entecavir is not indicated during pregnancy and tenofovir is the recommended first-line antiviral drug to be used in pregnancy.*[11] It is a category B drug given in dose of 300 mg/day. However, in most people, the treatment does not cure hepatitis B infection, but only suppresses the replication of the virus. Therefore, most people who start treatment must continue it lifelong.[1]

Intrapartum management: Hepatitis B infection should not alter the mode of delivery and cesarean section should be reserved for usual obstetric indications.[3]

Invasive procedures like fetal scalp electrodes and fetal blood sampling during labor should be avoided.

Postpartum management and immunoprophylaxis to the neonate:
- Universal precautions related to handling of blood and body fluid should be observed.
- In addition to routine vaccination, infants born to HBsAg-positive mothers should receive passive immunization with HBIg (0.5 mL intramuscular) at birth, preferably within 12 hours and certainly within 48 hours.
- Anti-HBs antibody and HBsAg levels should be measured in infants born to mothers of chronic hepatitis B infection at least 3–12 months after completing the primary vaccination course.[3] Absence of HBsAg and presence of anti-HBs indicate that the child is protected.
- The Indian National Guidelines for diagnosis and management of viral hepatitis suggests that if the baby needs to be tested for hepatitis B, this should be done only after 1 year of age. Any positivity before this age is difficult to interpret and may resolve spontaneously over time.[11]

Breastfeeding: A mother who has hepatitis B may breastfeed her baby, unless there is an exuding injury or disease of the nipple or surrounding skin. The advantages of breastfeeding far outweigh the risk, if any, of transmission of hepatitis B to a baby who has received hepatitis B vaccine.[11]

Breastfeeding is also not contraindicated even in those cases where mother is receiving tenofovir (grade B evidence).

TAKE HOME MESSAGE

- Universal screening of pregnant women for HBsAg during each pregnancy
- Screening all HBsAg-positive pregnant women for HBV DNA to guide the use of maternal antiviral therapy during pregnancy. Maternal antiviral therapy to be started when HBV DNA is >200,000 IU/mL.

- All HBsAg-positive patients should have their partners and other household members screened and vaccinated, if they are HBsAg negative.
- Hepatitis B in a pregnant woman is not a reason for considering termination of pregnancy.
- Similarly, cesarean delivery is reserved for obstetric indications only.
- Provision of immunoprophylaxis for infants born to infected mothers, including hepatitis B vaccine and hepatitis B immunoglobulin within 12 hours of birth
- Routine vaccination of all infants with the hepatitis B vaccine series, with the first dose administered within 24 hours of birth
- Breastfeeding is not contraindicated in HBsAg-positive mothers.

REFERENCES

1. World Health Organization. (2019). Hepatitis B. [online] Available from: https://www.who.int/news-room/fact-sheets/detail/hepatitis-b. [Last accessed June, 2020].
2. Ray G. Current scenario of Hepatitis B and its treatment in India. J Clin Transl Hepatol. 2017;5(3):277-96.
3. Sheshadri L, Arjun G. Hepatitis B: Hepatobiliary and Gastrointestinal Disorders. Essent Obstet. 2016;780-1.
4. RANZCOG. (2016). Management of Hepatitis B in pregnancy. [online] Available from: https://ranzcog.edu.au/RANZCOG_SITE/media/RANZCOG-MEDIA/Women%27s%20Health/Statement%20and%20guidelines/Clinical-Obstetrics/Management-of-Hepatitis-B-in-pregnancy-(C-Obs-50).pdf?ext=.pdf. [Last accessed June, 2020].
5. Mahoney FJ, Kane M. Hepattis B vaccine. In: Plotkin SA, Orenstein WA (Eds). Vaccines, 3rd edition. Philadelphia, Pa: WB Saunders Company; 1999. pp. 158-82.
6. Hollinger FB, Liang TJ. Hepatitis B Virus. In: Knipe DM, Howley PM, Griffin DE, Lamb RA, Martin MA, Roizman B, Straus SE (Eds). Fields Virology, 4th edition. Philadelphia, Pa: Lippincott Williams & Wilkins; 2001. pp. 2923-69.
7. Robinson WS. Hepatitis B virus and hepatitis D virus. Principles and practice of infectious diseases, 4th edition. New York, NY: Churchill Livingstone; 1995. pp. 1406-39.
8. Centre for Disease Control and Prevention. (2015). Perinatal Transmission. [online] Available from: www.cdc.gov/hepatitis/hbv/perinatalxmtn.htm#section1. [Last accessed June, 2020].
9. Perinatology.com. (2015). Hepatitis B in pregnancy. [online] Available from: http://perinatology.com/exposures/Infection/HepatitisB.htm#:~:text=%22The%20rate%20of%20neonatal%20hepatitis,be%20as%20high%20as%2016%25. [Last accessed June, 2020].
10. Dionne–Odom J. Hepatitis B in pregnancy screening, treatment, and prevention of vertical transmission. Am J Obstet Gynecol. 2015;(15):121-44.
11. Ministry of Health and Family Welfare, Government of India. (2018). National Guidelines for Diagnosis and Management of Viral Hepatitis. [online] Available from: https://www.inasl.org.in/diagnosis-management-viral-hepatitis.pdf. [Last accessed June, 2020].

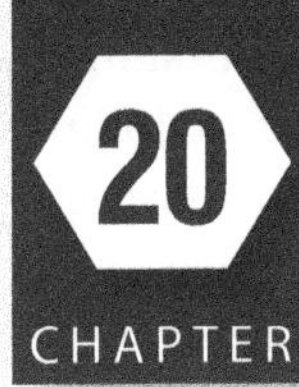

HIV-positive Discordant Couple

Madhuri Chandra

INTRODUCTION

Human immunodeficiency virus (HIV)/acquired immunodeficiency syndrome (AIDS) is one of the world's most dreaded and challenging infections. Since the first reported case in 1981, about 35.4 million people have died from AIDS-related illnesses.[1] HIV infects cells of the immune system and results in the progressive deterioration of the immune system, breaking down the body's ability to fend off infections and other diseases. Without treatment, HIV infection may progress to an advanced disease stage, known as AIDS or acquired immunodeficiency syndrome, with opportunistic infections or related cancers. The risk of HIV infection is more among men who have sex with men, people who inject drugs, transgender, and female sex workers.

In 2017, globally, there were 36.9 million people living with HIV, of which 75% were aware of their status and 21.7 million or 59% of people living with HIV were receiving antiretroviral treatment.[1] 80% of pregnant women living with HIV had access to antiretroviral medicines to prevent transmission of HIV to their babies.[1] New infections and deaths related to HIV infections have reduced drastically. Advances in HIV prevention and access to antiretroviral therapy have resulted in HIV-positive persons living longer and healthier lives.

In India, there are estimated 2.1 million people living with HIV, of which 0.88 million are women. 79% known their HIV status and 56% PLHIV are receiving first-line antiretroviral therapy (ART).[2] The policy has recently been modified to treat all HIV-positive with ART regardless of CD4 count.

SERODISCORDANT COUPLES

"Sero" for blood serum and "discordant" meaning different, hence, serodiscordant couples are those with differing HIV status. One partner is HIV positive, while other is HIV negative. The majority of people living in stable relationships are unaware of their partner's status, and many people with an HIV-positive partner are not aware of their own status.[3] There is possibility that this unawareness may lead to HIV transmission to uninfected partner or to an infant born from the relationship. Discordant couples are now recognized as a priority for HIV interventions, HIV counseling, and testing. Couples must be counseled together and in one-to-one sessions regarding reproductive and sexual health matters. Sessions must include safe sex practices, use of contraceptives, adherence to ART, and pre-exposure prophylaxis (PrEP). Their reproductive desires and options must be discussed along with the correct time to conceive keeping in view their viral load status.

Serodiscordant Couple in Reproductive Age not Desiring Pregnancy

Couple HIV Testing and Counseling

Couples now in a long-term relationship, who have had high risk behavior in past or are desirous of starting a family are advised to undergo couple HIV testing and counseling (CHTC).[3] This approach encourages mutual disclosure, eases tension, and tendency to a blame game. CHTC helps the counselor to share information about prevention and treatment and check understanding of the couple. It encourages joint decision making and adherence to ART and has proved a success in prevention of parent-to-child transmission (PPTCT) programs. HTC (HIV testing and counseling) should also be offered to all partners of people with known HIV positivity.

Antiretroviral Therapy

People with HIV in serodiscordant couples and who are started on ART (antiretroviral therapy) for their own health should be advised that ART is also recommended to reduce HIV transmission to the uninfected partner.[3] HIV-positive partners with CD4 count >350 cells/μL in serodiscordant couples should be offered ART to reduce HIV transmission to uninfected partners.[3] The HPTN 052 randomized controlled trial found a 96% reduction in HIV transmission in serodiscordant couples where the partner with HIV with a CD4 count between 350 and 500 cells/μL had started ART early.[3]

Condoms

Consistent and correct use of male and female condoms to prevent acquisition of other sexually transmitted infections (STIs) and transmission of HIV is advocated.

Screen for STI and Reproductive Tract Infections

Reproductive tract infection (RTI) and genital tract inflammation increase the risk of viral shedding and HIV transmission. Ulcerative STI, e.g., syphilis, also increase the risk of HIV transmission. Testing and prompt treatment of RTI and STIs are advised to prevent HIV acquisition and transmission.

Contraception

While barrier contraceptives are adequate in prevention of HIV transmission, women who do not desire pregnancy are advised to additionally use

TABLE 1: Drug interaction antiretrovirals (ARVs) and hormonal contraceptives.[4]

Contraceptive	ARV drug	Possible interaction effect
Combined oral contraceptives (COCs)	Protease inhibitor (PI) Efavirenz (EFV)	↓Contraceptive efficacy
	Elvitegravir/cobicistat	↓Contraceptive efficacy
Injectable contraceptive (DMPA)	EFV, lopinavir/ritonavir (LPV/r), nevirapine (NVP), nelfinavir, or NRTI	No significant interaction
Contraceptive implants (etonogestrel)	EFV	Contraceptive failure
Contraceptive implants (levonorgestrel)	EFV	Decreased bioavailability of levonorgestrel
	NVP and LPV/r	No change
Use effective contraception	Dolutegravir	Risk of teratogenicity and neural tubal defects. Avoid, if trying for pregnancy and in first 12 weeks of pregnancy

(NRTI: nucleoside reverse transcriptase inhibitor)

hormonal contraception. There are some studies reporting an increased risk of HIV acquisition with use of hormonal contraception, linked to a higher genital HIV RNA concentration in women using hormonal contraception (mostly injectable DMPA). However, WHO recommends use of all existing hormonal contraceptive methods without restriction.[4] Intrauterine contraceptive devices (IUCDs) appear to be a safe and effective contraceptive option for individuals with HIV.[4] Drug interaction between hormonal contraceptives and antiretroviral (ARV) drugs may decrease the efficacy of either with reduced contraceptive efficacy or increased risk of adverse effects **(Table 1)**. However, these concerns should not prevent prescribing the hormonal contraceptives to individuals who prefer this contraceptive method. The potential association of hormonal contraception use and HIV transmission, in the absence of ART, underscores the importance of ART-induced viral suppression to reduce transmission risk.[4]

Pre-exposure Prophylaxis

Pre-exposure prophylaxis or PrEP with ARVs (oral tenofovir or tenofovir plus emtricitabine) taken by HIV-negative partner in serodiscordant couples and by men who have sex with men helps to prevent sexual acquisition of HIV.[5]

Male Circumcision

Circumcision helps to prevent HIV transmission from females to their uninfected male partners.

Infection Prevention

Test the HIV-positive partner for tuberculosis and opportunistic infection. Vaccination against hepatitis B, HPV, influenza, Tdap (tetanus, diphtheria, and pertussis), meningococcal, and pneumococcal infection is advised for the couple.

Serodiscordant Couple in Reproductive Age-desiring Pregnancy

Serodiscordant couples should be informed about importance of adhering to ART to achieve maximal viral suppression of positive partner before considering pregnancy. They should be advised to practice consistent and correct use of condoms to avoid sexual transmission of HIV while attempting conception. Interventions include screening and treating both partners for STIs, use of PrEP by the partner without HIV, male circumcision and self-insemination with the semen of male partner without HIV during the periovulatory period, in case of HIV-positive women.[4]

Female Partner HIV Positive, Male Partner Negative

In case of HIV-positive female with HIV-negative man, preconception counseling with emphasis on adherence to ART to achieve maximal viral suppression in order to avoid HIV transmission to partner and child. The use of barrier contraceptives, improvement of general health, folic acid supplements, screening, and treatment of RTIs and STIs are necessary. They should maintain a monogamous relationship. The male partner undergoes HTC, is advised circumcision, and may be offered PrEP.

If the HIV-positive partner has achieved undetectable plasma viral load on ART, sexual intercourse without a condom limited to the 2–3 days before and the day of ovulation (peak fertility) is not associated with a risk of sexual HIV transmission to the partner without HIV.[5]

However, if maximal viral suppression is not achieved or the HIV viral load status is not known PrEP with oral tenofovir, or tenofovir and emtricitabine, 1 month prior to and 1 month after attempt at conception is recommended.[5] Expecting the periovulatory (fertile period), they should continue consistent and correct use of condoms for the rest of the month. HIV-negative partner should be tested for HIV every 3 months while attempting conception without condoms.

To further decrease the risk of HIV transmission, assisted or self-insemination of semen from male partner during the periovulatory phase is advised.

Once pregnant, she should be shifted to the PPTCT program.

Male Partner HIV Positive, Female Partner Negative

The coupe is advised to use condoms; male partner should achieve maximum viral suppression on ART and maintain a monogamous relationship. Both partners should be screened and treated for genital tract infections before attempting to conceive.

For conception, the options available are:

- If maximum viral suppression is achieved on ART, sexual intercourse without condom in the periovulatory phase with consistent correct use of condoms for the rest of the month is advised.
- When the partner living with HIV has not been able to achieve viral suppression or when the viral status is not known, PrEP to the partner without HIV is recommended to reduce the risk of sexual transmission of HIV.[5]
- When the man is living with HIV, the use of donor sperm from a man without HIV is an option for conception that eliminates the risk of HIV transmission to the partner without HIV.[5]
- Intrauterine insemination (IUI) of washed semen sample from male partner is also considered to decrease risk of transmission.

In cases where conception fails to occur over a 6-month period, workup for infertility including semen analysis is required. HIV and possibly ART may be associated with a higher prevalence of sperm abnormalities, such as low sperm count, low motility, a higher rate of abnormal forms, and low semen volume.[5]

During Pregnancy

Serodiscordant couples with HIV-positive female should be encouraged to seek antenatal care services early and register for PPTCT.

Pregnant serodiscordant women with HIV-positive partners should be offered HIV counseling and testing. Women who are tested HIV seropositive should receive appropriate evaluation and interventions to reduce perinatal transmission of HIV, including immediate initiation of appropriate ART.[5] She should maintain optimal viral suppression, throughout pregnancy in order to prevent vertical transmission to fetus and newborn.

Women who are tested HIV seronegative and have partners who are living with HIV should be counseled regarding consistent condom use. Condom use during pregnancy should be continued because of increased risk of HIV acquisition during pregnancy. Fresh acquisition of HIV in pregnancy or lactation by mother has maximum risk of vertical or perinatal transmission to baby.

They should also be counseled on the importance of their partner's adherence to ART and the need for achievement of sustained viral suppression by partner.[5] HIV testing must be repeated at least once in every trimester.

◼ REFERENCES

1. UNAIDS. (2019). Fact Sheet—World AIDS Day 2019. [online] Available from: https://www.unaids.org/sites/default/files/media_asset/UNAIDS_FactSheet_en.pdf. [Last accessed June, 2020].
2. World Health Organization. (2019). HIV AIDS Data and Statistics, HIV Country Profile India. [online] Available from: https://cfs.hivci.org/country-factsheet.html. [Last accessed June, 2020].

3. World Health Organization. (2012). Guidance on couples HIV testing and counselling including antiretroviral therapy for treatment and prevention in serodiscordant couples: recommendations for a public health approach. [online] Available from: https://www.who.int/hiv/pub/guidelines/9789241501972/en/. [Last accessed June, 2020].

4. A Working Group of the Office of AIDS Research Advisory Council; AIDSinfo. (2017). Guidelines for the Use of Antiretroviral Agents in Adults and Adolescents Living with HIV. [online] Available from: https://aidsinfo.nih.gov/contentfiles/AdultandAdolescentGL003510.pdf. [Last accessed June, 2020]

5. A Working Group of the Office of AIDS Research Advisory Council; AIDSinfo. (2014). Recommendations for the Use of Antiretroviral Drugs in Pregnant Women with HIV Infection and Interventions to Reduce Perinatal HIV Transmission in the United States. [online] Available from: https://aidsinfo.nih.gov/contentfiles/perinatalgl003381.pdf. [Last accessed June, 2020].

CHAPTER 21

Interpretation of TORCH Test

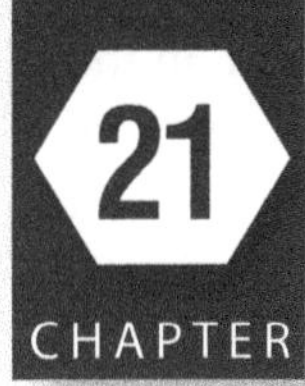

Charmila Ayyavoo

INTRODUCTION

Traditionally, TORCH (toxoplasmosis, rubella, cytomegalovirus, herpes simplex, and other organisms including syphilis, parvovirus, and Varicella zoster) testing was advised for recurrent pregnancy losses, but it is no longer recommended.[1,2]

UNIVERSAL SCREENING

The Federation of Obstetric and Gynecological Societies of India (FOGSI) GCPR guidelines on screening and management of TORCH in pregnancy reviewed in 2014 have made the following recommendations regarding routine universal screening for TORCH infections.[3]

- Routine full "TORCH panel" screening is not recommended in low-risk asymptomatic pregnant women.
- Routine screening for TORCH is unhelpful and should not be done for investigation of recurrent miscarriage; since, TORCH infections are not responsible for recurrent miscarriage.

TORCH PANEL RESULTS

Enzyme-linked immunosorbent assay (ELISA) detects the specific immunoglobulin M (IgM) and IgG antibodies. ELISA tests are the most cost-effective tests.[3] Positive results should be combined with IgG avidity tests. Avidity refers to the strength with which an antibody binds with an antigen. Increasing avidity is due to a progressive maturation of an immune response.

If both IgM and IgG are negative, then the mother is not infected and is also not exposed to the infection.

If IgM is positive and IgG is negative, then the mother is exposed for the first time to the infection. Sometimes, there may be a cross-reaction between organisms, which can cause occurrence of false-positive IgM antibodies. In these cases, a history of fever with rash should be elicited.

If IgG becomes positive with reduced IgM antibodies in a repeat sero-logical testing after 4 weeks, then the mother is interpreted to have suffered from a recent infection.

If IgG antibodies are present and IgM antibodies are absent, it means that the mother had a past infection. The time of occurrence of the maternal infection can be identified by doing the avidity test for that infection. In the early stages of the infection, IgG antibodies show low avidity for the antigen. *A high-avidity report indicates that the infection must have occurred >3 months before. A low-avidity test report is interpreted as an infection of <3 months duration.*

Avidity testing will help in the interpretation of the possibility of vertical transmission to the fetus. A report of high avidity in the first trimester is reassuring as there is reduced chance of any harm to the fetus. A high-avidity report in second or third trimester does not exclude the possibility of a vertical transmission to the fetus.

CLINICAL SITUATIONS WARRANTING TORCH PANEL TESTING

There are certain clinical presentations where TORCH testing is warranted even though routine screening is not advised.[4] They are as follows:

- Pregnant woman is exposed to or is at risk of TORCH infections
- A previously healthy pregnant woman with symptoms of TORCH infections
- A previously healthy pregnant woman with fetal abnormalities identified during routine ultrasound screening
- After delivery, identification of signs consistent with congenital infections in the newborn
- Unexplained intrauterine death and/or stillbirth.

Healthy Pregnant Woman Exposed to Potential TORCH Infections[4]

Toxoplasma Gondii[4]

If the mother is exposed to infection, toxoplasma IgG is tested. IgG develops 2–3 weeks after infection and persists for life. IgM antibodies develop 10 days after infection and usually become negative in 3–4 months. IgM antibodies alone cannot detect acute toxoplasmosis.

If IgG antibodies are present, no further testing is required, if it is only a single exposure.

If not present, repeat testing is done after 4 weeks. If present now, IgM testing is done. If IgM is not detected, no intervention is necessary.

If IgM is detected, IgM is repeated again to confirm and IgG avidity test should be performed.

If the report is high avidity, it is interpreted as infection of >3 months duration. Further testing is needed, if there is a clinical suspicion or there is an abnormality on ultrasound.

If the report is low avidity IgG, it indicates a recent infection.

Polymerase chain reaction (PCR) of amniotic fluid or fetal blood has high sensitivity and specificity for confirmation of vertical transmission and fetal infection.[5]

Presence of intracranial calcifications, hydrocephaly, liver calcifications, ascites, placental thickening, hyperechoic bowel, and growth restriction in ultrasound contributes to the diagnosis.

Rubella or German Measles[4]

Rubella infection is caused by a RNA Togavirus. It usually causes a minor maternal infection. The mother can develop a mild, febrile illness with a generalized maculopapular rash, which begins in the face and spreads to the trunk and extremities. Transmission is through nasopharyngeal secretions.

Diagnosis: Serological analysis will help in diagnosis. If IgG is detected, no further intervention is needed.

If IgG is not detected or the reports are equivocal, oral fluid and blood should be taken from the index patient and rubella virus can be isolated. This will confirm the diagnosis. The mother should now be followed up with the help of a fetal medicine specialist.

Serum IgM antibodies are detected using ELISA 4–5 days after the onset of the clinical illness and they can persist for 6 weeks after onset of rash.[6] Rubella reinfection can cause a transient increase in IgM antibodies.

The IgG avidity testing should be done along with the other antibodies. A high-avidity IgG antibodies report should be interpreted as an infection beyond 2–3 months.

Serological samples are best collected within the first few days of the onset of rash. If the specimen is collected 10 days after the rash, presence of IgG antibodies cannot differentiate between recent disease and past immunity.

Cytomegalovirus[4]

The virus is transmitted through person-to-person contact. Saliva, semen, urine, blood, nasopharyngeal, and cervical secretions can transmit the infection.

Serological testing of both acute and convalescent serum should be done **(Flowchart 1)**. IgM antibody levels will not reflect seroconversion, as they will be elevated for at least 1 year after infection. IgM antibodies can be seen with reactivation of the disease or when there is infection with a new strain.

Avidity testing for IgG antibodies should be performed along with routine testing. If there is high avidity for IgG antibodies, it indicates primary maternal infection >6 months before testing.[7]

Herpes Simplex Virus[4]

The IgM testing is not useful for detection of the disease. Type specific ELISA tests for IgG antibodies should be done to differentiate between the two types of herpes simplex virus (HSV). IgG antibodies are detected 1–2 weeks after a primary infection. The interpretation of IgG antibody and avidity reports will be similar to other TORCH infections.

Flowchart 1: Algorithm for serology in TORCH infections in pregnancy [e.g., *Cytomegalovirus* (CMV)].[4]

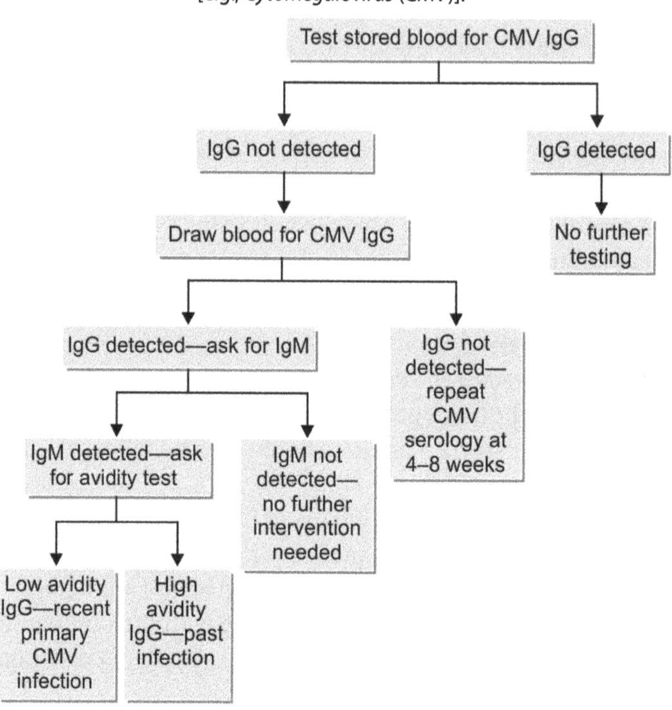

Other Infections in TORCH Group[4]

Varicella zoster virus (VZV): The incubation period is 10–21 days. The infected person is contagious from 1 day before onset of rash until crusting of the lesions.

If a pregnant woman has been exposed to an infected individual, a history of shingles or rash must be elicited. If there is clinical history, no further testing is required. If there is no clinical finding, blood is checked for VZV IgG. If IgG is detected, no further testing is required. If IgG is not detected, VZIg (varicella zoster immunoglobulin) should be administered within 10 days of exposure.

Parvovirus B19 (slapped cheek syndrome):[4] The mode of transmission is by respiratory or hand-to-mouth contact. The disease is also called erythema infectiosum or fifth disease.

- If a pregnant woman is exposed to the disease, blood should be checked for IgG and IgM.
- If IgG is detected and IgM is not detected, no further testing is required.
- If IgG and IgM are detected, serology should be repeated and *Parvovirus B19* DNA testing is done.
- If IgG and IgM are not detected, blood tests should be repeated after 4 weeks for evidence of seroconversion.

All pregnant women with recent *Parvovirus B19* infection should be followed up by a fetal medicine specialist.

Measles:[4] Transmission of the virus is by respiratory droplets. Measles does not cause a congenital syndrome. It is associated with an increased risk of spontaneous abortion and premature delivery. There is an increased risk of pneumonia, if the disease is acquired in the third trimester and peripartum period. This contributes to an increased morbidity and mortality in the mother.

The clinical illness is characterized by fever, coryza, conjunctivitis, and cough. A erythematous maculopapular rash develops on the face and trunk and spreads to the back, trunk, and extremities. Small white lesions with surrounding erythema called as Koplik spots can be visualized in the oral cavity.

Serology testing in measles:
Immunoglobulin G should be tested. If detected, no further intervention is needed. If IgG is not detected, human normal immunoglobulin (HNIg) should be administered within 6 days. If IgG is equivocal, HNIg should be given within 6 days.

Oral fluid should be collected from the index case and measles IgM and RNA should be done to confirm the diagnosis.

If a pregnant woman is not immune to measles, MMR vaccine should be administered after delivery and at least 3 months after receiving HNG.

Previously Healthy Pregnant Woman with Clinical Illness[4]

Presence of vesicular rash should be checked.

If rash is present, the most likely diagnosis will be VZV infection.

If there is no rash, the consideration will be for a diagnosis of *Measles, Enterovirus, Rubella,* and *Parvovirus* (MERP).

- Blood testing for measles, rubella, and *Parvovirus* IgM should be done.
- Oral fluid should be sent for measles and rubella IgM and RNA.
- Nose and throat swab, stool sample should be sent for *Enterovirus* RNA and culture.

In MERP infection, the following factors should be taken into consideration:

- For measles infection, no specific antiviral treatment is needed. The increased risk for pneumonia in the third trimester should be kept in mind.
- Enterovirus infection does not require any therapy. It is caused by Enterovirus or Coxsackie A virus. The disease is also called hand, foot, and mouth disease. The infection does not cause any congenital disease. But, infection in the first trimester can be associated with an increased risk of miscarriage. Infection in the third trimester can cause vertical transmission to the baby. There is no available serological test to confirm the diagnosis.

- There is no specific treatment for rubella infection in the mother. The patient should be followed up by a fetal medicine specialist.
- *Parvovirus B* infection of the mother does not need any treatment. The pregnancy should be followed up by a fetal medicine specialist with special attention toward monitoring for hydrops fetalis.

If there is rash and varicella is suspected, management will depend on the gestational age of the fetus.

- Infection in the first and early second trimester poses a great risk of acquiring congenital varicella syndrome. The incidence is 1–2%, if infection occurs before 20 weeks of gestation.
- The pregnancy should be followed up by a fetal medicine specialist.
- If infection occurs after 20 weeks or if the mother is immunocompromised, there is an indication for antiviral therapy in the form of acyclovir.
- Varicella zoster immunoglobulin (VZIg) therapy is not needed in treatment of maternal infection.
- Pregnant women have a higher risk for pneumonia particularly in the third trimester.

Pregnant Woman with Abnormalities Detected in Ultrasound[4]

If the abnormalities, which are described in **Table 1**, are identified in ultrasound, serological testing for the particular suspected infections must be done. If infections are confirmed, the pregnancy should be followed up by the fetal medicine specialist.

If suspected syphilis infection, maternal blood should be checked for antibodies to *Treponema pallidum*. If diagnosis is positive, RPR (rapid plasma reagin) should be done. This will be needed to confirm a recent infection. The pregnancy should be followed up by a venereologist.

TABLE 1: Abnormalities detected in ultrasound.

Abnormality in ultrasound	CMV	Parvovirus B19	Rubella	Toxoplasma	Treponema pallidum (syphilis)
Micro- or microcephaly	Yes		Yes	Yes	
IUGR	Yes	Yes	Yes	Yes	Yes
Intracranial calcifications	Yes		Yes	Yes	
Echogenic bowel	yes				
Ventriculomegaly	Yes			Yes	
Structural heart defects			Yes		
Hydrops		Yes			

(CMV: *Cytomegalovirus*; IUGR: intrauterine growth restriction)

TABLE 2: Neonatal abnormalities at birth.

Abnormality at birth	CMV	HSV	Parvovirus B19	Rubella	Toxoplasma	Treponema pallidum	VZV
Hepatitis/ jaundice/ hepatomegaly	Yes	Yes			Yes	Yes	
Rash	Yes	Yes				Yes	Yes
Thrombocytopenia	Yes		Yes			Yes	
Anemia	Yes	Yes	Yes	Yes		Yes	
IUGR	Yes		Yes			Yes	
Microcephaly	Yes			Yes	Yes		
Hydrocephalus	Yes				Yes		
Failed newborn hearing test	Yes						
Patent ductus arteriosus (at term)				Yes			
Intracranial calcification	Yes			Yes	Yes		
Congenital cataracts or microphthalmia				Yes			
Hydrops			Yes			Yes	

(CMV: *Cytomegalovirus*; HSV: herpes simplex virus; IUGR: intrauterine growth restriction; VZV: varicella zoster virus)

Neonatal Abnormalities at Birth[4]

If the neonatal abnormalities, which are given in **Table 2**, are identified at birth, confirmatory further testing for the particular infection should be done in the mother and the neonate. If the results are positive for recent infection, there should be a referral to the infectious diseases specialist.

Intrauterine Death/Stillbirth[8]

Transplacental infections associated with intrauterine fetal death (IUFD) include:

- Cytomegalovirus[9] (evidence level 2+)
- Syphilis[10,11] (evidence level 1+)
- *Parvovirus B19*[12,13] (evidence level 2++)
- *Listeria*[14,15] (evidence level 2+)
- Rubella[16] (evidence level 3)
- Toxoplasmosis[12,17,] (Evidence level 2+)
- Herpes simplex[9] (evidence level 2+)
- *Coxsackievirus, Leptospira,* Q fever, and Lyme disease[18]
- Malaria parasitemia has also been associated with stillbirth[19] (evidence level 2++)

Maternal Serology Testing in IUFD

There could have been occult maternal–fetal transmission of TORCH infections, which can be the reason for the fetal death in utero (Evidence 2+).[9] Blood collected at antenatal booking can be screened for serology of TORCH infections or a serology screening for viral infections can be done within 48 hours of fetal death in maternal blood. This will provide a baseline serology profile.[11-14] The infections, which need to be screened in a case of stillbirth/IUFD, are syphilis, *Parvovirus B19*, rubella (if nonimmune at booking), CMV, herpes simplex, and *Toxoplasma gondii* as a routine measure.

Fetal and Placental Tissue Testing (Evidence 2+)[12,13]

Testing in fetus and placenta for infections is more informative than maternal microbiology[3] and serology for detecting viral infections. The sample for testing is either fetal cord blood or cardiac blood (if possible). The samples, which can be utilized are swabs from the fetus and placenta, which should be placed in lithium heparin. Written consent from the parents should be obtained before taking cardiac blood of the fetus for analysis.

TAKE-HOME MESSAGE

For the interpretation of TORCH panel tests, there are certain conditions, which need to be adhered to. These are the following:[4]

- A pregnant woman presenting with the test results or has a diagnosis from another doctor should have a repeat serology testing so that the diagnosis is confirmed. This should be done before any intervention.
- Maternal infection does not automatically mean that the fetus is also infected or affected by the infection.
- The babies born to mothers who had infection during the pregnancy period should be screened at birth to rule out congenital infection.
- False-positive IgM results are not rare in pregnancy. But, all IgM results should not be presumed to be false positive without doing a confirmatory testing.
- Positive and unusual results warrant a detailed discussion with an infectious diseases specialist.

REFERENCES

1. Neu N, Duchon J, Zachariah P. TORCH infections. Clin Perinatol. 2015;42(1): 77-103.
2. Carp HJ. Investigation protocol for recurrent pregnancy loss. Recurrent Pregnancy Loss: Causes, Controversies and Treatment, 2nd edition. New York: CRC Press; 2007. pp. 269-80.
3. Pandit S (2014). Screening and management of TORCH in pregnancy. Reviewed at the Consensus group meeting at Hotel Tunga. [online] Available from: https://www.fogsi.org/wp-content/uploads/2015/11/smtp.pdf [Last accessed June 2020]..

4. Gascun CD, Knowles S. TORCH testing in Obstetrics and Neonatology. National Laboratory Handbook, volume 1. pp. 49-59. [online] Available from: https://www.hse.ie/eng/services/publications/clinical-strategy-and-programmes/guideline-10-torch-testing-in-obstetrics-and-neonatology.pdf [Last accessed June, 2020].

5. Sterkers Y, Pratlong F, Albaba S, Loubersac J, Picot MC, Pretet V, et al. Novel interpretation of molecular diagnosis of congenital toxoplasmosis according to gestational age at the time of maternal infection. J Clin Microbiol. 2012;50(12): 3944-51.

6. Muscat M, Zimmerman L, Bacci S, Bang H, Glismann S, Mølbak K, et al. Toward rubella elimination in Europe: an epidemiological assessment. Vaccine. 2012; 30(11):1999-2007.

7. Kanengisser-Pines B, Hazan Y, Pines G, Appelman Z. High cytomegalovirus IgG avidity is a reliable indicator of past infection in patients with positive IgM detected during the first trimester of pregnancy. J Perinat Med. 2009;37(1):15-8.

8. Royal College of Obstetricians and Gynaecologists (2010). Late Intrauterine Fetal Death [IUFD] and Stillbirth (Green–top Guideline No. 55). [online] Available from: https://www.rcog.org.uk/en/guidelines-research-services/guidelines/gtg55/#:~:text=Update%2026%20July%202011%3A%20The,gestational%20age)%20when%20inducing%20labour [Last accessed June, 2020].

9. Syridou G, Spanakis N, Konstantinidou A, Piperaki E, Kafetzis D, Patsouris E, et al. Detection of *cytomegalovirus, parvovirus B19* and herpes simplex viruses in cases of intrauterine fetal death: association with pathological findings. J Med Virol. 2008;80(10):1776-82.

10. Zhang XM, Zhang RN, Lin SQ, Chen SX, Zheng LY. [Clinical analysis of 192 pregnant women infected by syphilis]. Zhonghua Fu Chan Ke Za Zhi. 2004;39(10):682-6. Article in Chinese.

11. Osman NB, Folgosa E, Gonzales C, Bergström S. Genital infections in the aetiology of late fetal death: an incident case referent study. J Trop Pediatr. 1995;41(5):258-66.

12. Moyo SR, Tswana SA, Nyström L, Bergström S, Blomberg J, Ljungh A. Intrauterine death and infections during pregnancy. Int J Gynaecol Obstet. 1995;51(3):211-8.

13. Tolfvenstam T, Papadogiannakis N, Norbeck O, Petersson K, Broliden K. Frequency of human *parvovirus B19* infection in intrauterine fetal death. Lancet. 2001;357: 1494-7.

14. Smerdon WJ, Jones R, McLauchlin J, Reacher M. Surveillance of listeriosis in England and Wales, 1995–1999. Commun Dis Public Health. 2001;4:188-93.

15. Smith B, Kemp M, Ethelberg S, Schiellerup P, Bruun BG, Gerner Smidt P, et al. Listeria monocytogenes: maternal-foetal infections in Denmark 1994–2005. Scand J Infect Dis. 2009;41:21-5.

16. Andrade JQ, Bunduki V, Curti SP, Figueiredo CA, de Oliveira MI, Zugaib M. Rubella in pregnancy: intrauterine transmission and perinatal outcome during a Brazilian epidemic. J Clin Virol. 2006;35:285-91.

17. Moyo SR, Hägerstrand I, Nyström L, Tswana SA, Blomberg J, Bergström S, et al. Stillbirths and intrauterine infection, histologic chorioamnionitis and micro-biological findings. Int J Gynaecol Obstet. 1996;54(2):115-23.

18. Goldenberg RL, Thompson C. The infectious origins of stillbirth. Am J Obstet Gynecol 2003;189:861-73.

19. Poespoprodjo JR, Fobia W, Kenangalem E, Lampah DA, Warikar N, Seal A, et al. Adverse pregnancy outcomes in an area where multidrug-resistant *Plasmodium vivax* and *Plasmodium falciparum* infections are endemic. Clin Infect Dis. 2008;46:1374-81.

After Glucose Intolerance: What Next?

Susheela Rani

INTRODUCTION

Diabetes is a major health problem in India and has a high prevalence even in pregnancy. Gestational diabetes mellitus (GDM) is defined as glucose intolerance that develops or is first recognized during pregnancy. Owing to the placental hormones that oppose the actions of insulin, pregnancy is apparently a diabetogenic condition. Normally, the pregnant physiology adapts itself to maintain an euglycemic status. However, when this compensation is inadequate, gestational diabetes is unmasked.

It is estimated that the prevalence of GDM is 4 million women at any given time in the Indian population.[1]

At an estimated prevalence rate of 10–14.3% or even higher in women from urban population, the incidence of GDM is expected to increase up to 20%.[2] So, one in every five pregnant woman can be affected by this condition.

A pan-India study conducted by Federation of Obstetric and Gynecological Societies of India (FOGSI) and Diabetes in Pregnancy Study Group in India (DIPSI) showed that about one-third of the pregnant women are diagnosed with GDM during the first trimester and over quarter of them have a history of fetal loss in the previous pregnancies.

According to global statistics, offsprings of either uncontrolled pre-existing or gestational diabetes are 4–8 times more likely to develop diabetes in later life compared to their siblings born to the same parents in a non-GDM pregnancy.[3] However, the effects of pregnancy on diabetes, including fetal and maternal morbidity, are lesser than in cases of pregnancies with pre-existing diabetes mellitus.

It is the need of the hour to address this public health concern with a multipronged approach, which entails defining diagnostic criteria, creating awareness among general population and healthcare providers, training and disseminating information, sensitizing policy makers, and ensuring that the morbidity and mortality to mother and baby are curtailed.

DIAGNOSIS OF GLUCOSE INTOLERANCE

Who?

Universal screening ensures all pregnant women irrespective of presence or absence of any risk factor ought to be screened for diabetes in pregnancy.

Universal screening detects more cases and ensures better maternal and fetal outcomes when compared to selective screening.[4,5]

When?

Screening of pregnant women is done at *first visit/booking* and even if normal, repeated at *24–28* weeks and[6] then may be repeated at *32–34* weeks.[7-9] There should be a gap of at least 4 weeks between the two testings. However, if it has not been ever done, glucose challenge test (GCT) can be done at any time of gestation that a woman presents with. If the woman presents after 28 weeks, a single screening at the time of first visit is sufficient.[6]

How?

A single step testing (endorsed by The Diabetes in Pregnancy Study Group in India and recommended by WHO) involves the 75 g oral GCT.[7,10] Irrespective of the last meal, *GDM* is diagnosed if 2-hour plasma glucose (venous blood sample, GOD–POD method of laboratory estimation) is more than 140 mg/dL. Patients with values between 120 and 140 mg/dL are classified as belonging to gestational glucose intolerance (GGI).[7]

75 g of glucose is dissolved in 300 mL of water and is to be consumed over 5 minutes. The test is done irrespective of the last meal and woman need not be fasting. If vomiting occurs within 30 minutes of ingestion, the test has to be repeated. However, the test can continue, if the woman vomits 30 minutes after drinking glucose.[7]

If premeasured 75 g of glucose is not available, 5-level teaspoons (not heaped teaspoons) of glucose from 100 g glucose packet may be used.

The rationale for doing the test in nonfasting state is that glucose concentrations are affected little by the time since the last meal in a normal glucose tolerant woman unlike in a woman with GDM.[10] Normal pregnant physiology ensures brisk and appropriate insulin response after a meal or glucose load; whereas in GDM, the glucose levels increase after a meal and further exaggerate after a glucose load.

Terminology and Definitions

Glycemic criteria for diagnosis of different categories of glucose intolerance by 75 g, 2-h oral glucose challenge test (OGCT) are discussed in **Table 1**.[7,10]

Glycemic cutoff for impaired glucose tolerance (IGT) outside pregnancy is the same for diagnosis of GDM.[7] Hence, the term IGT is to be used outside pregnancy and not for any abnormality occurring during pregnancy.

Patients with values between 120 and 140 mg/dL are classified as belonging to GGI.[7]

Advantages of this method include:
- Patient need not be fasting and hence can be done at the time of antenatal visit.
- It is both a screen as and a diagnostic test.

TABLE 1: Glycemic criteria for diagnosis of different categories of glucose intolerance by 75 g, 2-h oral glucose challenge test.

Criteria	FPG (mg/dL)	2-h PG (mg/dL)
Normal glucose tolerance	<100	<140
Impaired fasting glucose	100–125	—
Impaired glucose tolerance	—	140–199
Diabetes mellitus	≥126 and/or	≥200

(FPG: fasting plasma glucose; PG: plasma glucose)

- Recognizing GGI is important as fetal morbidity and macrosomia can occur when 2-h postprandial sugars are 120–140 mg/dL also. These women need follow-up.[9]
- In limited resource settings, the GOI recommends testing with calibrated glucometer with the same reference values as above.[6]

If the 2-h glucose is over 200 mg/dL in the early weeks of pregnancy, she may be a case of pre-existing diabetes mellitus and glycosylated hemoglobin (HbA1c) of over 6 is confirmatory.[11]

Glycosylated Hemoglobin

This reflects the average blood glucose level over the last 3 months. Normal HbA1c during pregnancy is 5.3–6.[11]

The HbA1c level will be helpful to differentiate between a pregestational diabetic and GDM when impaired glucose metabolism is diagnosed early in pregnancy. If more than 6%, it indicates that the patient is likely to be pre-existing diabetic than GDM.[11]

Though HbA1c is useful in monitoring the glucose control during pregnancy and might be of prognostic value, it cannot be helpful in day-to-day management.

Postpartum Screening

The 75-g OGCT is performed 6 weeks after delivery.[6]

Cutoff for normal plasma and abnormal blood sugar levels for the 75-g OGCT are:

- *Fasting blood sugar (FBS):* ≥126 mg/dL
- *2-h blood sugar:*
  - Normal: <140 mg/dL
  - IGT: 140–199 mg/dL
  - Diabetes: ≥200 mg/dL.

Rationale for Recognizing and Treating GDM/GGI

Abnormal glucose metabolism not only impacts the current and future health of the mother and fetus, but also places a strain on the family, society, and finances, if it is not duly recognized and managed appropriately.

Risks for the mother with GDM:[6]
- Polyhydramnios
- Pre-eclampsia
- Prolonged labor
- Instrumental delivery and cesarean section
- Obstructed labor and shoulder dystocia
- Uterine atony and postpartum hemorrhage (PPH)
- Infections
- Future risk of type 2 diabetes

Risks to the baby:[6]
- Spontaneous miscarriage
- Fetal malformations
- Intrauterine death and stillbirth
- Shoulder dystocia and birth injuries
- Large for gestation with attended complications
- Respiratory distress syndrome
- Future risk of diabetes and obesity.

■ MANAGEMENT CHALLENGES POSED BY GDM/GGI

Gestational glucose intolerance/GDM poses the following challenges:
- Education about diet, nutrition, and exercises, self-monitoring of glucose, awareness of hypoglycemia, and ensuring compliance
- Initiating drug therapy [insulin or oral hypoglycemics (OHGs)] when diet and exercise are insufficient
- Monitoring for euglycemia and fetal well-being with appropriate fetal surveillance
- Timing of delivery
- Neonatal management

Various studies have proved that appropriate management of gestational diabetes (nutritional therapy, self-blood glucose monitoring, diet, and/or Insulin) has resulted in reductions in pre-eclampsia, birth weight >4,000 g, and shoulder dystocia.

Guiding Principles in Management of Abnormal OGCT

Gestational diabetes mellitus is best managed with a multidisciplinary team of obstetrician, dietician, diabetologist, diabetes educator, and pediatrician.

A mean plasma glucose level between 105 and 110 mg/dL with fasting sugar around 90 mg/dL and 2-h postprandial sugar around 120 mg/dL has been proven to have the best perinatal outcomes.[12-14]

Medical Nutrition Therapy

All women who test positive for GGI/GDM for the first time should be started on medical nutrition therapy (MNT) for 2 weeks. This includes women with GGI whose plasma sugar values after GCT are 120–139 mg/dL.[6]

Goals of MNT are:
- To ensure adequate nutrition for the mother and fetus
- To ensure sufficient calories for appropriate maternal weight gain
- To help to maintain normal blood sugar levels and hence prevent complications
- To avoid ketosis
- To minimize insulin/American Diabetes Association (ADA) requirement

After 2 weeks on MNT, a 2-h postprandial sugar should be done. If this is <120 mg/dL, it must be repeated once in 2 weeks in the second trimester and once a week in third trimester. MNT may be continued, if the desired sugar levels are achieved.

If, however, when the fasting glucose is over 90 mg/dL and/or the 2-h postprandial glucose is ≥120 mg/dL; medical management (insulin therapy preferably or oral hypoglycemics) has to be started as per guidelines.

Education about Diet, Nutrition, and Exercises[6,10,15]

Meal plan guidelines: Not to skip a meal—
- Three meal + 3 snack pattern with not more than 2½–3-h interval between meals
- *Breakfast to include low glycemic food:* Splitting the breakfast into two equal portions and consuming them at a gap of 2 h ensures that peak sugar levels are avoided after a complete meal. The rationale for splitting breakfast is that that the peaking of plasma glucose is high with breakfast (due to dawn phenomenon) than with lunch or dinner. In normal persons, the secretion of insulin is higher after breakfast than with lunch or dinner, but this is impaired in GDM. Hence, to match this deficiency, the challenge of quantity of food at one time must be avoided.
- Millets are better choices while nonvegetarians must opt for leaner cuts of meat.
- *Caloric requirements:*

Generally, women in reproductive age group have a caloric requirement between 1,900–2,800 kcal/day depending on weight and activity **(Table 2)**.

There is no increase in calories recommended in first trimester. An increase of 340 kcal/day over the normal requirements in second trimester and around 450 kcal/day over the normal requirements in third trimester is often recommended.

TABLE 2: Caloric requirement of women in reproductive age group depending on weight and activity.

Level of activity	Energy requirement during pregnancy (kcal/day)	Total energy requirement (kcal/day)
Sedentary work	1,900+350	2,250
Moderate work	2,230+350	2,580
Heavy work	2,850+350	3,200

The general increase in caloric recommendations for GDM pregnancy is:

- If body weight is ideal: 30 kcal/day
- For overweight women: 22–25 kcal/day
- For underweight women: 35–40 kcal/day
- For morbidly obese: 12–14 kcal/day

  Obese women should consume a minimum of 1,800 kcal/day to prevent ketosis.

- *The right diet should contain*:
  - A low-carbohydrate (60–65%) meal with 20–25% proteins and 10–15% fats achieves good glycemic control.
  - "My Plate Planner"—half a plate of vegetables, quarter plate of carbohydrates, and quarter of proteins.
  - *Choice of carbohydrates*: Complex carbohydrates (millet/whole grain cereals such as oats, bajra, jowar, ragi, whole pulses, vegetables, and fruits with skin) have fiber-rich bran layer and are slow to digest. Hence, they do not cause sudden rise of glucose levels. Millets and small grains are rich in fiber and are considered as nutri-rich cereals. Sugars and sweet foods and those made from refined flour are simple carbohydrates (white bread, cakes, naan, puddings, pizza, juice, soft drinks, etc.) and are best avoided, as they cause a spike in the sugars. Artificial sweeteners can be used as sugar substitutes in moderation (3–4 servings per day).
  - *Proteins*: Pregnancy demands an additional 23 g/day of protein over and above the routine requirements in order to allow for fetal growth. Milk and milk products, meat, seafoods, eggs, poultry, and pulses and legumes are good sources of protein. One protein food in each meal flattens the glycemic response and hence every meal ought to contain one protein food. Hence, three servings of proteins are required every day to meet the demands in pregnancy.
  - *Fats*: Saturated fats are ghee, butter, coconut and palm oil, red meat, organ meat, etc. The saturated fats must constitute less than 10% of total calories and the dietary cholesterol must be <300 mg/dL.

    Fried food is calorie dense and causes a sudden surge in sugar levels and is hence best avoided. Using less fat in cooking, low-fat dairy products instead of whole milk or cream, lean meat instead of red meat ensure that the fat content in meals is kept at the desire levels. High-fat snacks like pastries, fried foods, cakes may be substituted with low-fat snacks like fresh fruits, baked and steam food.

    Cooking method also matters. While steaming, boiling, roasting, and grilling with less fat are good, deep-frying with oil, sugar, and cream dressing make the food unhealthy.

    Use of color signals for food to demarcate healthy from unhealthy is used to educate women and their families about diet **(Fig. 1)**.

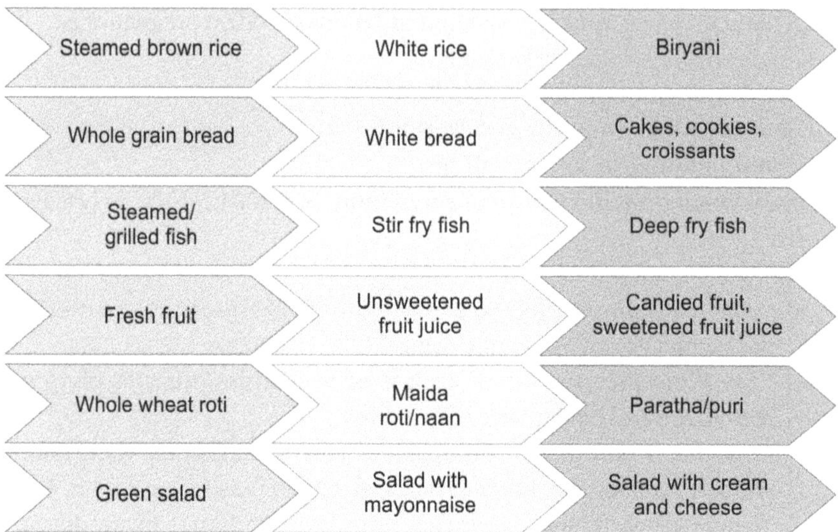

Fig. 1: Signal System: An empowering tool for healthy food choices. *Courtesy*: Kavita Kapur and Anil Kapur, Diabetes Voice, 2005.

- *Fibers*: Foods rich in fibers delay the gastric emptying time, slow the entry of glucose into blood, and reduce the postprandial surge in glucose. Flax seed, oat bran, dried beans of all peas and lentils (legumes) and pectins from fruits like apples and root vegetables such as carrot are also recommended.

  Fats consumption (in all forms) should not exceed 3–4 teaspoons oil per day, as this is the recommended dose. The rate of weight gain may be slowed down in the obese and overweight women who adopt lower-fat diet.

Exercises

Exercise increases muscle mass to improve glycemic control primarily from increased tissue sensitivity to insulin. Hence, both fasting and postprandial blood glucose concentrations can be reduced. Moderate exercise should be a part of the treatment plan for women with GDM, if there are no medical or obstetrical contraindications to this level of physical activity **(Table 3)**.

Glucose Monitoring[6,10]

- Targets recommended by the *Fifth International Workshop-Conference on GDM* include: Fasting <95 mg/dL (5.3 mmol/L) and either 1-h postprandial <140 mg/dL (7.8 mmol/L) or 2-h postprandial <120 mg/dL (6.7 mmol/L).
- Self-monitoring with a calibrated glucometer is recommended, as it obviates the need for repeated laboratory visits and gives the woman a sense of being in control.

TABLE 3: Ideal weight gain in pregnancy.

Prepregnancy weight	BMI (kg/m²)	Total weight gain range
Underweight	<18.5	12.5–18 kg
Normal weight	18.5–24.9	11.5–16 kg
Over weight	25–29.9	7–11.5 kg
Obese (Class I, II, and III)	≥30	5–9 kg

BMI: body mass index

- *Frequency of monitoring*: There is yet no optimal approach. At the initial diagnosis, fasting and 2-h blood sugars after each meal (breakfast, lunch, and dinner) are done.

  Blood glucose must be measured on awakening and after meals throughout pregnancy because fasting and preprandial glucose levels alone may not predict the need for insulin therapy. Postprandial blood glucose can be measured 1 or 2 hours after the beginning of each meal.

  Frequency of testing can be reduced when good glycemic control is achieved. Continuous glucose monitoring or pre- and postprandial monitoring after every meal has been shown to better pregnancy outcomes in some studies but more research is needed to validate this stand.
- Glycosylated hemoglobin (HbA1c) may be a helpful ancillary test in assessing glycemic control during pregnancy, but it is not clear how often it should be monitored in women with apparently well-controlled GDM.
- Monitoring for ketonuria—not routinely recommended in GDM.

Pharmacologic Therapy

When euglycemia is not achieved with MNT, medications must be started. The two pharmacologic options in GDM are insulin (and some insulin analogs) and selected oral antihyperglycemic agents (metformin and glyburide).

Society guidelines differ regarding the first choice of medications. American guidelines prefer insulin as the treatment of choice and OHGs reserved for women who refuse or are noncompliant with insulin. National Institute for Health and Care Excellence (NICE) guidelines (UK) and International Federation of Gynecology and Obstetrics (FIGO), however, recommend the use of OHGs as the first line of choice for some women with GDM, e.g., women with low-fasting blood glucose levels, as oral agents are more likely to prevent hyperglycemia in them.

International Federation of Gynecology and Obstetrics recommends insulin as the first-line treatment in:

- Women in whom diabetes is diagnosed before 20 weeks of gestation.
- Pharmacologic therapy is needed >30 weeks.
- Fasting blood glucose is >110 mg/dL (6.1 mmol/L).
- 1-hour postprandial glucose is >140 mg/dL (7.8 mmol/L).
- Pregnancy weight gain is >12 kg.

Insulin Therapy[6,9,10,12,13]

- *Initiation*: When MNT and exercises are insufficient to control sugars, it is the time for pharmacotherapy with insulin being the first choice.
- *General principles*:
  - Women with GDM often require less than 20 units per day but women with type 1 and type 2 DM may require more.
  - Insulin dosages have to be individualized and adjusted according to glucose levels and there is no fixed dosage for a weight or period of gestation.
  - A drop in insulin requirements may indicate increased utilization of maternal glucose by the supercharged beta cells of macrosomic fetus or placental insufficiency.
  - MNT must be continued along with insulin therapy also.
- *Dosing*: Insulin requirement is variable and depends on weight, ethnic characteristics, degree of hyperglycemia, and other demographic criteria. Also, the dose and type of insulin used is calculated based upon the specific abnormality of blood glucose noted during monitoring.

  Often women are started on premix insulin 30/70. The total insulin dosage per day can be divided as two-thirds in the morning and one-third in the evening. Insulin can be started as 4 units before breakfast with an increment of 2 units every 4th day until 10 units are reached. If the fasting glucose remains over 90 mg/dL, 6 units before breakfast and 4 units before dinner may be given.

  If the 2-h postprandial sugar is over 200 mg/dL at diagnosis, a starting dose of 8 units of premixed insulin before breakfast can be initiated immediately.

  Normally, a total insulin dose of 0.7–2 units per kg (present pregnant weight) achieves glucose control. Slightly lower doses maybe needed in early pregnancy.

  Further as a rough guide, if glucose elevations are mostly postprandial, then a starting dose of 10–20 units of intermediate-acting insulin and 6–10 units of rapid-acting insulin are prescribed in the morning before breakfast, based on the degree of elevations. If diabetes is diagnosed early in pregnancy, slightly lower doses are used.

  If the postdinner glucose level is elevated, then an additional injection of rapid-acting insulin is given just prior to dinner. If fasting glucose is elevated, the intermediate-acting insulin is preferably given at bedtime or before dinner.
- *Self-monitoring of glucose*: Hospitalization or laboratory visits is not required and the patient is taught to monitor glucose with the help of glucometers and document the results for future consultations.
- *Self-administering insulin*: Using insulin pens with suitable cartridges ensures compliance, self-dependence, and even easy adjustments of dosage, if the patient is well-educated about it.

- *Awareness and management of hypoglycemia*: Hypoglycemia in pregnancy is defined as a blood glucose <60 mg/dL and is rare in GDM.
  The woman and her family must be educated to recognize early symptoms of hypoglycemia that include tremors, sweating, palpitations, irritability, and discomfort. Hypoglycemia is a potentially dangerous situation especially in early pregnancy when she has nausea and vomiting. The woman is advised to take in 2 tablespoons sugar or 10–20 g of a mixed protein and carbohydrate snack immediately. 8 ounces or 230–240 mL of skim or low fat milk may also be taken to counter hypoglycemia. The sugars in milk release more slowly into the bloodstream than those in juice or white sugar.
- *Insulin analogs*: The three rapid-acting insulin analogs (lispro, aspart, and glulisine) are comparable in immunogenicity to human regular insulin. Aspart (NovoRapid) and Lispro (Humalog) have been found to be safe and effective in achieving targeted postprandial glucose values. They have been investigated in pregnancy and have been shown to have acceptable safety profiles. Long-acting insulin analogs (insulin glargine and insulin detemir) have not been studied extensively in pregnancy.

Oral Hypoglycemic Agents[6,10]

Metformin: Metformin is an insulin sensitizer and may be used when MNT has failed to control blood sugars. Started at a dose of 500 mg/day, a maximum of 2 g can be given. If sugars are not controlled with MNT and metformin, insulin injections need to be started.

There is yet no consensus, if metformin has to be continued in euglycemic patients if the woman was on metformin before pregnancy because of polycystic ovarian syndrome (PCOS). However, incidence of hypoglycemia and weight gain is less with metformin when compared with insulin. Metformin has also been shown to reduce the incidence of pregnancy-associated hypertension. Metformin, however, crosses the placenta with higher concentrations in fetus than glyburide. The common side effects that can occur with metformin are—diarrhea, nausea, heartburn, and bloating sensation. Lactic acidosis is sometimes a serious side effect, especially in patients with impaired renal functions.

Glyburide is the other OHG drug but is associated with greater incidence of hypoglycemia and hence must be carefully balanced with snacks and meals.

If OHGs cannot achieve euglycemia then supplemental insulin must be added and dual OHGs are not recommended.

ANTENATAL CARE[6]

General Principles

Hyperglycemia detected very early in pregnancy in the first trimester: The following investigations need to be done along with routine investigations done at booking. The rationale is that the patient could be a case of pre-existing diabetes and not just GDM. Such patients merit:

- *HbA1c*: Values >6 suggest pre-existing diabetes
- Blood urea nitrogen (BUN), serum creatinine, and protein-to-creatinine ratio (repeat in each trimester)
- Fundoscopic examination for retinopathy
- Thyroid-stimulating hormone-associated endocrinal deficiency.

Ultrasound

- *Early pregnancy*: Dating scan and for fetal viability, as many women may have previous irregular cycles
- *Combined screening for Down's syndrome*: At 11–14 weeks, an ultrasound for measurement of nuchal translucency (NT) and presence of nasal bone (NB) and the tricuspid regurgitation (TR) with biochemical markers for detection of trisomies 18, 13, and 21
- Fetal anomaly scan at 18–20 weeks
- Fetal cardiac evaluation by scan at 22–24 weeks
- *Growth scans*: As a part of fetal surveillance, growth scans are recommended at 28–30 weeks and repeated at 34–36 weeks.

  However, serial measurements of abdominal circumference and biometry in the third trimester do not improve the prediction of fetal macrosomia. History of a previous large for gestational age (LGA) baby, maternal obesity, and a fasting blood glucose greater than 100 mg/dL at diagnosis of GDM are risk factors for an LGA baby in current pregnancy. When such risk factors exist, but if two serial scans done at 24–27 weeks and 28–31 weeks are normal, we can predict that the newborn would be normal and not macrosomic with a reliability of 79% and the reliability would be a high 94%, if the risk factors are absent.

Challenges in Biochemical Screening for Aneuploidy and Neural Tube Defects in Diabetics

- Median levels of maternal serum α-fetoprotein (MSAFP) are about 15% lower in women with impaired glucose metabolism, but the prevalence of neural tube defect is higher. Hence, a lower threshold of MSAFP value, e.g., 1.5 MoM, is considered for cutoff.
- Levels of MSAFP, unconjugated estriol (uE3), and inhibin A, which are components of some second trimester Down's syndrome screening tests, are significantly reduced in women with diabetes, thereby mimicking the pattern suggestive of Down's syndrome. Hence, MoM values should be adjusted in women with diabetes and interpreted with caution.

Challenges in Ultrasonography

- Increased NT is a marker for congenital heart disease (which can occur in diabetics) as well as for Down's syndrome. Hence, a detailed fetal

echocardiogram must be done at 22–24 weeks even if and especially if the aneuploidy screen is normal.
- Obesity with thick maternal abdomen makes the scans suboptimal.
- *Doppler studies*: Fetal Doppler studies are less reliable as methods of fetal surveillance in diabetics, unless there is an associated fetal growth restriction.

ANTENATAL SURVEILLANCE

Apart from glucose monitoring and adjusting the doses of medications, the patient is assessed for hypertension and anemia. Incidence of urinary tract infections, asymptomatic bacteriuria, may be increased. MNT as per above recommendations is continued with a watch over the weight gain and exercises of the patient.

Growth scans are recommended at 28–30 weeks and again at 34–36 weeks.

Women who have the risk of preterm delivery may be given steroids for fetal lung maturity as per recommendations and under glucose monitoring. Insulin may have to be given for control of glucose over the next 72 hours. Injection dexamethasone 6 mg, intramuscular, every 12th hourly for four doses is recommended.

Timing of Delivery[6,10]

Gestational diabetes mellitus is not an indication for early delivery. Women with well-controlled sugars may be induced at or after 39 weeks, if there are no other confounding risk factors.

However, timing of delivery should be individualized in case of poor control and presence of risks like hypertension, previous intrauterine death, etc.

Route of Delivery

Vaginal delivery is preferred but cesarean is done for other obstetric indications only.

In cases of fetal macrosomia (estimated fetal weight over 4 kg), an elective cesarean section at 39 weeks may be considered in order to avoid shoulder dystocia.

INTRAPARTUM MANAGEMENT

Management includes:
- Obstetric management
- Glycemic management.

Obstetric Management

Diabetes in pregnancy is a high-risk situation. Fetal monitoring needs to be intense. The most dreaded complication in labor is that of shoulder dystocia with its attendant complications both in the mother and in the fetus.

Glycemic Management

Because of changes in glucose and insulin requirements during labor, frequent monitoring of capillary blood glucose concentration is required. The standard approach is every 2-4 hours during the latent phase, every 1-2 hours during the active phase, and every hour during insulin infusion.

However, women with gestational diabetes whose sugars are well-controlled with diet and exercise rarely require insulin in labor and their sugars can be checked at admission and every 4-6 hours only. In women undergoing induction of labor, the morning dose of insulin or metformin is withheld. Oral intake can be permitted during the process of induction till the patient goes into active labor. Thereafter, a dextrose saline infusion will provide the necessary glucose to sustain the intense exercise of labor while insulin can be given as an insulin infusion or as subcutaneous doses based on the sugar levels.

Intrapartum glucose targets: The American College of Obstetricians and Gynecologists' and the American College of Endocrinology's goal for intrapartum glycemic control is glucose levels between 70 and 110 mg/dL.

Insulin in Labor

The requirement and dosage of insulin depend on the type of diabetes and the phase of labor. Women with type 1 and type 2 diabetes require lower doses of insulin in labor. GDM on MNT will generally not need insulin since the intense exercise of labor will preclude any need for insulin.

Insulin can be administered in one of the two forms—a separate IV insulin infusion apart from a 5% dextrose infusion; or, as a single IV infusion of 5% dextrose normal saline with 5 units of regular insulin or rapid acting insulin given at the rate of 100–125 mL/h (**Flowchart 1 and Table 4**).

Flowchart 1: Insulin administration in labor.

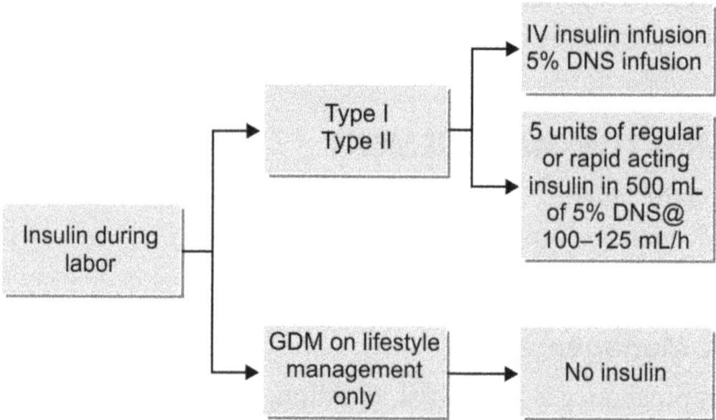

(DNS: dextrose normal saline; GDM: gestational diabetes mellitus; IV: intravenous)

TABLE 4: Guide to glucose levels and insulin.[6,10]

Blood sugar levels	Insulin units in 500 mL
90–120 mg/dL	0
120–140 mg/dL	4
140–180 mg/dL	6
>180 mg/dL	8

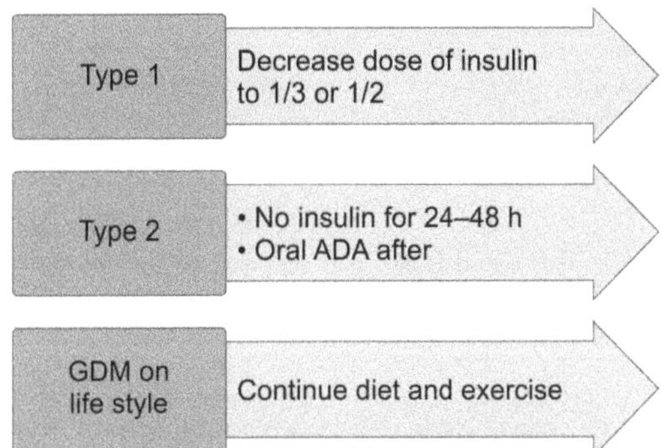

Fig. 2: Management Guide of GDM.
(GDM: gestational diabetes mellitus; ADA: American Diabetes Association)

Following delivery, the insulin requirement drops to one-third to one-half of the antenatal dose in women with type 1 diabetes. Insulin can be stopped for 24–48 hours in women with type 2 diabetes. Glycemic levels can be evaluated and appropriate antidiabetic agent started. Women with GDM need to have their glycemic status evaluated 6 weeks after delivery and managed accordingly **(Fig. 2)**.

MANAGEMENT IN THE POSTPARTUM PERIOD

Following delivery, discussion about diet, exercise, breastfeeding, weight loss, contraception, and subsequent GCT are mandatory **(Flowchart 2)**.

Risk of developing DM is highest between 6 months and 5 years. Fifty percent of them develop diabetes in the next 5–10 years. In South Asians, conversion to diabetes happens rapidly, usually within a year.

Lifestyle changes including diet and exercise are very useful in maintaining optimum sugars. In women with type 1 and type 2 diabetes, these changes help in decreasing the dose of antidiabetic agents and in women with gestational diabetes, they help to prevent or delay development of type 2 diabetes.

In the National Diabetes Prevention Program, participants who lost 5–7% of their body weight and added 150 minutes of exercise per week cut their risk of developing type 2 diabetes by up to 58%. Women should be encouraged to reach their pre-pregnancy weight 6–12 months postpartum. If still overweight, they need to lose at least 5–7% of weight slowly, over time, and keep it off.

Flowchart 2: Management algorithm.

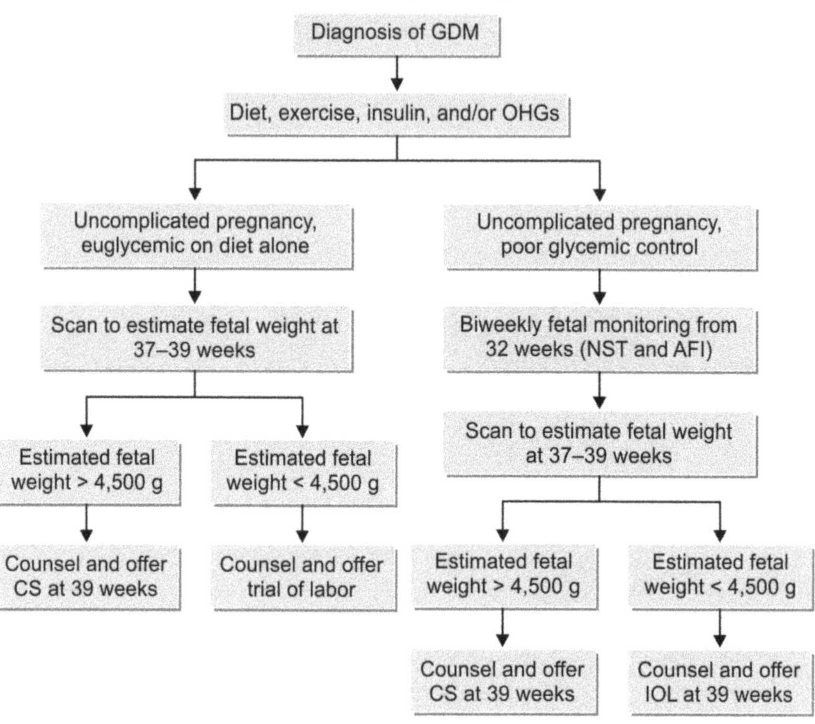

(GDM: gestational diabetes mellitus; OHGs: oral hypoglycemics; NST: nonstress test; AFI: amniotic fluid index; CS: cesarean section; IOL: induction of labor)

Postpartum Screening for Diabetes

To date, postpartum follow-up has been found to be inadequate in a number of studies including the findings from a recent systematic review, which reported only half of women in most populations are screened.

Counseling

Even in the antenatal period, the woman should be educated about the significance of postpartum screening. Counseling sessions should include important family members like the mother-in-law, husband, or any member who plays a crucial role in the life of pregnant woman.

Strategies that can be adopted to improve postpartum screening:
- Who should follow-up?
- When to call the woman for follow-up?
- How to send reminders?
- Which test to do?
- How to integrate screening in our health system?

Who should follow-up?
Gestational diabetes mellitus follow-up is a team effort and all those concerned in providing healthcare to the woman and her baby should

be involved. Obstetrician, endocrinologist, physician, family physician, and even the pediatrician should work together with sufficient overlap in providing postpartum screening.

When to call the woman for follow-up?
- 6 weeks to 6 months
- Once in 6 months, if IGT
- Once in a year, if normal

The conversion rates to diabetes mellitus in subsequent 5 years have been found to be 34–37% and 42% IGT in our country. The high rates of conversion warrant a much more frequent screening as compared to the ADA guidelines.

How to send reminders?
Text messages sent to the patient and her family members will help in improving the postpartum follow-up. Women who do not respond to this could be followed-up with telephone calls. Test could also be done when she visits the pediatrician for her baby's follow-up. In the rural settings, a visit to her house by the healthcare provider to provide the test at her doorstep could prove beneficial.

Which test to do?
The gold standard test is WHO OGT test.

75 g OGT test including fasting and 2 hour postprandial is performed at 6 weeks postpartum. Interpretations are given in **Table 5**.

However, the test for postpartum screening for glucose intolerance has to be simple, doable, and evidence based. In Asian Indians due to high insulin resistance, the postprandial blood glucose is high, which is advantageous for postpartum screening. The public healthcare ASHA workers are already performing GDM screening by "A Single step Procedure" of diagnosing GDM with 2-h PG > 140 mg/dL after 75 g oral glucose load without regard to the last meal timing, which is recommended by Ministry of Health Government of India. This same test procedure can be followed to detect glucose intolerance in the postpartum period also. The advantages are women need not be fasting and it causes least disturbance in their routine activities. The mothers would not refuse this test procedure, as they have already undergone this test in the antepartum period. Further, the above suggestion would avoid confusion among the healthcare workers, if the same procedure is followed both in the antepartum and postpartum period to diagnose glucose tolerance.

TABLE 5: Interpretations of oral glucose tolerance test.

Plasma glucose	Interpretation
2 h ≥ 200 mg/dL and/or FBS >120 mg/dL	Diabetes
2 h ≥ 140 mg/dL and ≤199 mg/dL	IGT
2 h < 140 mg/dL	Normal
(IGT: impaired glucose tolerance; FBS: fasting blood sugar)	

The test can be made easier by the use of plasma-calibrated glucometers, which have been approved by The Ministry of Health Government of India and WHO.

Integrating postpartum screening into the existing RCH program including the Janani Suraksha Yojana could make a world of difference to postpartum screening at the grass root levels.

Contraception: Among women with history of GDM other than long-acting progesterone, all contraceptive choices are applicable.

Key issues to be addressed in counseling are:
- The difficulty in accurately predicting birth weight by any method
- Estimated fetal growth between ultrasound examination and delivery
- The risks of shoulder dystocia and associated complications
- The risks of a cesarean delivery in the current pregnancy
- The implications of cesarean delivery in the management and outcome of future pregnancies.

CONSEQUENCES OF GDM[9,12,13]

Short-term

- *Large for gestational age (fetal or neonatal weight at or above the 90th centile) and macrosomia (birth weight ≥4,500 g):* Accelerated fetal growth may begin by 20–28 weeks of gestation and maternal hyperglycemia increases the risk of LGA or macrosomia. Maternal weight gain of over 18 kg doubles the risk.

  Macrosomia is associated with an increased risk of operative delivery (cesarean or instrumental vaginal) and adverse neonatal outcomes, such as shoulder dystocia and its associated complications—brachial plexus injury, fracture, and neonatal depression.
- *Pre-eclampsia and gestational hypertension*
- *Polyhydramnios*
- *Stillbirths:* Higher stillbirth rates are associated with poor glycemic controls.
- *Neonatal morbidity:* Multiple, often transient, morbidities, such as hypoglycemia, hyperbilirubinemia, hypocalcemia, hypomagnesemia, polycythemia, respiratory distress, and/or cardiomyopathy, might occur.

Long-term

- *For the offspring:* Risk of developing obesity, IGT, or metabolic syndrome
- *For the woman:* GDM is a strong marker for maternal development of type 2 diabetes, including diabetes-related vascular disease.

PRECONCEPTIONAL CARE AND COUNSELING IN FUTURE PREGNANCIES

Women with history of GDM have increased risk of developing GDM in future pregnancies. Also, the abnormal glucose control might persist as IGT or type 2 diabetes. Hence, these women are advised blood sugar estimations and optimization, if abnormal. The target sugars ought to be FBS—100 mg/dL and PPBS < 140 mg/dL and HbA1c levels of <6. The recurrence of diabetes in subsequent pregnancy also depends on the prepregnancy weight. Exercise decreases the prepregnancy weight, helps in glycemic control, and improves outcome. Women with BMI >27 kg/m^2 should be encouraged to reduce weight.

All women should receive 400 µg of folic acid. It is important to ensure safety of the drugs used for management of medical conditions associated with diabetes.

NPH (isophane) insulin, the short-acting insulin, and some rapid-acting analogs are safe.

Angiotensin-converting enzyme inhibitors and angiotensin-II receptor antagonists should be changed to α-dopa, labetalol, or calcium antagonists. Statins should be discontinued.

DIABETES WITH RETINAL DISEASE

Retinal assessment is mandatory.

Those likely to do well include those with minimal background retinopathy, who have had laser therapy, who are well-controlled, and whose eyes are stable.

Women with severe background or pre-proliferative retinopathy can have a rapid progression of retinal disease during pregnancy, even risking blindness.

DIABETES WITH NEPHROPATHY

Nephropathy is likely to progress with progressive proteinuria and hypertension. However, when nephropathy is not associated with hypertension, fetal outcome is not affected unless kidney function is more than 50% impaired.

CONCLUDING REMARKS

Gestational diabetes is a common condition among Indian women. Management includes early detection, patient education, diet and exercises with/without medications, appropriate fetal surveillance, timing of delivery, and follow-up postpartum for persisting hyperglycemia.

Gestational diabetes mellitus, though a challenges, can be surmounted satisfactorily with the above methods to ensure the best maternal and fetal outcomes.

REFERENCES

1. Kayal A, Anjana RM, Mohan V. (2013). Gestational diabetes—An update from India, 2013. [online] Available from: http://mdrf-eprints.in/860/1/Gestational_diabetes.pdf. [Last accessed June, 2020].

2. Maternal Health Division, Ministry of Health and Family Welfare Government of India. (2014). National Guidelines for Diagnosing and Management of Gestational Diabetes. [online] Available from: http://www.nrhmorissa.gov.in/writereaddata/Upload/Documents/National%20Guidelines%20for%20Diagnosis%20&%20Management%20of%20Gestational%20Diabetes%20Mellitus.pdf. [Last accessed June, 2020].

3. Damm P. Future risk of diabetes in mother and child after gestational diabetes mellitus. Int J Gynaecol Obstet. 2009;104 Suppl 1:S25-6.

4. Cosson E. Screening and insulin sensitivity in gestational diabetes. Abstract volume of the 40th Annual Meeting of the EASD. Munich, Germany: 2004; A 350.

5. Griffin ME, Coffey M, Johnson H, Scanlon P, Foley M, Stronge J, et al. Universal vs risk factor-based screening for gestational diabetes mellitus: detection rates, gestation at diagnosis and outcome. Diabet Med. 2000;17(1):26-32.

6. Maternal Health Division, Ministry of Health and Family Welfare Government of India. (2018). Diagnosis & Management of Gestational Diabetes Mellitus: Technical and Operational Guidelines. [online] Available from: https://nhm.gov.in/New_Updates_2018/NHM_Components/RMNCH_MH_Guidelines/Gestational-Diabetes-Mellitus.pdf. [Last accessed June, 2020].

7. Misra S. Screening for Gestational Diabetes. [online] Available from: https://www.fogsi.org/screening-for-gestational-diabetes/. [Last accessed June, 2020].

8. Seshiah V, Cynthia A, Balaji V, Balaji MS, Ashalata S, Sheela R, et al. Detection and care of women with gestational diabetes mellitus from early weeks of pregnancy results in birth weight of newborn babies appropriate for gestational age. Diab Res Clin Pract. 2008;80(2):199-202.

9. Seshiah V, Balaji V, Balaji MS, Paneerselvam A, Arthi T, Thamizharasi M, et al. Gestational Diabetes Mellitus manifests in all trimesters of pregnancy. Diabetes Res Clin Pract. 2007;77(3):482-4.

10. Seshiah V, Sahay BK, Shah S, Das AK. (2009). Gestational Diabetes Mellitus–Indian Guidelines. [online] Available from: https://www.researchgate.net/publication/44599204_Gestational_Diabetes_Mellitus_-_Indian_Guidelines. [Last accessed June, 2020].

11. Balaji V, Madhuri BS, Seshiah V, Ashalata S, Sheela R, Suresh S. A1C in gestational diabetes mellitus in Asian Indian women. Diabetes Care. 2007;30(7):1865-7.

12. Balaji V, Seshiah V, Balaji MS, Mukundan S, Datta M. Maternal glycemia and neonates birthweight in Asian Indian women. Diabetes Res Clin Pract. 2006;73(2):223-4.

13. Langer O, Levy J, Brustman L, Anyaegbunam A, Merkatz R, Divon M. Glycemic control in gestational diabetes mellitus—how tight is tight enough: small for gestational age versus large for gestational age? Am J Obstet Gynecol. 1989;161(3):646-53.

14. Kitzmiller JL, Block JM. Glycemic control & Perinatal Outcome. In: Kitzmiller JL, Jovanovic L, Brown F, Coustan D, Reader DM (Eds). Managing preexisting Diabetes & Pregnancy—Technical Reviews and Consensus Recommendations for Care. Arlington County, Virginia, United States: ADA; 2008. p. 3.

15. Joseph M, Shetty S, Thomas N. (2017). Diet in a pregnant mother with diabetes mellitus. [online] Available from: http://www.cmijournal.org/article.asp?issn=0973-4651;year=2017;volume=15;issue=3;spage=222;epage=226;aulast=Joseph. [Last accessed June, 2020].

Promotive Antenatal Care

- **Nutrition and Nutrients in Pregnancy**
  Ruchika Garg, Urvashi Verma

- **Vaccination in Pregnancy**
  Mousumi Das Ghosh

- **Safe Drugs in Pregnancy: An Update**
  Vidya Thobbi, Prabhat Agrawal, Ruchika Garg

- **Positive Pregnancy Experience: WHO Update**
  Pratima Mittal

Ruchika Garg, Urvashi Verma

23 | Nutrition and Nutrients in Pregnancy

CHAPTER

▮ INTRODUCTION

Nutrition in pregnancy refers to the nutrient intake and dietary planning that is undertaken before, during, and after pregnancy.

Nutrition consists of two parts: (1) macronutrition and (2) micronutrition. Macronutrients consist of carbohydrates, fat, and proteins; whereas, micronutrients are vitamins and minerals. Macronutrients serve as building blocks and energy sources for the body and micronutrients are essential as chemical partner for enzyme involved in metabolism, cell production, tissue repair, and other processes.

▮ CALORIES INTAKE DURING PREGNANCY

During pregnancy, additional energy is required to support the growth of the fetus, placenta, and maternal tissue as well as to meet the needs for the increased basal metabolic rate (BMR). Hence, National Advisory Committee (NAC) has recommended an additional 300 kcal/day in second and third trimester.[1]

If calories intake is insufficient, protein is metabolized rather being spared for its vital role in fetal growth and development. This is more so in pregnancies complicated with diabetes, renal disorder, hypertension, hyperemesis, anemia, or fetal growth restrictions. *Hence, an increase in carbohydrate consumption is preferred during pregnancy and lactation.*

Estimated energy requirement (EER) for pregnant women:
- First trimester—nonpregnant EER + 0
- Second trimester—nonpregnant EER + 340
- Third trimester—nonpregnant EER + 452

Protein Requirement

The fetus receives continuous stream of amino acids from the mother via the placenta, which play an important role in nitrogen metabolism. Shift in protein metabolism are complex and changes gradually throughout gestation so that nitrogen conservation for fetal growth can achieve full potential during the last trimester of pregnancy.

Safe level of additional protein required during pregnancy:[2]
- First trimester—1.2 g/day
- Second trimester—6.1 g/day
- Third trimester—10.7 g/day

Sources:
- *Animal sources*: Eggs, milk mutton, fish, and poultry
- *Plant sources*: Pulses, legumes, and cereals. The protein content of pulses is twice that of cereals (20–25%) and almost equal to that of meat and poultry. Pulses are lacking in amino acid methionine as compared to animal protein but the lysine content is more. This limitation can be overcome by combining pulses with cereals. WHO guidelines recommend balanced protein energy supplementation with <25% calories of energy from protein during pregnancy.

  Extra protein intake during lactation is about 16 g/day for first 6 months, 12 g/day for next 6 months and 11 g/day thereafter.[3]

Fat and Fatty Acid (DHA) Requirement during Pregnancy

Fat an essential component of diet is concentrated source of energy, carrier of fat-soluble vitamins, and provides palatability to diet. Fatty acids are of two types:
1. Saturated fatty acid (SFA)
2. Unsaturated fatty acid (USFA)

   Unsaturated fatty acids are further subdivided into monounsaturated fatty acid (MUFA) and polyunsaturated fatty acid (PUFA). PUFAs are indispensable for human development and health but cannot be synthesized by body in adequate amount to be provided by diet. They are of two subtypes— (1) Omega 6 (ω6) and (2) Omega 3 (ω3). ω3 is finally metabolized in body to docosahexaenoic acid (DHA).

   Long-chain PUFAs (LCPUFAs) are required component of the rapidly growing perinatal CNS.[4] The DHA is predominant structural fatty acid in brain, retina, and sperms.[5] It constitutes 40% of PUFA of brain and 60% of PUFA of retina. DHA is metabolized to docosanoids (DPA), comprising of several families of potent hormones. As human and mammals are able to make their own DHA from other, fatty acid deficiency is not common. Due to low conversion rate of alpha-linoleic acid (ALA) to DHA, it is important to directly consume DHA, especially during pregnancy and lactation.

Food source:
ω3 PUFAs are basically present in:
- Plant food and vegetables oils
- Animal foods such as meat
- Mustard, soya bean, green leafy vegetables, walnut, and wheat
- Fish-tuna fish, blue fish, mackerel, swordfish, sardines, and caviar, fish oil, and algae

Docosahexaenoic acid plays an important role in preventing preterm birth, improvement in birth weight, preventing pre-eclampsia, and decreasing incidence of postpartum depression.[4,6]

At birth, babies are only 5% of adult weight yet the brain size is almost 70% of the adult brain. There is a definite growth spurt (70%) in the human brain during the last trimester of pregnancy and the first postnatal month, which is appropriate time to ensure adequate DHA intake. Brain growth continues by a further 15% during the first year of life and an additional 10% during preschool years. High levels of DHA are found in gray matter of cerebral cortex.[7]

Higher level of ω3 fatty acid is associated with better hand eye co-ordination, language, and motor skills in childhood. Baby born to mother who eat recommended quantity of DHA during pregnancy are 32% less likely to develop obesity.[8,9]

Iron Requirement

- *Menstruating females*: 1–2 mg/day
- *Pregnancy females*: 1.5–2.5 mg/day
- *Children*: 1 mg/day

Total iron requirement is 900 mg in pregnancy (700–1,400 mg). During pregnancy, iron requirement increases by 4 g% in early pregnancy to 5.5 g% in 20–32 weeks and 6–8 g% 32 weeks onward.[5]

Calcium Requirement during Pregnancy

About 99% of body calcium, which amount to about 1,100–1,200 g, is in bone and 10–15% of bone is remodeled actively at any point of time. Hence, any deficiency leads to decrease in density of calcium in bones. During pregnancy and lactation, there is an increased bone turnover in order to meet fetal or infant need for calcium as well as increase urinary excretion of calcium, which is about 200 mg/day.[2]

The fetal calcium requirement in first 20 weeks is 50 mg/day, which increases to 330 mg/day at 35 weeks and continues 300 mg/day during lactation. The fetal calcium level is higher than maternal calcium level, with the total fetal accretion of calcium being 30 g. There is also an increase in dietary calcium absorption, i.e., 27% in nonpregnant women, 54% at 5–6 months, and 42% at term.

During pregnancy, a reduction in total bone mineral density (BMD) has been detected up to the values of 3.6%. This reduction is more at lumber region, femur neck, distal radius and trochanter. Bone loss can be 0.5–7% at spine level. The rate of bone loss during pregnancy and lactation is greater than the annual rate of loss in postmenopausal women. During pregnancy with history of pre-eclampsia or chronic use of heparin or steroid, calcium supplementation in the dose of 2,000 mg/day is recommended.[10]

Vitamin D

The current recommended dietary requirement of vitamin D of 200 IU/day may not be sufficient many times and sometimes may actually be as high as 6,000 IU/day.[11] Taking vitamin is safe and effective in preventing preterm labor, premature births, and infections. If dietary vitamin D supplements throughout pregnancy can be taken, the amount given should be 400 IU/day (10 µg/day). When delayed, 1,000 IU/day (25 µg/day) in last trimester of pregnancy should be given.[12,13]

■ MICRONUTRIENTS DURING PREGNANCY (TABLE 1)

Micronutrients are nutritional components, frequently referred to vitamins and minerals, which although required in little amounts; the consequences of their absence are severe.[7]

Folic Acid

A water-soluble vitamin B_9 is required for synthesis, repair, and methylation of DNA as well as to act as a cofactor in biological reactions. Folic acid itself is biological inactive, but its derivative tetrahydrofolate and other derivative after its conversion to dihydrofolic acid in the liver are important for rapid cell division and growth in pregnancy and infancy. It is an important nutrient during periconceptional period because of its proven preventive properties against neural tube defects (NTDs).[14]

A healthy individual has about 500–2,000 µg of folate in body stores, thus folic acid deficiency may not manifest for 4 months.[5] However, in high requirement state such as pregnancy, the folic acid utilization is much more hence recommended preconceptionally to build up the stores and 3-month postconception when organogenesis takes place.

The reference daily intake (RDI) for folate equivalents in pregnancy is 600–800 µg, twice the normal RDI of 400 µg in nonpregnant women.[5]

Folate deficiency may lead to increase in homocysteine level in blood, which may lead to spontaneous abortion, preterm delivery, abruption of placenta, pregnancy-induced hypertension, preterm delivery, intrauterine growth retardation, mental retardation, and NTDs. Folic acid supplementation also reduces the risk of congenital heart defect, cleft lips, limb defects, and urinary tract anomalies.

Preventive Measure

The folic acid used in fortified foods is a synthetic form called pteroylmonoglutamate.

Source: According to the nutritive value Indian foods (NVIF), a publication of the National Institute of Nutrition (NIN), Indian Council of Indian Research (ICMR), spinach (palak or pasalai keerai/Palang saag), eggs, and goat, or

TABLE 1: Daily dietary reference intake during pregnancy (RDI for micronutrients during pregnancy).

Nutrients	Age ≤ 18	Age 19–50 years
Biotin	30 µg/day	200–300 mg (RDI)
Folate	600 µg/day (4 mg/day h/o NTD)	200 µg/day (4mg/day h/o NTD)
Niacin (B$_3$)	18 mg/day	18 mg/day
Pantothenic acid	6 mg/day	6 mg/day
Riboflavin (B$_2$)	1.4 mg/day	1.4 mg/day
Thiamine (B$_1$)	1.4 mg/day	1.4 mg/day
Cyanocobalamin (B$_{12}$)	2.6 µg/day	2.6 µg/day
Vitamin A	750 µg/day (2,500 IU/day)	770 µg/day
Vitamin B$_6$	1.9 mg/day	1.9 mg/day
Vitamin B$_{11}$	2.6 mg/day	2.6 mg/day
Vitamin C	80 mg/day	85 mg/day
Vitamin D	5 µg/day (200 IU/day)	5 µg/day (200 IU/day)
Vitamin E	15 mg/day	15 mg/day
Vitamin K	75 µg/day	90 µg/day
Calcium	1,300 mg/day	1,000 mg/day
Chromium	29 µg/day	30 µg/day
Copper	1 mg/day	1 mg/day
Fluoride	3 mg/day	3 mg/day
Iodine	220 µg/day	220 mg/day
Iron	27 mg/day	27 mg/day
Magnesium	400 mg/day	360 mg/day
Manganese	2 mg/day	2 mg/day
Molybdenum	50 µg/day	50 µg/day
Phosphorus	1,250 mg/day	700 mg/day
Potassium	4,700 mg/day	3–4 g/day
Selenium	60 µg/day	60 µg/day
Sodium	1,500 mg/day	1,500 mg/day
Zinc	12 mg/day	11 mg/day
Choline	450 mg/day	450 mg/day
Chloride	–	2–1.3 g
Water	3 L	3 L
Carbohydrate	175 g/day	175 g/day
Protein	71 g/day	71 g/day
Fiber	28 g/day	28 g/day

(h/o: history of; NTD: neural tube defect)

sheep liver. Whole cereals, legumes, and green leafy vegetables are also good source while milled cereals, other vegetables, milk, and fruits are fair source of natural folate.[15]

Biotin (Vitamin B₇ or Vitamin H)

Biotin is required as a cofactor for carboxylase enzymes and for attachment of biotin to molecules, such as protein, for "biotinylation". Rapidly proliferating cells of the developing fetus require biotin for synthesis of indispensable carboxylase enzymes plus for histone biotinylation. Thus, the biotin requirement is increased during pregnancy. At present, it is projected that at least one-third of women develop marginal biotin depletion is not severe enough to cause diagnostic signs or symptoms; subclinical biotin deficiency has been shown to cause natal defects in several animal species.

The potential risk for teratogenesis due to biotin insufficiency makes it prudent to ensure adequate biotin intake preconceptionally and throughout pregnancy. Supplementing biotin (at least 30 µg/day) in the form of a multivitamin that also contains at least 400 µg of folic acid can be a helpful step.[16,17]

Riboflavin (Vitamin B₂)

Vitamin B_2 is a constituent of flavoenzymes concerned in energy metabolism and antioxidant function. The food and nutrition board of the institute of medicine recommends that all pregnant women should take 1.4 mg of vitamin B_2 every day.[16,17] Vitamin B_2 deficit has been connected to pre-eclampsia. Even though the exact causes of pre-eclampsia are not recognized, reduced intracellular levels of flavoenzymes could result in mitochondrial dysfunction, augment oxidative stress, and get in way with nitric oxide release and consequently blood vessel dilation.

Vitamin B₆

Vitamin B_6 has diverse roles in the body, including nervous system function, red blood cells formation and function, steroid hormone role, nucleic acid synthesis, and niacin formation. The RDI of vitamin B_6 during pregnancy is 1.9 mg/day.[17] Supplementation with high-dose vitamin B_6 may help to mitigate nausea and vomiting in pregnancy/morning sickness.

Vitamin B₁₂

Inadequate dietary intake of vitamin B_{12} causes elevated homocysteine levels, which have been associated with adverse pregnancy outcomes, including pre-eclampsia, premature delivery, low birth weight (<2,500 g), very low birth weight (<1,500 g), NTDs, and stillbirth.[15,17] Moreover, low serum levels of vitamin B_{12} during pregnancy has been directly linked to an increased risk for NDTs, and there is some concern that folic acid supplementation during pregnancy may mask the clinical diagnosis of vitamin B_{12} deficiency. After iron deficiency anemia, megaloblastic anemia is the second most prevalent cause of anemia in India. For these reasons, adequate vitamin B_{12} intake during pregnancy (RDI = 2.6 µg/day) is important. Because vitamin B_{12} is found only in foods of animal origin, vegans and lacto-ovo vegetarians are prone to suffer from vitamin B_{12} deficiency, making its supplementation even more important in countries like India.

MINERALS

Zinc

Zinc is an indispensable element of more than 200 metalloenzymes participating in carbohydrate and protein metabolism, nucleic acid synthesis, antioxidant role (through Cu/Zn SOD), and other vital function such as cellular division and differentiation, making it necessary for productive embryogenesis.[18] It was estimated in 2002 by the World Health Organization that suboptimal zinc nutrition affected nearly half the world population. During pregnancy, zinc is also used to help the fetus to develop the brain as well as to be a support to the mother in labor. Alternation in zinc homeostasis possibly will have disturbing effects on pregnancy result, together with prolonged labor, fetal growth restriction, embryonic or fetal death, and eclampsia.

Iodine

Iodine requirement becomes greater by >45% at the time of pregnancy. Adequate intake of iodine is needed for maternal thyroid hormone production, and thyroid hormone is needed for myelination of the central nervous system and is thus essential for normal fetal brain development. Iodine deficiency disorders (IDDs) constitute the single largest cause of preventable brain damage worldwide. Majority of consequences of IDD are invisible and irreversible but, at the same time, these are preventable. Maternal iodine deficiency has been associated with increased incidence of miscarriage, stillbirth, and birth abnormalities. Extreme iodine deficiency during pregnancy can result in congenital hypothyroidism and neurocognitive deficits in the offspring. A severe form of congenital hypothyroidism may lead to a condition that is occasionally referred to as cretinism and produces permanent mental retardation. Even mild forms of maternal iodine deficiency possibly will have unfavorable effects on cognitive maturity in the offspring, and iodine deficiency is now accepted as the main universal reason for avoidable brain damage in the world. Iodization of salt may be the world's simplest and most cost-effective measure available to improve health.

Recommendation from Various International Bodies

International Federation of Gynecology and Obstetrics (FIGO, 2015) states that even with use of iodized salt and eating seafood 2–3 days per week, a woman's daily iodine intake would be approximately half the amount recently recommended during pregnancy and lactation.

Organization such as American Academy of Pediatrics recommends that all the pregnant and breastfeeding women should seek out prenatal supplements that contain iodine. American Thyroid Association and Endocrine Society, 2011 guidelines recommend that all the women attempting to conceive and pregnant women should take a prenatal vitamin containing 150 µg of iodine while IOM (institution of medicine) recommends daily iodine intake of 220 µg during pregnancy and 290 µg during lactation; and the WHO recommends iodine intake of 250 µg for both pregnant and lactating women.[19]

Magnesium

Maternal magnesium deficiency has been linked to premature labor as well as implicated in the pathogenesis of sudden infant death syndrome (SIDS). Magnesium is thought to alleviate cerebral blood vessel spasm, increasing blood flow to the brain, and, hence, has a unique role in management of eclampsia and pre-eclampsia.[20]

Chromium

Chromium is identified to improve the effect of insulin as a result; several studies have investigated the utility of chromium supplementation for the management of plasma glucose levels in type 2 diabetes. However, its use in gestational diabetes is not well studied and more randomized controlled trials (RCTs) are needed.

Others

Copper

It is an essential cofactor for a number of enzymes involved in metabolic reactions, blood vessel formation, oxygen carrying, and antioxidant protection, including catalyse, superoxide dismutase (SOD), and cytochrome oxidase. Copper is essential for embryonic development. Maternal dietary deficiency can result in both temporary outcomes, together with early embryonic fatality and gross structural abnormalities, and long-term consequences such as increased risk of cardiovascular disease and reduced fertilization rates.

Selenium and Manganese

These are antioxidant trace elements important of various body functions.

The WHO group agreed that policymakers in population with a high prevalence of nutritional deficiencies might consider the benefit of multiple micronutrients supplements on maternal health to outweigh the disadvantages (toxicity) and may choose to give multiple micronutrient supplement that include iron folic acid.[21]

■ REFERENCES

1. World Health organization (2013). Energy and protein requirements. Report of a joint FAO/WHO ad hoc expert committee [meeting held in Rome from 22 March to 2 April 1971] (WHO Technical Report Series, No. 522). [online] Available from: https://apps.who.int/iris/handle/10665/41042 [Last accessed June, 2020].
2. Tripathy SN. Nutrition in pregnancy: An overview. Nutrition and Pregnancy ECAB Clinical Update: Obstetrics and Gynecology. Gurgaon, India: Elsevier; 2011. p. 5.
3. Pardesi R, Mane A. Nutrition supplements in pregnancy-optimal use. FOGSI FOCUS Preconception and Antenatal Care Update. Mumbai, India: FOGSI Focus. pp. 29-35.
4. Food and Agriculture Organization of the United Nations (2010). Chapter 7: Fat and Fatty Acid during Pregnancy and Lactation. Fat and fatty acid in human nutrition: Report of an expert consultation; FAO Food and nutrition Paper 91. [online] Available from: http://www.fao.org/3/a-i1953e.pdf [Last accessed June, 2020].
5. Rao DA. Maternal Nutrition. Melbourne, Australia: GlaxoSmithKline Consumer healthcare Ltd.; 2004.
6. Makrides M, Gibson RA, Mcphee AJ, Yelland L, Quinlivan J, Ryan P, et al. Effect of DHA supplementation during pregnancy on maternal depression and neurodevelopment of young child—a randomized controlled trial. JAMA. 2010;304(15):1675-83.
7. Hininger I, Favier M, Arnaud J, Faure H, Thoulon JM, Hariveau E, et al. Effects of a combined micronutrient supplementation on maternal biological status and newborn anthropometrics measurements, a randomized double blind placebo controlled trial in apparently healthy pregnant women. Eur J Clin Nutr. 2004; 58(1):52-9.
8. Tanentsapf I, Heitmann BL, Adegboye AR. Systematic review of clinical trials on dietry interventions to prevent excessive weight gain during pregnancy among normal weight, overweight and obese women. BMC Pregnancy Childbirth. 2011;11:81-93.
9. Donahue SM, Rifas-Shiman SL, Gold DR, Jouni ZE, Gillman MW, Oken E. Prenatal fatty acid status and child adiposity at age 3 years-results from a US pregnancy cohort. Am J Clin Nutr. 2011;93(4):780-8.
10. Chotboon C, Soontrapa S, Buppasiri P, Muktabhant B, Kongwattanakul K, Thinkhamrop J. Adequacy of calcium intake during pregnancy in a tertiary centre. Int J Womens Health. 2018;10: 523-7.
11. Sanyal SC. Role of calcium and vitamin D in Fetomaternal Well Being. Nutrition and pregnancy ECAB Clinical update: Obstetrics and Gynecology. Gurgaon, India: Elsevier; pp. 81-98.
12. Salle BL, Delvin EE, Lapillonne A, Bishop NJ, Glorieux FH. Perinatal metabolism of vitamin D. Am J Clin Nutr. 2000;71 (5 Suppl):1317S-24S.
13. Thomson K, Morley R, Grover SR, Zacharin MR. Postnatal evaluation of vitamin D and bone health in women who were vitamin D-deficient in pregnancy and in their infants. Med J Aust. 2004;181(9):486-8.
14. Park H, Kim YJ, Ha EH, Kim KN, Chang N. The risk of folate & vitamin B12 deficiencies associated with hyperhomocysteinemia among pregnant women. Am J Perinatol. 2004;21(8):469-75.
15. Jain M. Importance of folate in conception and periconception. AICOG Manual on Nutrition in Pregnancy, 1st edition. New Delhi, India: Jaypee Brothers Medical Publishers (P) Ltd; 2016. pp. 12-5.

16. Franca M, Cetin I, Verduci E, Canzone G, Giovannini M, Scollo P, et al. Maternal diet and nutrients requirement in pregnancy and breastfeeding. Nutrients. 2016;8(10):629.

17. Aya M, Naqash A, Lim S. Macronutrient and micronutrient intake during pregnancy: An overview of recent evidences. Nutrient. 2019;11(2):443.

18. Hambridge M. Human zink deficiency. J Nutr. 2000;130:1344-9.

19. Glinoer D. Iodine nutrition requirement during pregnancy. Thyroid. 2006;16:947-8.

20. Khera R. Critical micronutrients in pregnancy: role of zink, choline magnesium, iodine & vitamin D during pregnancy. AICOG Manual on Nutrition in Pregnancy, 1st edition. New Delhi, India: Jaypee Brothers Medical Publishers (P) Ltd.; 2016. p. 60.

21. World Health Organization; e-Library of evidence for Nutrition Action (eLENA). Multiple Micronutrient Supplementation during pregnancy. [online] Available from: https://www.who.int/elena/titles/micronutrients_pregnancy/en/ [Last accessed June, 2020].

CHAPTER 24

Vaccination in Pregnancy

Mousumi Das Ghosh

INTRODUCTION

Vaccination during pregnancy is an integral part of obstetric care. Pregnancy increases susceptibility to many bacterial and viral infections, which lead to morbidity and mortality of both mother and fetus. Many vaccine preventable diseases can be avoided by immunizing the mother.[1]

Vaccine is a biological preparation that works by inducing active immunity and by providing immunological memory. When exposed to a natural infection after vaccination, the immune system recognizes and helps to prevent or modify the course of the disease.[1] Inactivated vaccines and toxoids are considered safe during pregnancy.

Vaccination during pregnancy protects the mother as well as the newborn from infections, as the antibodies are passed to the neonate who is protected for the first few months of life until it is time for his own vaccination.[2] Maternal IgG antibodies are actively transferred to fetus, mainly after 32 weeks of gestation. Hence, there is a high level of protection due to these antibodies in fetus born at term compared to preterm. Other factors influencing the transfer of maternal IgG are placental integrity, total maternal IgG and its subtype, and timing of immunization compared to delivery.[3]

Traditionally, vaccination was the responsibility of pediatricians and physicians. Obstetricians also have a key role to play for both the mother and neonate in the most vulnerable moments in the life. Immunization history should be obtained and vaccines advised as part of antenatal care. The success story of maternal and neonatal tetanus through immunization adds hope for many diseases in future.[4]

The use of vaccine is recommended in pregnancy, especially for developing countries **(Table 1)**. Expanded Program on Immunization (EPI), 1983 included tetanus toxoid (TT) immunization for pregnant women. In 2006, WHO position paper on tetanus recommended three doses of diphtheria-tetanus-pertussis (DTP) vaccine in infancy, with boosters in childhood and adolescence and a sixth dose at first pregnancy.[5] When the immunization status is unknown, the mother should receive two doses of vaccine 4 weeks apart and preferably 2 weeks before delivery. If a mother received two doses in her last pregnancy and conceives within 3 years, only one booster dose is recommended. WHO also recommends a third dose of

TABLE 1: Vaccines recommended for all pregnant women.

Vaccine	Vaccine type	Pregnancy recommendation
T-dap	• Tetanus and diphtheria—inactivated toxoids • Acellular pertussis—inactivated subunit • Inactivated toxoids	One dose T-dap from 27 to 36 weeks, regardless of previous immunization
Tetanus toxoid/tetanus diphtheria (incomplete immunization/unknown status)		Two doses 4 weeks apart (2nd dose can be T-dap)
Influenza	Inactivated viral subunit	1st dose during flu season, any gestational age
Vaccines recommended under special circumstances		*Vaccines contraindicated in pregnancy*
• Hepatitis A • Hepatitis B • Pneumococcal • Meningococcal • Yellow fever • Japanese encephalitis • Typhoid • Rabies • Anthrax		• Measles Mumps Rubella (MMR) • Varicella • Human papillomavirus (HPV) • Bacillus Calmette-Guérin (BCG)

(T-dap: tetanus-diphtheria-acellular pertussis)

TT 6 months after the second one to extend protection for at least 5 years.[6] A serum antibody titer of >0.01 U/mL provides protection. Elimination of neonatal tetanus is monitored, as it is linked to immunization status of mothers. This is defined as less than one case per 1,000 live births in every district of every country. India was finally free of maternal and neonatal tetanus in 2015.[2] Eradication of tetanus is not possible because the spores are widespread in the environment. If a case of neonatal tetanus is identified, the mother should be given tetanus toxoid as early as possible and the baby to be treated as per national guidelines. The mother should receive second dose of toxoid 4 weeks after the first and a third dose 6 months after the second.[7]

DIPHTHERIA

Diphtheria is an acute infectious disease caused by *Corynebacterium diphtheria*.

Though the disease burden has declined due to childhood vaccination, India still contributes substantially to the global scenario. India is gradually moving toward tetanus diphtheria vaccine, instead of only tetanus. In pregnancy, this will benefit both mother and the neonate against two diseases.

PERTUSSIS (WHOOPING COUGH)

Pertussis is a highly prevalent acute respiratory infection caused by *Bordetella pertussis*. The disease burden is not exactly known; however, it leads to significant mortality and morbidity. The highest risk of complications and hospitalizations is among the neonates who are too young to be vaccinated. Adolescents and adults act as reservoirs for disease transmission, as the immunity imparted by the vaccine wanes off. Family members and caregivers transmit the infection to the baby. Antenatal vaccination prevents pertussis in mothers and their infants by passive transfer of maternal antipertussis antibodies. This also diminishes the probability of the mother infecting her newborn.[8]

TETANUS-DIPHTHERIA-ACELLULAR PERTUSSIS VACCINE

The tetanus-diphtheria-acellular pertussis (T-dap) vaccine includes tetanus toxoid, reduced diphtheria toxoid, and acellular pertussis. This provides protection against three bacterial infections—tetanus, diphtheria, and pertussis. Antenatal immunization protects both the mother and the baby. The recommendation is to immunize all pregnant women with a single dose of T-dap in the third trimester, preferably between 27 and 36 weeks of gestation irrespective of prior Td or T-dap vaccination.[9,10] This maximizes passive transfer of antibody to the infant. However, it may be given at any time during pregnancy. This has to be repeated in every pregnancy regardless of previous immunization status, as the protection against pertussis is short lived.

The T-dap vaccine can be considered instead of the second dose of TT to extend protection against diphtheria and pertussis in addition to tetanus.

Family members are usually the source of pertussis transmission in infants.[11] Hence, T-dap is also important for healthcare professionals and any person (siblings, grandparents, and childcare providers) having close contact with an infant aged <1 year. This is termed as cocooning and a good strategy against infantile pertussis.[12] Postpartum vaccination with T-dap, if missed during pregnancy, also offers some protections to the infant.[13]

INFLUENZA IN PREGNANCY

Influenza (flu) is an RNA (ribonucleic acid) virus with A and B serotypes. Both serotypes can cause endemic flu, whereas type A is responsible for pandemic flu as a result of antigenic drift of its surface proteins hemagglutinin and neuraminidase.[14] The virus is unique and undergoes frequent antigenic change.

Influenza is a neglected disease in pregnancy with considerable mortality and morbidity. Various studies have shown that pregnant women with influenza virus infection are seven times more likely to be hospitalized and four times more likely to need ICU care. A 2011 Lancet meta-analysis reports 20 million influenza-related acute lower respiratory infections. Also, there is increase in miscarriage rates, stillbirths, and early neonatal deaths. There is increased risk of premature and complicated birth.[2] The best solution for flu prevention is immunization. The CDC recommendation is to immunize all pregnant women with inactivated influenza vaccine during flu season. There is no place for live attenuated vaccine in pregnancy. The influenza vaccination is beneficial for both seasonal influenza and influenza pandemics.[15] It is recommended for mothers from 26 weeks onwards and in case of pandemic, the vaccine can be given earlier to protect the mother.[12] This benefits both mother and her baby through transfer of maternally derived antibodies.

The strains included in the vaccine are selected based on epidemiologic and virological surveillance by WHO's Global Influenza Surveillance and Response System (GISRS). WHO monitors the evolution of viruses and recommends the viruses to be included in the vaccines twice a year (Northern and Southern hemisphere formulations). Influenza vaccine formulations change up to twice annually. The global vaccine action plan suggests moving toward universal influenza vaccine by 2020.[16,17]

VACCINES IN PREGNANCY UNDER SPECIAL CONDITIONS

Hepatitis A

Hepatitis A is an RNA picornavirus and the vaccines are formalin inactivated. The safety of vaccination during pregnancy is not known. However due to the fact that the vaccine is inactivated, the risk to the fetus is expected to be low. The vaccine is indicated in special circumstances when the benefits outweigh the risks—chronic liver disease, hemophilia, intravenous (IV) drug abuse, working with primates, and travel to endemic regions.

Finally, if exposed to hepatitis A infection, immunoglobulin should be administered.[6] It is highly effective and prevents acute infection.

Hepatitis B

Hepatitis B is an DNA (deoxyribonucleic acid) virus and the vaccine is recombinant formulation based on hepatitis B surface antigen envelope protein. A series of three doses is highly effective in disease prevention. The vaccine is recommended for pregnant women who are at high risk during pregnancy.[6] As it is an inactivated subunit vaccine, the risks to the baby is very low.

High-risk groups are women with multiple sex partners during the previous 6 months, those who inject drugs/partner injects drugs, regular blood transfusion, liver disease, chronic kidney disease, and women travelling to high-risk countries.[18] The vaccine is also advisable for women at risk of contact with body fluids such as doctors, nurses, and laboratory staff and those who are evaluated or treated for sexually transmitted disease (STD). The vaccine is highly immunogenic and the antibodies protect the newborn.[13]

Meningococcal Disease

Meningococcal disease is caused by *Neisseria meningitidis*, a bacterium. It has a high mortality rate, despite treatment and the survivors have significant sequelae and a poor quality of life. Two inactivated vaccines are effective against meningococcal disease—conjugate vaccine and a polysaccharide vaccine. The meningococcal vaccine is recommended during pregnancy to mothers at high risk for the disease. The risk factors[1] are living in close contact such as dormitories, functional and anatomical asplenia, immunosuppression, complement deficiency, and travel to high-risk endemic areas. The vaccine is safe during breastfeeding.

Pneumococcal Disease

Pneumococcal disease is caused by *Streptococcus pneumonae* and is responsible for pneumonia, bacteremia, meningitis, and otitis media. Valent pneumococcal conjugate vaccine and 23-valent polysaccharide vaccines are recommended for mothers who have risk factors.[1] The vaccine can be given during breastfeeding.

The risk factors, which recommend vaccine usage, are chronic heart disease, chronic lung disease, asthma, diabetes mellitus, congenital or acquired immunodeficiencies, sickle cell disease and other hemoglobino-pathies, anatomic or functional asplenia, chronic liver disease, smoking, alcoholism, cirrhosis of liver, and chronic renal failure.[13]

Travel Vaccinations

International travel is increasing and the specialty of travel medicine is emerging to protect the health of travelers through the use of immunization and appropriate drugs.[14] Hence, diseases and health conditions relevant to each destination including disease outbreaks should be checked.

Pregnant women planning international travel need to fulfill country-specific recommendations.[19] Centers for Disease Control and Prevention (CDC) travel website helps and should be checked. The vaccine preventable diseases encountered are yellow fever, Japanese encephalitis, and typhoid fever.

Yellow Fever

Yellow fever is caused by an RNA flavivirus and spread by mosquitoes. The disease spectrum varies from mild symptoms to severe, which include multiorgan failure, hemorrhage, and death. The disease is endemic in South America and sub-Saharan Africa. Yellow fever vaccine is live-attenuated. It is safe and effective.

Center for Disease Control and Prevention recommends vaccination during pregnancy, if her risk of exposure and infection is high and the advantages outweigh the risks of vaccine.[1] Nonpregnant women of reproductive age group are advised to avoid conception for 4 weeks postvaccination. In countries where yellow fever vaccine is an entry requirement but the disease is not endemic, pregnancy constitutes medical grounds for exemption from the vaccination requirement.

Japanese Encephalitis

Japanese encephalitis is also caused by an RNA flavivirus and spread by mosquitoes. The disease is prevalent in Asia. The mortality rate is high and the survivors have neurocognitive and psychiatric sequelae.

Center for Disease Control and Prevention recommends inactivated Japanese encephalitis vaccine for pregnant women planning longer duration travel to endemic areas, where immunization is more beneficial compared to the risk of infection.

Typhoid Fever

Typhoid fever is a bacterial disease caused by *Salmonella typhi*. The disease is prevalent in developing countries. Two vaccines are available—a live-attenuated vaccine and a polysaccharide vaccine. In cases of travel to endemic areas, the inactive parenteral vaccine may be administered.[1]

Rabies

Rabies is caused by *rhabdovirus* and the infection is spread through saliva or central nervous system tissue of an infected animal.[14] The disease is fatal to both mother and baby. Pre-exposure prophylaxis is advised, if risk of exposure is high. Inactivated rabies vaccine is available. CDC recommends postexposure prophylaxis to any pregnant woman after a moderate or high-risk exposure to rabies.[1] This includes rabies vaccine and human rabies immunoglobulin.

Anthrax

Anthrax is caused by *Bacillus anthracis*, a spore-forming bacterium. The spores can be aerosolized and remain viable for long periods, considered a deadly biological weapon. Pre-exposure vaccination is not advised during pregnancy. However, postexposure vaccination with inactivated subunit should be recommended with anthrax exposure.

VACCINES CONTRAINDICATED DURING PREGNANCY

Live-attenuated vaccines are contraindicated during pregnancy. The virus can cross the placenta and infect the fetus.

Measles, Mumps, and Rubella

Measles and mumps are both caused by *paramyxovirus* and rubella by *togavirus*. The disease burden has decreased with childhood vaccination and adult booster dosing. *The vaccine is live-attenuated and possible teratogenic effects of vaccine on fetus exist.*[1] *This is not advisable during pregnancy.*

Hence, pregnancy status should be ruled out in women of childbearing age before vaccination. They must be advised contraception for 1 month postvaccination.[20] Accidental administration of measles, mumps, and rubella (MMR) vaccine, however, does not call for termination of pregnancy, as no evidence of harm has been documented so far. Preconception screening and MMR administration are advised to avoid congenital rubella syndrome in her subsequent pregnancy.[21] A single dose of vaccine produces antibody levels in 95% of susceptible persons.

Pregnant women who are susceptible to rubella are vaccinated postpartum, as it eliminates the risk in future pregnancies. The virus is excreted in breast milk and causes seroconversion and asymptomatic infection is reported in the neonate.

Varicella

Varicella is caused by *varicella zoster virus* of the herpes family. Pregnant women are usually immune to infection and have protective antibodies. Maternal varicella zoster virus infection is seen in 2–3 cases per 1,000 pregnancies.[22] Varicella immunization is not recommended during pregnancy, as the virus can harm the fetus. However, accidental administration during pregnancy does not call for termination.

Pre-pregnancy and postpartum period should be utilized to vaccinate all nonimmune women. In case of a possible exposure to varicella in antenatal period, the immunity should be checked by history of previous infection, immunization, or immunoglobulin G serology.[22] If immune status is not known and the serum status is negative, varicella zoster immunoglobulin should be administered as soon as exposure occurs. The patient and family must understand the maternal and fetal sequelae of varicella infection and the risk of transmission.

Human Papillomavirus

Human papillomavirus (HPV) is a small DNA virus and the vaccine is L1 major capsid protein of HPV, which form virus-like particles. The vaccine is not recommended during pregnancy and conception is avoided for 1 month postvaccination. However, if a vaccine series is started and then pregnancy is confirmed, vaccination should be delayed and completed after delivery.

Bacillus Calmette–Guérin

Bacillus Calmette-Guérin (BCG) vaccination should not be given during pregnancy, as it is a live vaccine and can harm the fetus.

BREASTFEEDING AND POSTNATAL VACCINATION

For breastfeeding mothers, almost all vaccines (inactivated, live, recombinant, subunit, conjugated vaccines, and toxoids) can be safely administered.[1] Rubella, hepatitis B, varicella, influenza, tetanus, and HPV vaccinations are advised to all nonimmunized postnatal mothers by FOGSI (Federation of Obstetric and Gynaecological Societies of India).

Yellow fever vaccination should be avoided, but if travel cannot be postponed to endemic areas, vaccination should not be withheld.

VACCINES: SIDE EFFECTS AND CONTRAINDICATIONS

The side effects of vaccine are as follows:[13]

- Immediate effects can be fainting and vasovagal reactions. Patients are usually advised to wait for 15–30 minutes after receiving a vaccine.
- Local effects include erythema and swelling (most common).
- Systemic effects can be malaise and fever.
- *Mild allergic reactions*: This may happen with yellow fever and influenza vaccine due to egg proteins.
  Anaphylactic reactions are very rare and should be treated immediately.

General contraindications are:

- Anaphylaxis to a vaccine or vaccine component
- Severe asthma
- History of Guillain-Barré syndrome (GBS) within 6 months of receiving a vaccine.

FUTURE

Vaccines beneficial during pregnancy are in various stages of research and development. Two examples are Group B *Streptococcus* (GBS) and respiratory syncytial virus.[23] GBS is the leading cause of neonatal sepsis and meningitis and the vaccine would be effective in preventing both early and late onset disease. A polysaccharide conjugate vaccine of GBS is in clinical trials in Europe and Africa. Respiratory syncytial virus causes bronchiolitis and pneumonia in infants and the vaccine would prevent hospitalization and infant mortality due to the disease. The infant will get protection during the first few months of life due to antibody transfer from the mother.

Other potential vaccines targeting *Cytomegalovirus*, herpes simplex virus, and Zika virus will have promising results in future.

OVERCOMING THE BARRIERS

Childbearing is a joyful but sensitive time. Vaccination during pregnancy raises lots of questions in the minds of the mother and the family regarding the safety concerns, particularly related to the fetus. Other barriers to antenatal vaccination include patients' misconceptions, complexity of the immunization schedules, religious beliefs, and cost.[19] These anxieties and hesitation should be addressed by providing adequate information to the family.

The supportive recommendation from the healthcare provider increases acceptance of the vaccine to the extent of 20–100 times. Various surveys have confirmed that the obstetrician plays an important role in the decision making and in overcoming the barriers and building this confidence. To overcome maternal immunization hesitancy, educational activities should target healthcare workers and government officials also along with mothers and their families. The vaccines with proven benefit such as T-dap and influenza should be added in national immunization schedule. Maternal immunization should be given a priority by researchers, public health officials, and healthcare workers.

CONCLUSION

Vaccination in pregnancy is an essential preventive measure in obstetrics to protect the mother, fetus, and the infant. Tetanus, diphtheria, pertussis, and influenza vaccines are recommended in pregnancy, whereas others are recommended in postnatal period or in special circumstances in the antenatal period. Obstetricians and healthcare workers should recommend the vaccines and educate the mothers and the families. In developing countries like India, where cost of vaccine is a barrier, the government should include these in routine immunization program.

TAKE-HOME MESSAGE

- Single dose of T-dap vaccine is recommended in the third trimester, preferably between 27 and 36 weeks of gestation irrespective of prior Td or T-dap vaccination.
- All pregnant women should be immunized with inactivated influenza vaccine during flu season at any gestational age, preferably from 26 weeks onwards.
- Women with risk factors and travel needs can be vaccinated with hepatitis A, hepatitis B, pneumococcal, meningococcal, Japanese encephalitis, yellow fever, typhoid, rabies, and anthrax vaccines.
- Women who have inadvertently received a live or live-attenuated vaccine during pregnancy should not be counseled for termination in view of teratogenic risks. Nonpregnant women receiving these vaccines should be advised to delay pregnancy for 4 weeks.

REFERENCES

1. Arunakumari PS, Kalburgi S, Sahare A. Vaccination in pregnancy. Obstet Gynaecol. 2015;17:257-63.
2. Rathi A. Is TT immunization in pregnancy enough in Indian settings? Int J Vaccine Res. 2017;2(1):1-4.

3. Bloom BR, Lambert PH. Chapter 10: Maternal Immunization: Protecting vulnerable populations. The Vaccine book, 2nd edition. 2016. pp. 183-203.

4. Englund JA. Maternal immunization—promises and concerns. Vaccine. 2015; 33(47):6372-3.

5. Schleiss MR. Chapter 238: Tetanus (Clostridium tetani). Nelson Textbook of Pediatrics, 21st edition. Philadelphia, PA: Elsevier; 2019. pp. 1549-52.

6. Verma R, Khanna P, Dhankar M. Vaccination during pregnancy: Today's need in India. Hum Vaccin Immunother. 2016;12(3):668-70.

7. World Health Organization (2006). Maternal immunization against tetanus. [online] Available from: https://www.who.int/reproductivehealth/publications/maternal_perinatal_health/immunization_tetanus.pdf [Last accessed June, 2020].

8. van Hoek AJ, Campbell H, Amirthalingam G, Andrews N, Miller E. Cost-effectiveness and programmatic benefits of maternal vaccination against pertussis in England. J Infect. 2016;73(1):28-37.

9. American college of Obstetricians and Gynaecologists. ACOG Committee opinion No 741: Maternal Immunization. Obstet Gynecol. 2018;131(6):e214-7.

10. Siddiqui M, Khan AA, Varan AK, Esteves-Jaramillo A, Sultana S, Ali AS, et al. Intention to accept pertussis vaccine among pregnant women in Karachi, Pakistan. Vaccine. 2017;35(40):5352-9.

11. American college of Nurse-Midwives (2014). Immunization in pregnancy and postpartum Position statement. [online] Available from: http://midwife.org/ACNM/files/ACNMLibraryData/UPLOADFILENAME/000000000289/Immunization-in-Pregnancy-and-Postpartum-May-2014.pdf [Last accessed June, 2020].

12. Medical Disorders in Pregnancy Committee, FOGSI (2014). Vaccination in women. [online] Available from: https://www.fogsi.org/wp-content/uploads/2015/11/vaccination_women.pdf [Last accessed June, 2020].

13. Castillo E, Poliquin V. No. 357-Immunization in pregnancy. J Obstet Gynaecol Can. 2018;40(4):478-89.

14. Neuzil KM, Ortiz JR. Influenza Vaccines and Vaccination Strategies. The Vaccine Book, 2nd edition. 2016. pp. 423-45.

15. World health Organization; Global Advisory Committee on Vaccine Safety. (2014). Safety of immunization during pregnancy: A review of the evidence. [online] Available from: https://www.who.int/vaccine_safety/publications/safety_pregnancy_nov2014.pdf?ua=1#:~:text=There%20is%20no%20evidence%20of,medically%20indicated%20(Table%201).&text=Live%20vaccines%20may%20pose%20a%20theoretical%20risk%20to%20the%20fetus. [Last accessed June, 2020].

16. Swamy GK, Heine RP. Vaccinations for pregnant women. Obstet Gynecol. 2015;125(1):212-26.

17. Taylor CM, Shelton CM. Vaccine recommendations in pregnancy and lactation. J Am Pharm Assoc. 2019;59(1):137-40.

18. Damitz BA. Immunization Practices. Section 20: Preventive health. In: Kellerman B (Ed). Conn's Current Therapy. Philadelphia, PA: Elsevier; 2018:1333-8.

19. Shrim A, Koren G, Yudin MH, Farine D. No. 274: Management of Varicella infection in pregnancy. Reaffirmed SOGC Clinical Practice Guideline. J Obstet Gynaecol Can. 2018;40(8):e652-7.

20. Larson HJ. Maternal Immunization: The new "normal" (or it should be). Vaccine. 2015;33(47):6374-5.

21. Dontigny L, Arsenault MY, Martel MJ. No. 203-Rubella in pregnancy. J Obstet Gynaecol Can. 2018;40(8):e615-21.

22. Abramson JS, Mason E. Strengthening maternal immunization to improve the health of mothers and infants. Lancet. 2016;388(10059):2562-64.

23. Castillo E, Sadarangani M. Immunization in pregnancy: The future for neonatal protection. J Obstet Gynaecol Can. 2018;40(4):387-8.

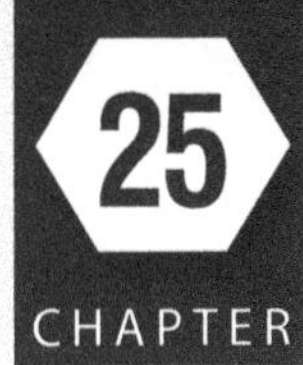

Safe Drugs in Pregnancy: An Update

Vidya Thobbi, Prabhat Agrawal, Ruchika Garg

INTRODUCTION

In order to simplify the criteria whether a drug can be used during pregnancy or not, United States Food and Drug Administration (US FDA) has classified all the drugs into five categories **(Box 1)**. Categories A and B medications usually are considered safe in humans. Category C drugs have not been definitively shown to be unsafe to human fetuses, but reasons exist to be cautious while prescribing them. Category D drugs are those with evidence of human fetal risk based on previous human studies, but the benefits of treatment prevail over the risks **(Fig. 1)**.

BOX 1: United States Food and Drug Administration Drug Classification System (US FDA).	
FDA category	*Pregnancy category definition*
A	• Controlled studies showed no risk to humans • Adequate, well-controlled studies in pregnant women have not shown an increased risk of fetal abnormalities
B	• No evidence of risk in humans • Animal studies have revealed no evidence of harm to the fetus. However, there are no adequate and well-controlled studies in pregnant women Or • Animal studies have shown an adverse effect, but adequate and well-controlled studies in pregnant women have failed to demonstrate a risk to the fetus
C	• Risks cannot be ruled out in humans • Animal studies have shown an adverse effect, and there are no adequate and well-controlled studies in pregnant women or • No animal studies have been conducted, and there are no adequate and well-controlled studies in pregnant women
D	• Clear evidence of risk in humans • Studies, adequate well-controlled or observational, in pregnant women have demonstrated a risk to the fetus. However, the benefits of therapy may outweigh the potential risk
X	• Drugs contraindicated in human pregnancy • Studies, adequate well-controlled or observational, in animals or pregnant women have demonstrated positive evidence of fetal abnormalities. The use of the product is contraindicated in women who are or may become pregnant

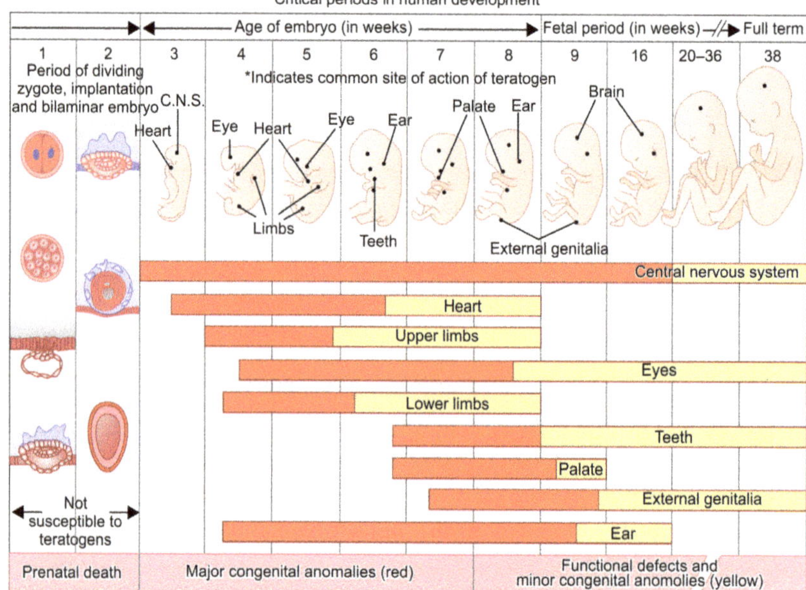

Note: *Red indicates highly sensitive periods when teratogens my induce major anomalies.

Fig. 1: Critical periods in human development.

The decision, whether to recommend a drug for a pregnant woman or not, must be made by the physician while considering many factors such as route of administration, gestational age of the fetus or embryo, absorption rate of the drug, whether the drug crosses the placenta or not, the necessary effective dose of the drug, molecular weight of the drug, whether monotherapy will suffice or if multiple drugs are required to be effective, and also the mother's genotype. Potential harm to the mother on stopping or not prescribing the drug at all is of utmost importance among these factors along with the risk to the fetus. The decision therefore totally depends upon—*"Does the benefit of the drug outweigh over its risks?"*

In the Indian setup, most of the pregnancies are complicated by infections and therefore deciding upon which antibiotic to use has always been a dilemma.

What makes antibiotic usage during pregnancy even trickier is the fact that there are marked and progressive physiological changes during pregnancy, and the drug disposition can be altered. Some of these are:

- Gastrointestinal motility is impaired and therefore drug absorption is reduced.
- Volume of drug administration is increased as plasma volume is expanded.
- Due to decrease in serum albumin and increase in alpha-1 acid glycoprotein, the unbound fraction of acidic drug increases while that of basic drugs decreases.

- Renal blood flow is markedly increased and hence increased clearance of the drugs
- Due to induction of the hepatic microenzymes, many of the drugs are cleared rapidly.

Drugs can affect the fetus at three stages:

1. *Before day 31:* During this phase, drug produces all or none effect. The conceptus either survives without anomalies or does not survive at all. As there are only few cells during this early stage, so any damage at this stage is either irreparable or lethal.
2. *Day 31 to day 71:* This is the most critical period for organ formation and most of the teratogenic effects are therefore precipitated during this phase.
3. *Day 71 onwards:* During this phase, growth of the organs formed during organogenesis occurs and teratogenic effects can occur but are less common than the second phase.

Although a large number of studies have been conducted by researchers and the pharmaceutical companies till date, the license to market the drug is usually obtained before its long-term effects have been studied. *Therefore, the usage of antibiotics must be individualized depending upon the patient requirements (Table 1).*

TABLE 1: Individual drug status and considerations during pregnancy.

Drug	Consideration	Teratogenicity	Category
Cephalosporins:			
Cefazolin			B
Cefadroxil			B
Cephalexin			B
Cefuroxime			B
Cefaclor	Safe	No teratogenicity	B
Cefotaxime			B
Ceftazidime			B
Cefixime			B
Ceftriaxone	• Safe • Can interfere with hemostasis due to its hypoprothrombinemic action	• No • Vitamin K should be given to infant, if given near to term	B
Cefoperazone	• Safe • Can derange liver enzymes and can interfere with hemostasis by having similar effect as that of ceftriaxone	No	B

Contd...

Contd...

Drug	Consideration	Teratogenicity	Category
Cefpirome	Can derange liver enzymes and can lead to eosinophilia and thrombocytopenia	No	B
Penicillins are considered safe Can be used with beta-lactamase inhibitors such as clavulanic acid and sulbactam			
Amoxicillin	Should be avoided in women at risk of preterm delivery due to increased risk of neonatal necrotizing enterocolitis	No	B
Ampicillin	Safe	No	B
Methicillin			B
Piperacillin			B
Mezlocillin			B
Cloxacillin			B
Carbenicillin	Safe to use; however, can lead to pregnancy-induced hypertension and interferes with platelet function	No	B
Meropenem	Safe	No human data; however, there is no evidence of increased risk of major congenital malformations with other beta-lactam antibiotic	B
Ertapenem			B
Sulfonamides	Contraindicated	association with neural tube defects (NTDs), cardiovascular malformations and facial cleft as a result of antifolate effect in third trimester, as they increase the risk of kernicterus in the fetus	C
Tetracyclines	Contraindicated Can lead to acute fatty liver of pregnancy	Can lead to yellowish discoloration of teeth and growth retardation due to its deposition in small bones	D
Chloramphenicol	Contraindicated	No	C

Contd...

Contd...

Drug	Consideration	Teratogenicity	Category
Macrolides:			
Azithromycin	Can be used	Not expected to increase risk of major congenital malformations	B
Clindamycin			B
Clarithromycin			C
Vancomycin	Should be avoided, associated with maternal nephrotoxicity and ototoxicity		C
Nitrofurantoin	Should be avoided	Papillary adenomas and growth retardation in neonates	C
Tigecycline	• No reports on use during human pregnancy • Tigecycline is structurally related to tetracycline and thus *should be avoided after 15 weeks of gestation*	Use of an alternate agent with a known safety profile would be preferred	D
Aminoglycosides:			
Amikacin		Theoretical risk of ototoxicity and nephrotoxicity	D
Gentamicin			D
Tobramycin	*Contraindicated*		D
Kanamycin			D
Streptomycin			D
Fluoroquinolones:			
Levofloxacin		Teratogenic effects have C	
Norfloxacin		Have been seen in experimental animals like decreased placental light, cartilage lesions, and embryonic losses	C
Ofloxacin	*Contraindicated*		C
Ciprofloxacin			C
Moxifloxacin			C
Linezolid	Can be used if benefits outweighs the risk	Not expected to increase risk of major congenital malformations	C
Antifungal agents:			
Miconazole	Safe if used topically	Syndactylia, oligodactylia, and dystocia have been seen in animals	C

Contd...

Contd...

Drug	Consideration	Teratogenicity	Category
5-flucytosine	Use only if the potential benefit outweighs the risk	Can lead to encephaloceles, macroglossia, and major skeleton defects	C
Ketoconazole	• Should be avoided • Local application is safe	Leads to increased placental weight. Has been associated with abortions, supernumerary ribs, renal pelvis dilatation and delayed ossification	C
Itraconazole	Should be avoided	Associated with increased CNS and skeletal abnormalities	C
Fluconazole	Inhibits estrogen synthesis in fetus		C
Griseofulvin	As it interferes with mitosis, it can lead to formation of conjoined twins if used in 1st trimester		C
Antivirals:			
Acyclovir	Contraindicated for systemic administration	Head and tail development in lower animal fetuses	B
Famciclovir			C
Ganciclovir			C
Amantadine	Use only if clearly indicated	At high doses may lead to cardiac malformations	C
Foscarnet	• No human data in 1st trimester • Case reports describe treatment in 2nd and 3rd trimester with no adverse effects in the neonates • Should be used only when the benefit outweighs the unknown risk to the fetus • Due to potential for renal toxicity, close follow-up of the fetus and monitoring of amniotic fluid volume is recommended		C

Contd...

Contd...

Drug	Consideration	Teratogenicity	Category
Antitubercular drugs:			
Isoniazid			C
Rifampicin	Safe	When used in last weeks of pregnancy, can lead to postnatal hemorrhage in mothers and infants	C
Rifabutin			B
Ethambutol		Optic neuritis has not been shown in infant	C
Pyrazinamide	*Should be avoided*		C
PAS	Has increased incidence of hepatotoxicity in mothers		C
Ethionamide	*Contraindicated*	Teratogenic effects have been shown in the animals	D
Cycloserine	*Contraindicated* Increased risk of psychosis in mothers		C
Streptomycin	*Contraindicated*		D
Antimalarials:			
Chloroquine		Not expected to increase risk of major congenital malformations	C
Quinine	Safe		C
Mefloquine			C
Primaquine	Contraindicated Prophylactic administration of this drug should be withheld until after delivery	Associated with hemolysis in newborn	C
Artesunate	• Limited human data, mostly on use in 2nd and 3rd trimester • Should be used only when the benefit outweighs the unknown risk to the fetus	Not expected to increase risk of major congenital malformations	
Drugs used for hyperuricemia:			
Allopurinol	Animal studies using high doses have revealed evidence of fetotoxicity and teratogenicity; it is not clear if these effects are a result of direct toxicity or maternal toxicity. There are no controlled data in human pregnancy	Allopurinol should only be given during pregnancy when benefit outweighs risk	C

Contd...

Contd...

Drug	Consideration	Teratogenicity	Category
Febuxostat	• Febuxostat was not teratogenic in animal studies at high human doses; however, increased neonatal mortality and a reduction in Febuxostat is only recommended for use during pregnancy when benefit outweighs risk		C
	• The neonatal body weight gain was observed when pregnant rats were treated with oral doses up to 40 times the human equivalent. There are no adequate and well-controlled studies in pregnant women		

COMMONLY USED DRUGS AND SAFER ALTERNATIVES (TABLE 2)

Antiepileptics in Pregnancy

No drug has been proven to be completely safe in pregnancy; however, as the seizure itself is harmful to the mother and fetus, it is advised that any patient on antiepileptic drugs should be continued on the same drugs as prescribed before conception. However, if possible, valproate should be avoided or switched to some other drugs if pregnancy is to be planned. Carbamazepine, lamotrigine, and levetiracetam are relatively safe.

If initiation of antiepileptics is required, phenobarbitone is the drug of choice.

Drugs used for Urinary Tract Infections

- Ampicillin and cotrimoxazole can be given
- *Meropenem and piperacillin*: Tazobactam can be given in resistant cases
- Nitrofurantoin and fluoroquinolones are better to be avoided.

Drugs used for Upper and Lower Respiratory Tract Infections

- Macrolides such as azithromycin and clarithromycin can be given safely.
- Cephalosporins and meropenem can be used, if associated with septicemia.

Drugs Used for Tuberculosis

- Isoniazid, rifampicin, and ethambutol can be given safely.
- Safety regarding pyrazinamide (PZA) cannot be assured, but when used for 6 months regimen, the benefits may outweigh the possible risks.

TABLE 2: Commonly used drugs and safer alternatives.

Condition/drug	Safety uncertain (strictly contraindicated drugs are marked with asterisk)	Safer alternative
Antiemetics	Domperidone and ondansetron	Promethazine, doxylamine, dicyclomine, and metoclopramide
Antacid	Cimetidine, cisapride, mosapride, and lansoprazole	Ranitidine and pantoprazole
Laxatives	Senna, bisacodyl, and docusate	Lactulose, ispaghula, and dietary fibers
Antidiarrheals	Diphenoxylate atropine and loperamide	ORS
Analgesics	Aspirin, COX-2 inhibitors, morphine, Tramadol	Paracetamol and ibuprofen (low dose)
Cold cough remedies	Codeine and dextromethorphan	Xylometazoline nasal drops and chlorpheniramine can be given safely
Antiallergics	Cetirizine, fexofenadine, and astemizole	Chlorpheniramine and promethazine
Antiamebic	Metronidazole and tinidazole	Diloxanide furoate and paromomycin
Anthelmintic	Albendazole, mebendazole, ivermectin, and diethylcarbamazine	Piperazine niclosamide and praziquantel
Antiretroviral	Didanosine, abacavir, indinavir, ritonavir, and efavirenz	Zidovudine, lamivudine, nevirapine, nelfinavir, and saquinavir
Antihypertensives	ACE inhibitors, ARBs, thiazides, furosemide, and propanolol	Methyldopa, hydralazine, atenolol, metoprolol, nifedipine, prazosin, and clonidine
Antidiabetics	Metformin, acarbose, sulfonylurea, pioglitazone, and gliptins	Preferably insulin to be used; however, metformin and glibenclamide have been given successfully in some trials
Antithyroid drugs	Carbimazole, methimazole, and radioactive iodine	Propylthiouracil
Antiasthmatics	Theophylline, montelukast, and systemic corticosteroids	Inhaled agents must be preferred.
Antipsychotics	Chlorpromazine, clozapine, olanzapine, and risperidone	Haloperidol and trifluoperazine
Antidepressants	Dothiepin, escitalopram, sertraline, trazodone, and venlafaxine	Amitriptyline, imipramine, and fluoxetine

(ACE: angiotensin-converting enzyme; ARB: angiotensin receptor blocker; COX: cyclooxygenase)

- Streptomycin may cause congenital deafness, as this drug interferes with the development of ear and must be avoided.
- Other injectables, such as amikacin, kanamycin, and capreomycin, may also cause fetal nephrotoxicity and ototoxicity and should be avoided.
- Ethionamide and prothionamide are contraindicated in pregnancy, as they are found teratogenic in animal studies.
- Cycloserine crosses placenta, and since its safety in pregnancy is not established, it should be avoided and used only if no other suitable alternatives are available.

Important Note

Readers may find it surprising that though certain drugs are placed in category C, yet the comment reads that they are safe since many infections during pregnancy have to be treated carefully and therefore even they are placed in category C, they can be used safely.

■ TERATOGENIC DRUGS

To date, very few drugs are proven teratogens. However, malformations induced by drugs are important because they are potentially preventable. Proper prescribing of drugs in pregnancy is a challenge and should provide maximal safety to the fetus as well as therapeutic benefit to the mother.

Placental Transfer

The rate of placental transfer is affected by metabolism and gestational age, and the protein binding, ionization, lipid solubility, and molecular weight of the drug. There is a misconception that there is a placental barrier providing protection to the fetus; however, almost all drugs are able to pass freely through the placenta, with only those with a molecular weight of >1,000 Da being unable to do so, e.g., insulin and heparin.

Teratogenicity

A drug is identified as a teratogen, if exposure *in utero* causes, directly or indirectly, structural or functional abnormalities in the fetus or in the child after birth.

Neuropsychological and behavioral abnormalities may also occur after drug exposure. Some antiepileptic drugs and drugs of abuse have been associated with learning and behavioral problems following *in-utero* exposure; however, the potential confounding effects of social factors and maternal illness can make ascertainment of causality difficult.

Timing of Exposure

During the preimplantation stage, in very early pregnancy, exposure to a drug is unlikely to produce a teratogenic effect due to an inbuilt "recovery process" in the conceptus.

If a teratogenic insult occurs and there is damage to only a small number of cells then "compensation" occurs whereby the remaining viable cells continue to divide to replace any that were damaged.

Timing of Exposure

During the preimplantation stage, in very early pregnancy, exposure to a drug is unlikely to produce a teratogenic effect due to an inbuilt "recovery process" in the conceptus. If a teratogenic insult occurs and there is damage to only a small number of cells then "compensation" occurs whereby the remaining viable cells continue to divide to replace any that were damaged.

However, if a large number of cells are damaged then implantation will not occur and the pregnancy will be lost. This is known as the *"all or nothing" or totipotent period.*

The 10 weeks following implantation are the most sensitive, as this is the time during which major structural changes and organogenesis are taking place. For example, it is during this period that the neural tube closes and major organs and limbs develop.

While the first trimester is the most sensitive period to structural malformations, some drugs may affect the fetus in the later stages of pregnancy, so care should be taken when prescribing throughout pregnancy.

For example, exposure to ACE inhibitors in the second and third trimesters can cause serious adverse effects such as oligohydramnios, growth retardation, lung and kidney hypoplasia, and hypocalvaria.

▮ GENERAL PRINCIPLES OF PRESCRIBING IN PREGNANCY

These involve the woman and her family, where appropriate, in all decisions about treatment:

- Not treating mental illness in pregnancy or the postpartum period may be associated with adverse outcomes
- Establish a clear indication for drug treatment
- Choose treatments with the lowest known risk
- In choosing, consider the implications for breast feeding and the benefits of avoiding the need to switch drugs
- Use treatments in the lowest effective dose for the shortest period necessary
- Be aware of potential drug interactions, particularly with nonpsychotropics, and aim for monotherapy
- Where there is no clear evidence base that one drug is safer than another; the safest option is not to switch. The only drug with a clear indication for switching on safety grounds is valproate.
- Be aware of the potential effects of pregnancy and childbirth on drug pharmacokinetics and pharmacodynamics
- Knowledge of teratogenic effects of psychotropic drugs is increasing, understanding of the long-term neurodevelopmental effects of such medications in pregnancy and breastfeeding is extremely limited.

- Close monitoring for change in mental state where a woman decides to cease her usual medication
- Where there is known risk, ensure that women are offered appropriate fetal screening and monitoring of the neonate for adverse effects
- Premature or ill babies are more at risk of harmful drug effects
- Monitor the infant for drug side effects, feeding patterns, growth, and development
- Caution women against sleeping in bed with the infant, particularly if taking sedative drugs

The risk posed by drug use in pregnancy can be minimized through prepregnancy counseling. When prescribing for a patient planning pregnancy or a patient who has become pregnant, consideration should be given whether drug is absolutely essential. When prescribing, it is important to balance the risk of treatment to the fetus against the risk to both mother and fetus from failing to treat the maternal condition. Each case should be individualized.

All drugs in pregnancy should be prescribed in the lowest possible dose for the shortest possible time.

Interpreting Pregnancy Outcome Data

Robust pregnancy outcome data especially for new drugs is lacking. This is partly due to ethical constraints of enrolling pregnant women into clinical trials.

Selected Drugs or Substances Suspected or proven to be Human Teratogens (Table 3)

TABLE 3: Selected drugs or substances suspected or proven to be human teratogens.	
Alcohol	Methimazole
ACE inhibitors	Methyl mercury
Aminopterin	Methotrexate
Androgens	Misoprostol
Bexarotene	Mycophenolate
Carbamazepine	Paroxetine
Chloramphenicol	Penicillamine
Chlorobiphenyls	Phenobarbital
Cocaine	Phenytoin
Corticosteroids	Radioactive iodine
Cyclophosphamide	Ribavirin
Danazol	Streptomycin

Contd...

Contd...

DES	Tamoxifen
Efavirenz	Tetracycline
Etretinate	Thalidomide
Leflunomide	Tobacco
Lithium	Tretinoin
Valproate	Warfarin

(DES: diethylstilbestrol)

Proven Teratogenic Drugs in Humans

Alcohol

The fetal alcohol syndrome is characterized by intrauterine growth restriction (IUGR), microcephaly, developmental delay, and dysmorphic faces. Cleft palate and cardiac anomalies may also occur. Thus, alcohol is one of the most frequent nongenetic causes of mental retardation as well as the leading cause of preventable birth defects in the United States.

Angiotensin-converting Enzyme Inhibitors (Captopril, Enalapril, and Lisinopril) and Angiotensin Receptor Blockers

There use in late pregnancy has been associated with renal insufficiency. IUGR, prematurity, and complications of oligohydramnios (fetal limb contractures and lung hypoplasia) have been reported with their use in late pregnancy. Teratogenic risk with first trimester use of them appears to be low.

Carbamazepine

Exposure causes 1% risk of neural tube defects (10 times their baseline risk).

Phenytoin

It causes fetal hydantoin syndrome (1993) with craniofacial dysmorphology, growth retardation, and cardiac defects.

Valproate

First-trimester exposure is associated with neural tube defects.

Cocaine

It is associated with abruption placentae, prematurity, fetal loss, decreased birth weight, microcephaly, and limb defects.

Coumarin Anticoagulants (Warfarin)

The critical period of exposure for the *fetal warfarin syndrome* appears to be between *6 and 9 weeks* of gestation. Second and third trimester exposure is associated with *hemorrhage* leading to disharmonic growth and deformation.

Diethylstilbestrol

Clear cell adenocarcinoma of vagina is associated with first trimester exposure. Hypoplastic and T-shaped uterine cavity and septa are also reported.

Antineoplastic Agents

Folic acid antagonists—aminopterin and methotrexate: Central nervous system (CNS) defects fascial anomalies and mental retardation occur following first trimester exposure. After a review of 20 first trimester exposure, Feldcamp and Carey (1993) calculated that a dose of 10 mg/week is necessary to produce abnormalities.

Cyclophosphamide

First trimester use is associated with missing and hypoplastic digits, cleft palate, and imperforate anus. Nurses who administer cyclophosphamide may be at increased risk for fetal loss, but there are no adequate epidemiological studies.

Isotretinoin

It is prescribed for acne and causes a pattern of anomalies called retinoic acid embryopathy.

Psychiatric Medications

- *Lithium:*
  Ebstein's anomaly (a rare malformation of tricuspid value) is caused by it.
- *Selective serotonin reuptake inhibitors:*

Paroxetine exposure is associated with congenital cardiac malformations and persistent pulmonary hypertension in the newborn. *American College of Obstetricians and Gynecologists* (2007) concluded that selective serotonin reuptake inhibitors (SSRIs) are not major teratogens and treatment must be individualized.

Misoprostol

First-trimester exposure is associated with limb defects with or without *Moebiu's sequence.*

Prescribing misoprostol in obstetrics and gynecology:

Routes of administration: Oral, vaginal, sublingual, buccal, or rectal.

Vaginal misoprostol is associated with slower absorption, lower peak plasma levels, and slower clearance, similar to an extended release preparation.

Vaginal misoprostol is also associated with a greater overall exposure to the drug [area under the curve (AUC)] and greater effects on the cervix and uterus. There is, however, a wide variation in the absorption of misoprostol through the vaginal epithelium among different women. *There is no clinically significant difference between vaginal misoprostol that is administered dry and vaginal misoprostol moistened with water, saline, or acetic acid.*

Misoprostol is considered a teratogen. The absolute risk of congenital malformations is 1.%.

Breastfeeding: Misoprostol is excreted into breast milk. Levels become undetectable within 5 hours of maternal ingestion. Women should be advised that misoprostol may cause infant diarrhea.

Tetracycline

Yellowish brown discoloration of teeth may occur with exposure of drug after 17 weeks of gestation.

Thalidomide

More than any other event, the thalidomide tragedy altered the world to the teratogenic potential of drugs. It produces limb reduction defects in fetuses exposed to it during *34–50 days menstrual age.*

Hormones

Androgenic progestins: Norethindrone (a progesterone only contraceptive) causes virilization of 1% of exposed female fetus.

Androgens

Exposure of a female fetus to anabolic steroids results in varying degrees of virilization.

Danazol

- Virilization of female fetus

Corticosteroids

First trimester exposure is associated with increased incidence of fascial clefts. However, they are not considered to represent a major teratogenic risk.

Methyl Mercury

Prenatal exposure is associated with developmental delay and neurological abnormalities. Ingestion of contaminated fish (enters the echosystem through industrial pollution) may expose the fetus to it.

Antivirals

- *Ribavirin*: It is highly teratogenic in all animal species studied.
- *Amantadine*: There is possible association with cardiac defects.

Possible Teratogenic Drugs in Humans

- *D-penicillamine*: Connective tissue disorders (Cutis laxa)
- *Methimazole*: Scalp defects (aplasia cutis congenita)
- *Diazepam*: First trimester exposure has been associated in small studies with a small increase in the incidence of cleft lip and palate. Larger studies did not confirm the association.

Fluconazole and Itraconazole

There have been several reports of skull abnormalities and limb defects with their exposure. Despite this, large cohort studies suggest that neither drug is teratogenic.

Leflunomide

It is used to treat rheumatoid arthritis. In animals, its use is associated with hydrocephalus and skeletal anomalies.

■ SUGGESTED READING

1. Cunningham F, Leveno K, Bloom S, Hoffman B. Williams Obstetrics, 24 edition. New York: McGraw Hill; 2014.
2. Drug Facts and Comparison. Philadelphia: Lippincott Williams & Wilkins; 2013.
3. Dutta DC. Textbook of Obstetrics, 6th edition. New Delhi: Jaypee Brothers Medical Publisher (P) Ltd.; 2018.
4. Medscape. Tigecycline (Rx.). [online] Available from: https://reference.medscape.com/drug/tygacil-tigecycline-342527. [Last accessed July, 2020].
5. Perinatology.com. Drugs in Pregnancy and Breastfeeding. [online] Available from www.perinatology.com/exposures/druglist.htm. [Last accessed July, 2020].
6. Tripathi KD. Essentials of medical pharmacology, 7th edition. New Delhi: Jaypee Brothers Medical Publisher (P) Ltd.; 2013.

Positive Pregnancy Experience: WHO Update

Pratima Mittal

■ INTRODUCTION

A magical time that every woman awaits to have in her lifetime to carry a soul within her, being pregnant is such an inspirational time for any woman. Pregnancy and childbirth are physiological events in the life of a woman. Though most pregnancies result in normal birth, it is estimated that about 15% may develop complications. It is estimated that in 2015 alone, an estimated 303,000 women died due to pregnancy-related issues and 2.6 million babies were stillborn.[1] Most of these complications can be averted by preventive care, skilled care at birth, early detection of risk, appropriate and timely management of obstetric complications, and postnatal care. Quality antenatal care (ANC) based upon scientifically sound evidence-based practices plays a major role in significantly reducing these adverse outcomes and improving the health of both mother and child.

2016 WHO ANC MODEL: IMPLEMENTATION OF GUIDELINES AND RECOMMENDATIONS

The ultimate goal of the 2016 WHO recommendations for ANC is to improve the quality of ANC and to improve maternal, fetal, and newborn outcomes related to ANC. These ANC recommendations need to be deliverable within an appropriate model of care that can be adapted to different countries, local contexts, and the individual woman The 2016 WHO ANC model stresses upon a holistic regimen of patient centered care, integrated clinical practices (interventions and tests), provision of useful information, psychological and emotional support by health practitioners working in an organized health system.

The WHO recommendations are not only aimed at ensuring mother and child survival but also to provide an enriching experience for the mother during her journey through pregnancy, institute a systematic ANC organization and delivery system practice, and emphasize upon individualistic care and well-being.

The major aims of these recommendations are:
- To provide a "positive pregnancy experience", which is defined by WHO as one in which the mother *maintains* optimum physical health and

sociocultural mindset, *enjoys* a healthy pregnancy (including prevention or treatment of risks, illness, and death), *experiences* a smooth transition to positive labor and birth and *accomplishes* a positive sense of motherhood (including self-esteem, competence, and autonomy).

- The recommendations are intended to complement (and not replace) existing WHO guidelines on the management of specific pregnancy complications with the overall theme being to improve the patient's experience of ANC.

A total of *49* recommendations related to five major interventions are made. The interventions being:

1. Nutritional interventions (14)
2. Maternal and fetal assessment (13)
3. Preventive measures (7)
4. Interventions for common physiological symptoms (6)
5. Health system interventions to improve utilization (9)

Including *10* recommendations relevant to routine ANC from other WHO guidelines.

The first four are the critical evidence-based practices that improve pregnancy outcome. The fifth intervention is concerned with improving healthcare quality and adopting the best ANC practices.

One of the *most significant recommendations* made by WHO is *raising the number of ANC contacts (visits) to a minimum of eight* as WHO believes that greater the number of ANC contacts, more is the degree of maternal satisfaction and reduction in perinatal mortality.[2] Thus, a minimum of one contact in the first trimester (up to 12 weeks of gestation), two contacts in the second trimester (at 20 and 26 weeks of gestation), and five contacts in the third trimester (at 30, 34, 36, 38, and 40 weeks) are desirable. However, it is important to consider the logistical and financial burden required for such a high number of ANC visits, especially in a resource-poor country like India. Each country is expected to adapt these recommendations based on their own core health needs and resources to provide the best possible ANC across all eight ANC contacts. Also, here the term *"contact"* is used—it implies an active connection between a pregnant woman and a healthcare provider that is not implicit with the word "visit". In terms of the operationalization of this recommendation, "contact" can take place at the facility or at community level.

In the new WHO ANC guideline, an ultrasound scan before 24 weeks of gestation is recommended for all pregnant women to—estimate gestational age, detect fetal anomalies and multiple pregnancies, and enhance the maternal pregnancy experience. An ultrasound scan after 24 weeks of gestation (late ultrasound) is not recommended for pregnant women who have had an early ultrasound scan. Ultrasound can also be used for other indications (e.g., obstetric emergencies) or by other medical departments.

The WHO recommendations have been categorized for ease of interpretation as:

- Universal recommendations (for all countries)
- Recommendations for specific contexts
- Recommendations for specific contexts in research
- Practices not recommended.

All the five major intervention groups will be discussed as per universal recommendation/recommendations for specific contexts/recommendations for specific contexts in research/practices not recommended.

NUTRITIONAL INTERVENTIONS

Nutrition plays a vital role for maternal and fetal well-being and development. Mother's nutrition is important before conception, throughout pregnancy and through breastfeeding period.

A healthy balanced adequate diet meeting daily need of energy, protein, vitamins, and minerals is one of the foremost requirements for a healthy and safe pregnancy. However, dietary intake often proves inadequate to meet these needs. On the other end of the spectrum, obesity and overweight are also associated with poor pregnancy outcomes and many women gain excessive weight during pregnancy.

Anemia is associated with iron, folate, and micronutrient deficiencies. It is estimated that anemia affects 38.2% of pregnant women globally, with the highest prevalence in the WHO regions of South-East Asia (48.7%) and Africa (46.3%), medium prevalence in the Eastern Mediterranean Region (38.9%) and the lowest prevalence in the WHO regions of the Western Pacific (24.3%), the Americas (24.9%), and Europe (25.8%).[3] Other micronutrient deficiencies (vitamin A and iodine) also constitute serious public health problems.

In resource-poor countries like India, besides adequate nutrition, counseling regarding increasing daily energy and protein intake along with proper dietary supplementation becomes important to avoid low birth weight and stillborn babies. Understanding of the relation between maternal nutrition and birth outcomes provides a basis for developing nutritional interventions that will improve birth outcomes and long-term quality of life and will reduce mortality, morbidity, and healthcare costs. Thus, nutritional interventions play a major role in this regard. These interventions include:

- *Universal recommendations*:
  - *Counseling on*:
    - *Healthy eating and physical activity to stay healthy and to prevent excessive weight gain*: A healthy diet contains adequate energy, protein, vitamins, and minerals and is obtained through the consumption of a variety of foods, including green and orange vegetables, meat, fish, beans, nuts, whole grains, and fruit.
    - A healthy lifestyle includes aerobic physical activity and strength-conditioning exercise aimed at maintaining a good level of fitness

throughout pregnancy, without trying to reach peak fitness level or train for athletic competition. Women should choose activities with minimal risk of loss of balance and fetal trauma.[4]

- Gestational weight gain occurs after 20 weeks of gestation and the definition of "normal" is subject to regional variations, but should take into consideration prepregnant body mass index (BMI). According to the Institute of Medicine Classification,[5] women who are underweight at the start of pregnancy (i.e., BMI < 18.5 kg/m^2) should aim to gain 12.5–18 kg, women who are normal weight at the start of pregnancy (i.e., BMI 18.5–24.9 kg/m^2) should aim to gain 11.5–16 kg, overweight women (i.e., BMI 25–29.9 kg /m^2) should aim to gain 7–11.5 kg, and obese women (i.e., BMI > 30 kg/m^2) should aim to gain 5–9 kg.
- Daily oral iron and folic acid supplementation with 30–60 mg of elemental iron and 400 µg (0.4 mg) of folic acid is recommended for pregnant women to prevent maternal anemia, puerperal sepsis, low birth weight, and preterm birth.[6,7]

- *Context-specific recommendations:*
  - Nutrition education on increasing daily energy and protein intake among the undernourished
  - Balanced energy and protein dietary supplementation in under-nourished population
  - Intermittent oral iron and folic acid supplementation with 120 mg of elemental iron and 2,800 µg (2.8 mg) of folic acid once weekly, if daily iron is not acceptable due to side effects
  - Daily calcium supplementation (1.5–2.0 g oral elemental calcium) is recommended to reduce the risk of pre-eclampsia
  - Vitamin A supplementation is only recommended in areas where vitamin A deficiency is a severe public health problem to prevent night blindness
  - Restricting caffeine intake in pregnant women with high daily caffeine intake (more than 300 mg per day).
- *Context-specific recommendation for research:* Zinc supplementation is only recommended in the context of rigorous research.
- *Not recommended:*
  - High protein supplementation to improve maternal and perinatal outcome
  - Multiple micronutrient supplementation to improve maternal and perinatal outcome
  - Vitamin B$_6$ (pyridoxine) supplementation to improve maternal and perinatal outcome
  - Vitamin C and E supplementation to improve maternal and perinatal outcome
  - Vitamin D supplementation to improve maternal and perinatal outcome.

■ MATERNAL AND FETAL ASSESSMENT

A general assessment of the pregnant woman's health status should be conducted during each antenatal visit. Regular monitoring of pregnancy allows early detection of health problems that could arise during pregnancy, and their treatment, thus increasing the chance for a normal pregnancy and the birth of a healthy baby.

Detection of three major conditions in pregnancy, viz., anemia, asymptomatic bacteriuria, and intimate partner violence is to be emphasized. In addition, existing WHO recommendations on diagnosing gestational diabetes mellitus (GDM) and screening for alcohol and substance abuse, tobacco smoking, TB, and HIV infection have also been incorporated by WHO.

Assessment of fetal growth and well-being constitutes an important part of ANC and the interventions meant to assess fetal growth and well-being in healthy pregnant women should be addressed at each antenatal visit.

- *Universal recommendations*:
  - *Gestational diabetes mellitus (GDM)*: Hyperglycemia first detected at any time during pregnancy should be classified as either gestational diabetes mellitus (GDM) or diabetes mellitus in pregnancy.

    Gestational diabetes mellitus should be diagnosed at any time in pregnancy, if one or more of the following criteria are met:[8]
    - Fasting plasma glucose 5.1–6.9 mmol/L (92–125 mg/dL)
    - 1-hour plasma glucose 10.0 mmol/L (180 mg/dL) following a 75 g oral glucose load
    - 2-hour plasma glucose 8.5–11.0 mmol/L (153–199 mg/dL) following a 75 g oral glucose load.

    Diabetes mellitus in pregnancy should be diagnosed, if one or more of the following criteria are met:
    - Fasting plasma glucose 7.0 mmol/L (126 mg/dL)
    - 2-hour plasma glucose 11.1 mmol/L (200 mg/dL) following a 75 g oral glucose load
    - Random plasma glucose 11.1 mmol/L (200 mg/dL) in the presence of diabetes symptoms.

    The usual window for diagnosing GDM is between 24 and 28 weeks of gestation. Risk factor for screening is used in some settings as a strategy to determine the need for a 2-hour 75 g oral glucose tolerance test (OGTT). These include a BMI of greater than 30 kg/m^2, previous GDM, previous macrosomia, family history of diabetes mellitus, and ethnicity with a high prevalence of diabetes mellitus. In addition, glycosuria on dipstick testing (2+ or above on one occasion, or 1+ on two or more occasions) may indicate undiagnosed GDM and, if this is observed, performing an OGTT could be considered:[9]
  - *Tobacco use*: Healthcare providers should ask all pregnant women about their tobacco use (past and present) and exposure to

second-hand smoke as early as possible in pregnancy and at every ANC visit. They should routinely offer advice and psychosocial interventions for tobacco cessation to all pregnant women who are either current tobacco users or recent tobacco quitters.

- *Substance use*: Healthcare providers should ask all pregnant women about their use of alcohol and other substances (past and present) as early as possible in the pregnancy and at every ANC visit.
    - For women identified as being dependent on alcohol or drugs, further recommendations include:
        - Healthcare providers should at the earliest opportunity advise pregnant women dependent on alcohol or drugs to cease their alcohol or drug use and offer, or refer them to, detoxification services under medical supervision, where necessary and applicable.
        - Healthcare providers should offer a brief intervention to all pregnant women using alcohol or drugs.
- *Human immunodeficiency virus (HIV)*: Provider-initiated testing and counseling (PITC) should be carried out routinely in high-prevalence settings. Human immunodeficiency virus (HIV) and syphilis testing in low-prevalence settings can be considered to eliminate HIV transmission from mother-to-child and to integrate HIV testing with syphilis. WHO recommends that ART should be initiated in all pregnant women diagnosed with HIV at any CD4 count and continued lifelong.[10]
- One ultrasound scan before 24 weeks of gestation (early ultrasound) is recommended for pregnant women to estimate gestational age, improve detection of fetal anomalies and multiple pregnancies, and reduce induction of labor for post-term pregnancy. Accurate gestational age dating is critical for the appropriate delivery of time-sensitive interventions in pregnancy, as well as management of pregnancy complications, particularly pre-eclampsia and preterm birth, which are major causes of maternal and perinatal morbidity and mortality, and early ultrasound is useful for this purpose.

■ *Context-specific recommendations*:
- *Anemia*: Full blood count is the optimal method of detection of anemia. Less favored methods like onsite hemoglobin testing with a hemoglobinometer and hemoglobin color scale can be used in low-resource settings.
- *Asymptomatic bacteriuria (ASB)*: Midstream urine culture is recommended for diagnosing asymptomatic bacteriuria in pregnancy. Less favored methods like onsite midstream urine Gram-staining can be used in low-resource settings.
- *Intimate partner violence (IPV)*: Routine enquiry about IPV can be implemented upon availability of well-trained healthcare providers.

A minimum condition for healthcare providers to ask women about violence is that it must be safe to do so (i.e., the partner is not present) and that identification of IPV is followed by an appropriate response. In addition, providers must be trained to ask questions in the correct way and to respond appropriately to women who disclose violence.[11] Examples of conditions during pregnancy that may be caused or complicated by IPV include:[11]

- Traumatic injury, particularly if repeated and with vague or implausible explanations
- Intrusive partner or husband present at consultations
- Adverse reproductive outcomes, including multiple unintended pregnancies and/or terminations, delay in seeking ANC, adverse birth outcomes, repeated STIs
- Unexplained or repeated genitourinary symptoms
- Symptoms of depression and anxiety
- Alcohol and other substance use
- Self-harm, suicidality, symptoms of depression, and anxiety.

- *Tuberculosis (TB)*: In settings where the TB prevalence in the general population is 100/100,000 population or higher, systematic screening for active TB should be considered for pregnant women as part of ANC. Systematic screening is defined as the systematic identification of people with suspected active TB in a predetermined target group, using tests, examinations or other procedures that can be applied rapidly. Options for initial screening include screening for symptoms (either for cough lasting longer than 2 weeks, or any symptoms compatible with TB, including a cough of any duration, hemoptysis, weight loss, fever, or night sweats) or screening with chest radiography. The use of chest radiography in pregnant women poses no significant risk but the national guidelines for the use of radiography during pregnancy should be followed.[12]
- *Symphysis-fundal height (SFH) measurement*: If routinely practiced in a particular ANC setting, it is recommended that SFH has no real advantage over abdominal palpation method.

- *Context-specific recommendation for research*: Daily fetal movement counting ("count to ten" kick charts) is only recommended in the context of rigorous research. While daily fetal movement counting is not recommended, healthy pregnant women should be made aware of the importance of fetal movements in the third trimester and of reporting reduced fetal movements.
- *Not recommended*:
  - Routine antenatal cardiotocography examination is not recommended to improve maternal and perinatal outcomes
  - Routine Doppler ultrasound is not recommended to improve maternal and perinatal outcomes.

■ PREVENTIVE MEASURES

World Health Organization recommends antenatal interventions for prevention of certain debilitating conditions impacting maternal health and perinatal outcome that include:

- *Universal recommendation:*
  - *Antibiotics for asymptomatic bacteriuria (ASB):* It is defined as true bacteriuria in the absence of specific symptoms of acute urinary tract infection. *Escherichia coli* is associated with up to 80% of isolates.[13] Other pathogens include *Klebsiella species, Proteus mirabilis,* and group B streptococcus (GBS). ASB is an often ignored condition that often predisposes to acute pyelonephritis. A 7-day antibiotic regimen is recommended for all pregnant women with asymptomatic bacteriuria (ASB) to prevent persistent bacteriuria, preterm birth, and low birth weight.
  - *Tetanus toxoid vaccination:* It is recommended for all pregnant women, depending on previous tetanus vaccination exposure, to prevent neonatal mortality from tetanus:
    - If a pregnant woman has not previously been vaccinated, or if her immunization status is unknown, she should receive two doses of a tetanus toxoid-containing vaccine (TT-CV) 1 month apart with the second dose given at least 2 weeks before delivery. Two doses protect against tetanus infection for 1–3 years in most people. A third dose is recommended 6 months after the second dose, which should extend protection to at least 5 years.
    - Tetanus vaccination and clean delivery practices are major components of the strategy to eradicate maternal and neonatal tetanus globally.[14]
- *Context-specific recommendation:*
  - *Preventive anthelmintic treatment:* In endemic areas, a preventive anthelmintic treatment is recommended for pregnant women after the first trimester as part of worm infection reduction programs. Preventive deworming, using single-dose albendazole (400 mg) or mebendazole (500 mg), is recommended as a public health intervention for pregnant women, after the first trimester, living in areas where both:
    1. The baseline prevalence of hookworm and/or *Trichuris trichiura* infection is 20% or more, and
    2. Where anemia is a severe public health problem, with prevalence of 40% or higher among pregnant women, in order to reduce the burden of hookworm and *T. trichiura* infection.
  - *Intermittent preventive treatment of malaria in pregnancy (IPTp):* In malaria-endemic areas in Africa, intermittent preventive treatment with sulfadoxine–pyrimethamine (IPTp-SP) is recommended for all pregnant women. Dosing should start in the second trimester and

dose should be given at least one month apart with the objective that at least three doses are received.

A package of interventions for preventing and controlling malaria during pregnancy includes promotion and use of insecticide-treated nets, appropriate case management with prompt, effective treatment, and administration of IPTp-SP in areas with moderate-to-high transmission of *Plasmodium falciparum*.[15]

- *Pre-exposure prophylaxis (PrEP) for HIV prevention*: In pregnant women at significant risk for HIV, oral PrEP containing tenofovir disoproxil fumarate (TDF) should be offered as an additional prevention choice. "Substantial risk" is provisionally defined as HIV incidence greater than 3 per 100 person-years in the absence of PrEP, but individual risk varies within this group depending on individual behavior and the characteristics of sexual partners.

- *Context-specific recommendation for research*:
  - Antibiotic prophylaxis to prevent recurrent urinary tract infections is recommended only in the context of rigorous research.
  - Antenatal anti-D immunoglobulin prophylaxis in nonsensitized Rh-negative pregnant women at 28 and 34 weeks of gestation is recommended only in the context of rigorous research.
- *Not recommended*: None in this intervention.

INTERVENTIONS FOR COMMON PHYSIOLOGICAL SYMPTOMS

Pregnancy-induced hormonal and mechanical effects lead to troublesome symptoms such as nausea and vomiting, low back and pelvic pain, heartburn, varicose veins, constipation and leg cramps that negatively affect their pregnancy experience. All the interventions in this regard are recommended in all settings and can be categorized as:

- *Universal recommendation*:
  - *Nausea and vomiting*: Nonpharmacological interventions for nausea and vomiting such as ginger, chamomile, vitamin B_6, and/ or acupuncture are recommended in early pregnancy, based on a woman's preferences and available options. Pharmacological options like doxylamine and metoclopramide are reserved only for those with unresponsive symptoms.
  - *Heartburn*: Advice regarding diet and lifestyle modifications such as avoidance of large, fatty meals, and alcohol, cessation of smoking, and raising the head of the bed to sleep is recommended to prevent and relieve heartburn in pregnancy. Antacid preparations such as magnesium carbonate and aluminum hydroxide preparations can be offered to women with troublesome symptoms that are not relieved by lifestyle modification.

- *Leg cramps*: Magnesium, calcium, or non-pharmacological options like muscle stretching, relaxation, heat therapy, dorsiflexion of the foot, and massage can be used for the relief of leg cramps in pregnancy.
- *Low back and pelvic pain*: Regular exercise throughout pregnancy is recommended; other options such as physiotherapy, support belts, and acupuncture can also be used to prevent low back and pelvic pain in pregnancy.
- *Interventions for constipation*: Dietary modification is the optimal method; however in unresponsive cases, wheat bran or other fiber supplements can be used to relieve constipation in pregnancy.
- *Varicose veins and edema*: Options such as compression stockings, leg elevation, and water immersion are recommended for the management of varicose veins and edema in pregnancy.

HEALTH SYSTEMS INTERVENTIONS TO IMPROVE THE UTILIZATION AND QUALITY OF ANC

This constitutes the "how of ANC" and consists of GDG recommendations to improve the utilization and quality of ANC depending on the context and setting. These interventions include:

- Women-held case notes (home-based records)
- Midwife-led continuity of care models
- Group ANC
- Community-based interventions to improve communication and support
- Task shifting
- Recruitment and retention of staff
- ANC contact schedules.
  These interventions can be categorized as:
- *Universal recommendations*:
  - *Women-held case notes*: Home-based records either in print or electronic form are recommended to be carried by all pregnant women to improve continuity, client provider communication, and improved accuracy of gestational age estimation.
  - *Task shifting components of ANC delivery*: Involving a broad range of medical personnel such as lay health workers, auxiliary nurses, nurses, midwives, and doctors in the promotion of maternal and newborn health-related behavior.
  - The distribution of recommended nutritional supplements and intermittent preventive treatment in pregnancy (IPTp) for malaria prevention is to be done by different categories of medical personnel such as lay health workers, auxiliary nurses, nurses, midwives, and doctors.
  - *Antenatal care contact schedules*: Antenatal care models with a minimum of eight ANC contacts are recommended to reduce perinatal mortality and improve women's experience of care.

- Antenatal care models with minimum of eight contacts are recommended for reduction of perinatal mortality and improved women's experience of care.
- *Context-specific recommendations*:
  - *Midwife-led continuity of care (MLCC)*: Midwives are the primary care providers in many ANC settings.[16] In countries with well-functioning midwifery programs, a known midwife or small group of known midwives supports a woman throughout the antenatal, intrapartum, and postnatal period.
  - *Community-based interventions to improve communication and support*: These include:
    - *Facilitated participatory learning and action (PLA) cycles with women's groups*: Participatory women's groups represent an opportunity for women to discuss their needs during pregnancy, including barriers to reaching care, and to increase support to pregnant women.
    - *Community mobilization and antenatal home visits*: These are applicable mainly to pregnant women in rural settings with poor accessibility to health services. Healthcare providers need initial and ongoing training in communication with women and their partners and also need training on group facilitation, in the convening of public meetings and in other methods of communication.

When considering the use of antenatal home visits, women's groups, partner involvement, or community mobilization, program planners need to ensure that these can be implemented in a way that respects and facilitates women's needs for privacy as well as their choices and their autonomy in decision making:

- *Recruitment and retention of staff in rural and remote areas*: For recruiting and retaining skilled health workers in rural and remote areas, policy makers need to provide educational, regulatory, financial, and personal and professional support.
- *Context-specific recommendation for research—Group ANC*: As an alternative to individual ANC, group ANC may be offered for pregnant women in the context of rigorous research as per their preference. With the group ANC model, the first visit for all pregnant women is an individual visit. Then at subsequent visits, the usual individual pregnancy health assessment, held in a private examination area, is integrated into a group ANC session, with facilitated educational activities and peer support.

DISSEMINATION, APPLICABILITY, AND LIMITATIONS OF THESE RECOMMENDATIONS

The large-scale reorganization and redistribution of healthcare resources required to achieve these objectives particularly in resource poor settings is one of the major challenges faced in implementation of the above recommendations.

The other hurdles faced in the implementation process include:

- Lack of skilled health personnel
- Lack of necessary infrastructure to support interventions
- Community misunderstandings regarding the new model of care, in particular regarding contact schedule and potentially longer wait times
- Meagre physical resources, e.g., equipment, test kits, supplies, medicines, and nutritional supplements
- Absence of effective referral mechanisms and care pathways for women identified as needing additional care
- Inadequate understanding of utility of these newly recommended interventions among healthcare personnel
- Lack of effective documentation and monitoring of recommended practices (e.g., client cards, registers, etc.)

The long list of these hurdles to implementation dictates a prudent, planned approach to the adoption and implementation of the guidelines and recommendations.

MONITORING AND EVALUATING THE IMPACT OF THE GUIDELINE

Monitoring the implementation and impact of these WHO recommendations needs to be performed at all levels whether it is at the local health center, district, state, or country. The WHO has constituted special monitoring and evaluation teams which collect data and study the impact of these guidelines on National policies individual states. It is proposed to utilize interrupted time series, clinical audits, or criterion-based audits to obtain the relevant data on the guideline interventions.

Hence, *the overall aim of this WHO ANC model 2016* is "To provide pregnant women with respectful, individualized, person-centered care *at every contact*, with implementation of effective *clinical practices* (interventions and tests), and provision of relevant and timely *information*, and *psychosocial and emotional support*, by practitioners with good clinical and interpersonal skills within a *well-functioning health system*."

REFERENCES

1. Alkema L, Chou D, Hogan D, Zhang S, Moller AB, Gemmill A, et al. Global, regional, and national levels and trends in maternal mortality between 1990 and 2015, with scenario-based projections to 2030: a systematic analysis by the UN Maternal Mortality Estimation Inter-Agency Group. Lancet. 2016;387:462-74.
2. World Health Organization. WHO recommendations on antenatal care for a positive pregnancy experience. Geneva, Switzerland: WHO; 2016.
3. World Health Organization (2015). The global prevalence of anaemia in 2011. [online] Available from: https://apps.who.int/iris/bitstream/handle/10665/177094/9789241564960_eng.pdf?sequence=1. [Last accessed June, 2020].

4. Royal College of Obstetricians and Gynaecologists (2006). Exercise in pregnancy (RCOG Statement No. 4). [online] Available from: https://www.rcog.org.uk/en/guidelines-research-services/guidelines/exercise-in-pregnancy-statement-no.4/#:~:text=Exercise%20in%20Pregnancy%20(Statement%20No,4)&text=This%20RCOG%20statement%20has%20now,be%20physically%20active%20during%20pregnancy. [Last accessed June, 2020].

5. Rasmussen KM, Yaktine AL; Institute of Medicine and National Research Council (2009). Weight gain during pregnancy: Re-examining the guidelines. [online] Available from: https://www.nap.edu/catalog/12584/weight-gain-during-pregnancy-reexamining-the-guidelines. [Last accessed June, 2020].

6. WHO; de Benoist B, McLean E, Egli I, Cogswell M (2008). Worldwide prevalence of anaemia 1993–2005. WHO global database on anaemia. [online] Available from: https://apps.who.int/iris/bitstream/handle/10665/43894/9789241596657_eng.pdf;sequence=1. [Last accessed June, 2020].

7. World Health Organization (2006). Iron and folate supplementation: integrated management of pregnancy and childbirth (IMPAC). Standards for maternal and neonatal care 1.8. [online] Available from: https://www.who.int/reproductivehealth/publications/maternal_perinatal_health/iron_folate_supplementation.pdf. [Last accessed June, 2020].

8. World Health Organization (2013). Diagnostic criteria and classification of hyperglycaemia first detected in pregnancy. [online] Available from: https://apps.who.int/iris/bitstream/handle/10665/85975/WHO_NMH_MND_13.2_eng.pdf?sequence=1. [Last accessed June, 2020].

9. National Institute for Health and Clinical Excellence (2008; updated 2016). Antenatal care for uncomplicated pregnancies: clinical guideline [CG62]. [online] Available from: https://www.nice.org.uk/guidance/cg62. [Last accessed June, 2020].

10. World Health Organization (2015). Guideline on when to start antiretroviral therapy and on pre-exposure prophylaxis for HIV. [online] Available from: https://apps.who.int/iris/bitstream/handle/10665/186275/9789241509565_eng.pdf?sequence=1. [Last accessed June, 2020].

11. World Health Organization (2013). Responding to intimate partner violence and sexual violence against women: WHO clinical and policy guidelines. [online] Available from: https://apps.who.int/iris/bitstream/handle/10665/85240/9789241548595_eng.pdf?sequence=1. [Last accessed June, 2020].

12. World Health Organization (2013). Systematic screening for active tuberculosis: principles and recommendations. [online] Available from: https://www.who.int/tb/tbscreening/en/. [Last accessed June, 2020].

13. Smaill FM, Vazquez JC. Antibiotics for asymptomatic bacteriuria in pregnancy. Cochrane Database Syst Rev. 2015;8:CD000490.

14. Thwaites CL, Loan HT. Eradication of tetanus. Br Med Bull. 2015;116(1):69-77.

15. World Health Organization (2015). Guidelines for the treatment of malaria, third edition. [online] Available from: http://apps.who.int/iris/bitstream/10665/162441/1/9789241549127_eng.pdf. [Last accessed June, 2020].

16. Ten Hoope-Bender P, de Bernis L, Campbell J, Downe S, Fauveau V, Fogstad H, et al. Improvement of maternal and newborn health through midwifery. Lancet. 2014;384(9949):1226-35.

Manage the Risk Situation

Anemia in Pregnancy

Garima Kachhawa, Asmita Kaundal, Alka Kriplani

INTRODUCTION AND EPIDEMIOLOGY

Anemia, commonly defined as low hemoglobin concentration in blood, is a major public health problem worldwide. It affects nearly one-third of the world's population and half of these cases are due to iron deficiency. According to global data, around 38% (32.4 million) of pregnant women were affected by anemia in year 2011.[1] The situation is more serious in low- and middle-income countries where 56% of the pregnant women are anemic.[2] *World Health Organization (WHO) estimated that, between 1993 and 2005, worldwide prevalence of anemia was 30.2% in women, and 41.8% in pregnancy.*[3]

It affects maternal and child health, physical performance, and referral to healthcare professionals. Associated with adverse maternal and fetal outcome anemia alone is identified as a direct cause of 20% of maternal deaths globally.[4]

DEFINITION

Anemia is a condition where the number and size of red blood cells or hemoglobin concentration is lower than the established cut off levels.

The WHO and American College of Obstetrician and Gynecologist define anemia in pregnancy as hemoglobin < 11 g/dL or hematocrit < 33% in first and third trimester and hemoglobin < 10.5 g/dL or hematocrit < 31% in second trimester.[5,6]

Indian Council of Medical Research further classifies anemia into mild (hemoglobin between 10 and 10.9 g/dL), moderate (hemoglobin between 7 and 9.9 g/dL), and severe (hemoglobin < 7 g/dL) and very severe (hemoglobin < 4 g/dL) anemia **(Table 1).**[7,8]

TABLE 1: Hemoglobin concentration in normal and anemic women (g/dL).[8]

Population	Normal range	Mild anemia	Moderate anemia	Severe anemia
Nonpregnant women	12 or more	11–11.9	8–10.9	<8
Pregnant women	11 or more	10–10.9	7–9.9	<7

What makes pregnancy at risk of developing anemia?

During pregnancy to meet the demands of women and growing fetus, the overall nutritional requirement of the women is more than a nonpregnant woman. On an average for a normal healthy pregnant woman, the iron requirement is increased by two- to threefold and folate by 10–20-fold. Certain symptoms of pregnancy such as nausea and vomiting make it difficult for the women to take proper diet or interfere with the absorption of the essential nutrients from the diet.

Causes of anemia:

- *Physiologic anemia*: Though there is increase in red cell mass (15–30%) but the plasma volume expansion that occurs during pregnancy is greater (30–50%) than the red cell mass increase leading to dilutional anemia also termed as physiological anemia of pregnancy
- *Nutritional anemia*: Iron deficiency, folate, and vitamin B12 deficiency, vitamin A and C deficiency, and protein deficiency anemia
- Acute or chronic blood loss (gastrointestinal bleeding and heavy menstrual cycles)
- *Infections*: Secondary bacterial infection, severe malaria, chronic inflammation (helminthic infections), and human immunodeficiency viruses (HIV)
- *Hemoglobinopathies*: Sickle cell anemia and thalassemia
- *Autoimmune disorders*: Systemic lupus erythematosus and acute viral infection
- *Hemolytic anemia*: Drugs, congenital
- Hypothyroidism
- Chronic kidney disease
- Neoplasia.

What are the risks associated with anemia during pregnancy?

Pregnancy with anemia is a high-risk condition where both women and baby are at risk. Anemia can pose a woman at risk of premature preterm labor, infection, pre-eclampsia, postpartum hemorrhage, congestive cardiac failure, and maternal death.[9,1] Babies born to the anemic mothers are at risk of premature births and complications related to prematurity, low birth weight, and perinatal death. Such babies are at risk of developing anemia later in life due to low iron stores.[10,11]

SIGNS AND SYMPTOMS

Clinical presentation of women with anemia varies according to the severity. Symptoms can be insidious or acute onset. A through history and examination here can be very important for two reasons—(1) for making the diagnosis and (2) to find the cause.

- *Chronic anemia*: Asymptomatic (mild-to-moderate anemia), dyspnea, palpitation, easy fatigability, loss of appetite, and lethargy. If the anemia remains untreated, these symptoms gradually progress from initially being present on exertion to be present at rest.

- *Acute blood loss*: Along with all the symptoms of chronic anemia, acute hemorrhage presents with postural hypotension, dizziness, altered sensorium, and shock depending upon the blood loss.
- Severe anemia may lead to confusion, dyspnea, arrhythmia, and congestive cardiac failure.[12]

Symptoms Specific to Cause

- Women with iron deficiency anemia can have strong urge to eat mud (Pica) or suck dry ice (Pagophagia).
- Soreness of tongue, graying of hair, loss of sensation to perceive one's own body parts and sense of movement (proprioception), and malabsorption leading to steatorrhea may be present in case of megaloblastic anemia.
- Paresthesia can also be present in the women with pernicious anemia.
- Episodic abdominal pain or back pain can be present in women with sickle cell anemia.
- History of recurrent fever with chills and rigor, prolonged cough with expectoration, and urinary complaints may be associated with infections such as malaria, tuberculosis, and urinary tract infection.
- History of repeated blood and blood component transfusion in self or family gives a clue about the presence of some hemoglobinopathy.
- Bleeding gums, piles, or passage of worms in stool may be related to chronic blood loss.
- Petechiae, easy bruisability, and ecchymosis may be associated with coagulation disorders.
- High-colored urine, discolored sclera, and drug intake may be associated with hemolysis.
- Dietary habits and cooking practices may be related to nutritional deficiencies.
- History of heavy or frequent cycles, history of repeated abortions, frequent pregnancies, intrauterine contraceptive device use, etc.

EXAMINATION

Examine conjunctiva, tongue, face, palms, and mucous membranes.

- *Look for pallor*: Pallor can be assessed by looking at the palpebral conjunctiva of the women or palms of her hand. Ask women to hyperextend her palm, if the skin surrounding the palmar crease is darker than hemoglobin is <8 g/dL. Though pallor as a predictor of degree of anemia is 20–70% sensitive[13]
- *Look for icterus*: Jaundice can be found, if the women have hemolytic anemia
- Look for any petechiae and ecchymosis
- Clubbing of nails, platonychia, or koilonychia

- Look for any lymphadenopathy, raised jugular venous pressure (JVP), and thyroid enlargement
- Pedal edema
- Chest examination should be done to see ant sternal tenderness, crepitus (fine basal or coarse apical), and any murmur (soft systolic murmur due to hyperdynamic circulation).
- Abdominal examination to rule out any abdominal wall edema, hepatosplenomegaly, and presence of free fluid. Obstetrics palpation to see height of uterus, tone of uterus, number of fetus, presentation, and fetal heart auscultation.

▊ EVALUATION OF ANEMIA (FLOWCHART 1)

Universal screening for anemia with complete blood count at first visit is recommended by ACOG and CDC.[6,3] Those who are found to be anemic should undergo full workup to ascertain the etiology. Initial workup of anemia aims at finding:

- *Severity of anemia*: Hemoglobin and hematocrit levels
- *Type of anemia*: Complete blood count with blood indices and peripheral smear
- *Cause of anemia*: Peripheral smear, liver function test, kidney function test, serum proteins, electrophoresis/high-performance liquid chromatography, stool examination for ova, cyst and occult blood, bone marrow examination for abnormal cells and iron stores
- *Bone marrow activity*: Reticulocyte count (normal 0.2–2%)

▊ MANAGEMENT OF ANEMIA IN PREGNANCY (FLOWCHART 2)

Management depends upon:
- Cause of anemia
- Severity of anemia
- Gestation age at presentation
- Compliance to the treatment
- Any symptom of congestive cardiac failure.

Treatment Guidelines for the Management of Anemia during Pregnancy

To achieve an adequate response to treatment, it is very important to first educate women about the diet, treatment options, and importance of adherence to the treatment and follow-up. Iron deficiency anemia (IDA) is the most common cause of anemia in India followed by dimorphic anemia due to combined deficiency of iron and folic acid.[14] So while treating a woman for anemia, folic acid supplementation should always be given with iron supplements, to supplement folic acid deficiency and also to compensate for increase erythropoiesis after iron supplementation.

Flowchart 1: Stepwise approach to the evaluation of anemia.

First step:
• Estimation of hemoglobin level
• Peripheral smear

Microcytic: IDA and thalassemia

Macrocytic: Megaloblastic anemia

Second step: Estimation of serum ferritin

<30 ng/dL: Low: Iron deficiency anemia

30–40 ng/dL: Borderline: Chronic illness (diabetes, chronic kidney disease), collagen vascular disease (SLE and rheumatoid arthritis)

Normal serum ferritin

Third step: Check blood indices:
MCV (80–100 fL)
• MCV < 80 fL: Thalassemia
• MCV > 100 fL: Vitamin B12 deficiency/folate deficiency/reticulocytosis due to hemolysis
MCH (27.5–33.2 pg):
• <21 beta-thalassemia minor confirm by HPLC
MCHC (30 g/dL od RBC):
• Low: IDA and thalassemia
• High: Congenital/acquired spherocytosis, congenital hemolytic anemia (sickle cell anemia, HbC disease)

Iron studies

Serum ferritin

Serum iron

Total iron binding capacity

Transferrin saturation <20% (even if S. ferritin in normal IDA)

Fourth step: RDW

Raised: Megaloblastic anemia

Low: IDA (with low ferritin)

Normal with low MCV and normal-to-high ferritin—thalassemia

Fifth step: Reticulocyte index

>2.5: Hemolytic anemia

Low: Hypoproliferative bone marrow

(SLE: systemic lupus erythematosus; IDA: iron deficiency anemia)

Dietary Advice

Dietary modification includes increasing the intake of diet rich in iron and folic acid and modifying practices to increase the absorption of iron.[15] Iron is present in diet in two forms—heme and nonheme, out of which heme iron is more bioavailable. Meat, poultry, fish, green leafy vegetables, and dry fruits are rich in heme iron and should be included in the diet. Around 60% of the animal food, almost all the plant food, and most of the supplements contain non-heme iron. To increase the absorption of iron, vitamin C-rich food such as citric fruits should be included in the diet along with iron-rich food.[16,17] Food items containing phytates, tannin (tea and coffee), calcium (milk and

Flowchart 2: Management of anemia during pregnancy.

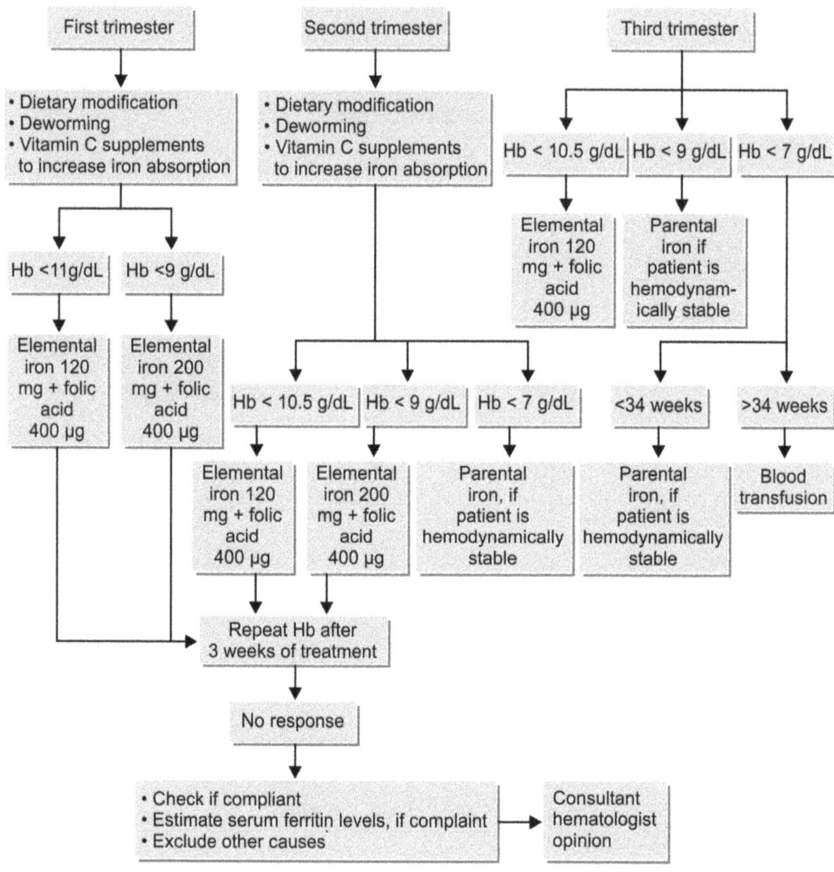

milk products), oxalate (vegetables), and phosphate (egg yolk) can inhibit iron absorption and should be avoided during and immediately after the meals.[18,19]

Deworming

All women with anemia should receive deworming therapy as tablet albendazole 400 mg single dose or mebendazole 100 mg twice a day for 3 days. WHO recommends chemoprophylaxis in all areas where the prevalence of helminthic infestation is more than 20%.[20]

Oral Iron Therapy (Box 1)

Iron therapy is the first line of management for mild-to-moderate iron deficiency anemia at early gestation. Before starting women on oral iron, it is very important to instruct the women about the intake of oral iron, check for compliance, and follow-up to see for response to the treatment. There are several preparations of oral iron available in the market containing

> **BOX 1:** Instructions for oral iron intake.
>
> - Iron tablet should be taken either empty stomach or 1 hour after the meals (in case of gastritis, nausea, and vomiting)
> - Avoiding consumption of tea, coffee or milk, or calcium tablets within 1 hour of iron intake
> - Avoid food-containing phytates (whole grain, lentils, and nuts) with or immediately after iron intake
> - Taking food rich in ascorbic acid (lemon juice) to promote iron absorption
> - Stool can be black in color during iron intake
> - Patient should follow-up in case of any side effect due to treatment so that alternate therapy can be planned

either ferrous sulfate, ferrous fumarate, succinate, gluconate, or ferrous ascorbate. Advantage of oral supplementation is its ease of intake and no supervision/admission is required. Still, most of the studies have reported poor compliance to the oral iron therapy owing to poor tolerability and side effects associated with oral prepration.[21] Nausea, vomiting, heartburn, and constipation are some of the common side effects of oral iron therapy. Some of the effective ways of dealing with the common side effects are as follows:[22]

- Take iron tablets with the meals, but it reduces the absorption to 40%.
- Take small doses two to three times between meals.
- Decrease the dose.
- Change the iron preparation to one with different salt.

Repeat Hb level after 3 weeks of starting the oral iron, if the women is complaint and still there is no/poor response, one should reconfirm the diagnosis or rule out other conditions which can interfere with iron absorption. Inflammatory bowel disease (limiting absorption), gastrointestinal disease (Crohn's disease and ulcerative colitis), infectious condition which affects erythropoiesis, drugs inhibiting erythropoiesis, and incorrect diagnosis of IDA are some of the reasons for no response to the oral iron therapy.

Parenteral Therapy

Parenteral therapy is another option for the management of mild-to-moderate anemia where time for replacement limits oral iron therapy or severe anemia where the women are hemodynamically stable and remote from term. Parenteral therapy is also an alternative to blood transfusion in hemodynamically stable women in postpartum period. Hence, provider should always discuss the option of parenteral iron therapy during postpartum period before blood transfusion if she is a suitable candidate. This would avoid unnecessary blood and blood product transfusion and risk associated with it. Women noncompliant to oral iron either due to lack of motivation to take the daily iron or due to side effects or women where the absorption of oral iron is affected by intestinal ailment leading to poor response to the therapy are also good candidates for parenteral iron therapy.[23] As the parenteral iron bypasses the first-pass metabolism, its absorption is rapid and no gastrointestinal upset is noted as with oral supplementation; but since it is available as free iron in circulation, it can damage the tissues due to its effects of peroxidation, hence, making it very important to know the iron status of women before parenteral therapy to avoid overload.

Parenteral iron can be given either intravenous or intramuscular. Due to the availability, safety, and less side effects of intravenous preparation, now most of the clinicians prefer intravenous iron therapy over intramuscular route. Iron sucrose, ferric gluconate, ferric carboxymaltose, and iron dextran are some of the common parenteral preparations available. Various studies have shown that intravenous iron preparations are safe during pregnancy with fewer side effects and rapid response as compared to oral therapy.[24,25] Erythroid response is one of the most common side effects of parenteral iron. Delayed adverse events such as fever with chills and rare anaphylactoid reactions can also be seen.

Parenteral iron therapy can be either given as single iron replacement therapy or as multiple dose therapy on alternate day with similar efficacy. Single parenteral dose is considered safe and effective to replenish the iron deficit and stores.[26]

How to give parenteral iron? (Box 2)
Calculate iron deficit as:

$$Iron\ requirement = (Normal\ Hb - Patient's\ Hb) \times weight\ (kg) \times 2.21 + 1,000$$

Where normal Hb = 14 g/dL, 2.21 is standard coefficient and 1,000 is added for the stores.

Though the anaphylactic reaction is less common, resuscitation measures should be in place before starting the infusion.

Ferric carboxymaltose (FCM): Maximum dose of FCM that can be infused in a single setting is 1,000 mg after diluting it in 200 mL of 0.9% normal saline intravenous over 30 minutes. If the iron requirement is more, then the subsequent dose can be given after 1 week.

Iron sucrose is another intravenous iron preparation available. 200 mg of iron sucrose is diluted in 200 mL of 0.9% normal saline. Initial 12.5 mL is given slowly and if no adverse reaction is noted, infusion is completed over 15–20 minutes. Subsequent doses can be repeated on alternate days. Dose should not exceed 600 mg/week.

BOX 2: Things to remember before considering parenteral iron therapy.

- Parenteral iron therapy should be given as an inpatient (daycare facility)
- Iron status should be known with certainty to avoid overload
- Emergency measures for resuscitations should be in place before giving parenteral iron
- Women should be instructed to stop oral iron before starting parenteral therapy

Blood Transfusion (Box 3)

Blood transfusion is reserved for women who are severely anemic and has no time for replacement therapy, e.g., those near term (after 34 weeks), in labor or women with severe anemia with signs and symptoms or congestive failure anytime during pregnancy, labor, or postpartum. The decision of blood transfusion should be taken after weighing its benefits against its risks. Carefully watch for the signs and symptoms of blood transfusion reaction and overload. Ideally, a properly cross-matched ABO Rhesus D (RhD) compatible unit should be transfused and the blood sample for cross-match should not be 3 days old. In rare situations of emergency where blood group is unknown and compatible blood is not available, O Rh-negative blood can be given. Transfusion should be given under Lasix cover to avoid overload.

Risks associated with blood transfusion:
- Risk of incompatible blood transfusion
- Risk of severe hemolytic transfusion reaction
- Transmission of HIV, hepatitis B, hepatitis C, malaria, and syphilis to the recipient

Monitoring of patient:
- Before blood transfusion
- Immediately after starting transfusion
- 15 minutes after starting the transfusion
- 1 hour after starting the transfusion
- At completion of transfusion
- 4 hours of transfusion

BOX 3: Indications of blood transfusion during pregnancy.[27,28]

Pregnancy < 34 weeks:
- Hb < 5 g/dL even without clinical signs of cardiac failure
- Hb between 5 and 7 g/dL in presence of impending heart failure

Pregnancy > 34 weeks:
- Hb < 7 g/dL even without clinical signs of cardiac failure
- Patient with severe anemia who is decompensated

Anemia not due to hematinic deficiency: Hemoglobinopathy or bone marrow failure syndromes. Consult a hematologist.

Acute hemorrhage:
- Always indicated if Hb < 6 g/dL
- If patient become unstable due to ongoing hemorrhage

Intrapartum: Hb < 7 g/dL (in labor) decision for blood transfusion should depend upon medical history or symptoms

Postpartum:
- Anemia with signs of shock/acute hemorrhage with signs of hemodynamic instability
- *Hb < 7 g/dL:* Decision for blood transfusion depends upon medical history or symptoms

Erythropoietin

Erythropoietin is usually given as an alternative method of treatment of iron deficiency anemia in renal or sucrose refractory anemia. Injection erythropoietin 100–150 IU/kg is given either intravenous or subcutaneous on alternate days along with intravenous iron therapy.[29] Measures for emergency resuscitation should be ensured before the administration for erythropoietin, as it is associated with hypertension.

Management of Anemia according to Gestational Age

Gestational age < 30 weeks:
- *Mild-to-moderate anemia*: Oral iron therapy should be considered as first-line management along with dietary modifications. If the patient is non-compliant or intolerant to oral iron, parenteral iron therapy should be considered.
- *Severe anemia with no signs of congestive cardiac failure*: Parenteral iron should be considered as first-line management.
- *Severe anemia with signs of congestive cardiac failure*: Blood transfusion.

Gestational age between 30 and 34 weeks:
- *Mild anemia*: Oral iron
- *Moderate-to-severe anemia (with no sign of cardiac failure)*: Parenteral iron should be considered as first line of management in these cases.
- *Severe anemia with signs of congestive cardiac failure*: Blood transfusion.

Gestational age > 34 weeks:
- *Mild anemia*: Parenteral iron therapy should be considered over oral iron.
- Blood transfusion should be considered as first line of management in the women with moderate-to-severe anemia.

During Labor (Flowchart 3)

Anemic patient in labor is at risk of congestive cardiac failure and postpartum hemorrhage. As the reserve is already poor blood loss which is considered normal to a normal healthy woman may not be tolerated by them, hence they require meticulous monitoring during labor.

Important points to be taken care of when a woman with anemia is in labor:
- Detailed history of any significant present or past medical or surgical history and any drug intake should be noted. Previous obstetric history and any history of postpartum hemorrhage are important. Examine patient to rule out any acute bleeding event such as antepartum hemorrhage concealed or revealed, check her vitals and rule out any sign and symptom suggestive of congestive cardiac failure.
- Patient should lie propped up.
- Oxygen by mask should be made available.
- Minimal vaginal examination should be done to avoid infection

Flowchart 3: Management of anemia during labor and postpartum.

Labor

First stage:
• Admit
• Secure intravenous line
• Blood group and cross-match
• Hb on admission
• Arrange blood and blood products
• Keep women propped up in comfortable environment
• Give oxygen by mask if needed
• Minimum vaginal examinations
• Restrict IV fluids
• No early ARM
• Avoid augmentation of labor, if not indicated
• Monitor vitals
• Monitor input/output
• Look of signs and symptoms of CCF

Second stage:
• Vaginal birth is preferred unless any contraindications
• Cut short second stage of labor
• Active management of third stage of labor
• Preparedness for management of postpartum hemorrhage

Postpartum

Full blood count and serum ferritin estimation on day 1 postpartum, if:
• Postpartum hemorrhage
• Uncorrected antenatal anemia
• Known IDA
• Any women with sign and symptom of anemia

Hb < 10 g/dL:
• Start oral iron replacement with elemental iron 200 mg in divided doses for 3 months
• Dietary advice
• Vitamin C supplements
• Repeat Hb and serum ferritin after 3 weeks

Hb < 8 g/dL:
• If hemodynamically stable: Consider total dose replacement
• Repeat Hb and serum ferritin after 10 days and 3 months

Hb < 7 g/dL:
• Discuss options of total dose intravenous iron replacement or blood transfusion
• Blood transfusion, if hemodynamically unstable, symptomatic anemia or heavy bleeding still continues

(ARM: artificial rupture of membranes; IDA: iron deficiency anemia; IV: intravenous)

■ Augmentation of labor only, if required.

■ Avoid early artificial rupture of membranes (ARM).

■ Monitor for any sign and symptom of congestive cardiac failure (breathlessness, tachycardia, raised JVP, and basal crepitation).

■ Keep blood and blood products arranged.

■ Keep oxytocics arranged (for the management of postpartum hemorrhage).

■ Cut short second stage of labor.

■ Active management of third stage of labor.

■ Patient should be monitored for any excessive blood loss, check vitals (PR, BP, and RR), check for signs of congestive cardiac failure.

Postpartum (Flowchart 3)

Monitor for vitals and bleeding for first 24 hours strictly to ensure any deterioration in patient condition in immediate postpartum period. Assess for Hb and serum ferritin on day 1 postpartum, if:

■ Postpartum hemorrhage (blood loss > 500 mg)

■ Signs and symptoms of anemia are present

■ Known iron deficiency anemia

■ Uncorrected antenatal anemia

Depending upon Hb level and women and patients' condition, iron therapy is decided. If the Hb is <10 g/dL, oral therapy is treatment of choice along with dietary modification. If Hb is <8 g/dL and patient is hemodynamically stable, total intravenous iron replacement is preferred. If the Hb is <7 g/dL and women are hemodynamically stable, care provider can discuss the option of blood transfusion and total intravenous iron replacement therapy. Repeat Hb and serum ferritin after 3 weeks to look for the replacement.

Irrespective of the treatment women received, all women are put on iron supplementation postpartum for 6 months to replenish the iron stores and provide for the increased demand during breastfeeding.

Management of Other Causes of Anemia

Folate deficiency: Established folic acid deficiency should be supplemented by folic acid 5 mg oral per day along with dietary modifications. Continue treatment for at least 4 weeks postpartum.

Vitamin B12 deficiency: Though anemia due to vitamin B12 during pregnancy is rare, pernicious anemia usually presents with infertility. Plus the daily requirement is also very low, which is easily met by the normal diet. In case the cause of anemia is due to vitamin B12 deficiency, parenteral cyanocobalamin 250 µg should be given as intramuscular injection monthly.

KEY MESSAGES

- Hemodynamic changes occur in pregnancy to prepare for expected blood loss at delivery.
- Physiologic anemia occurs in pregnancy because plasma volume increases more quickly than red cell mass.
- Anemia is most commonly classified as microcytic, normocytic, or macrocytic.
- Iron deficiency anemia accounts for 75% of all anemias in pregnancy.
- It is recommended to screen for and treat iron deficiency anemia in pregnancy because treatment to maintain maternal iron stores may be beneficial to neonatal iron stores.
- Oral iron supplementation is the recommended treatment of iron deficiency anemia in pregnancy.
- Parenteral iron should be encouraged in the management of anemia during pregnancy.

REFERENCES

1. Stevens G, Finucane M, De-Regil L, Paciorek C, Flaxman S, Branca F, et al.; Nutrition Impact Model Study Group (Anaemia). Global, regional, and national trends in haemoglobin concentration and prevalence of total and severe anaemia in children and pregnant and non-pregnant women for 1995-2011: a systematic analysis of population-representative data. Lancet Glob Health. 2013;1:e16-e25.

2. WHO. The global prevalence of anemia in 2011. Geneva: World Health Organization; 2015.

3. Centers for Disease Control and Prevention. Recommendation to prevent and control iron deficiency in the United States. MMWR Recomm Rep. 1998;47:1.

4. Dutta DC. Anaemia in pregnancy. Text book of Obstetrics including Perinatology & Contraception, 6th edition. Kolkata, India: New Central Book Agency (P) Ltd.; 2004. pp. 262-7.

5. World Health Organization. WHO recommendations on antenatal care for positive pregnancy experience. Luxembourg: World Health Organization; 2016.

6. American College of Obstetrician and Gynecologist. ACOG Practical Bulletin No. 95: anemia in pregnancy. Obstet Gynecol. 2008;112(1):201-7.

7. Indian Council of Medical Research. Evaluation of the National Nutritional Anaemia Prophylaxis Programme. Task Force Study. New Delhi: ICMR; 1989.

8. WHO. Haemoglobin concentrations for the diagnosis of anemia and assessment of severity. Vitamin and Mineral Nutrition Information System. Geneva: World Health Organization; 2011.

9. Black RE, Victora CG, Walker SP, Bhutta ZA, Christian P, de Onis M, et al. Maternal and child undernutrition and overweight in low-income and middle-income countries. Lancet. 2013;382(9890):427-51.

10. Levy A, Fraser D, Katz M, Mazor M, Sheiner E. Maternal anemia during pregnancy is an independent risk factor for low birth weight and preterm delivery. Eur J Obstet Gynecol Reprod Biol. 2005;122(2):182-6.

11. Gebre A, Mulugeta A. Prevalence of anemia and associated factors among pregnant women in north western zone of tigray, northern ethiopia: a cross-sectional study. J Nutr Metab. 2015;2015:165430.

12. Schrier SL, Leung LLK, Mentzer WC, Jennifer S, Kunins L (2018). Approach to an Adult with Anemia. [online] Available from https://www.uptodate.com/contents/approach-to-the-adult-with-anemia?search=anemia%20workup&source=search_result&selectedTitle. [Last accessed June, 2020].

13. Hung OL, Kwon NS, Cole AE, Dacpano GR, Wu T, Chiang WK, et al. Evaluation of the physician's ability to recognize the presence or absence of anemia, fever, and jaundice. Acad Emerg Med. 2000;7(2):146-56.

14. Centers for disease Control and Prevention. Criteria for anemia in children and childbearing aged women. MMWR Morb Mortal Wkly Rep. 1989;38(22):400-4.

15. Ahluwalia N. Intervention strategies for improving iron status of young children and adolescents in India. Nutr Rev. 2002;60:S115-7.

16. Thankachan P, Walczyk T, Muthayya S, Kurpad AV, Hurrell RF. Iron absorption in young Indian women: the interaction of iron status with the influence of tea and ascorbic acid. Am J Clin Nutr. 2008;87(4):881-6.

17. Walczyk T, Muthayya S, Wegmüller R, Thankachan P, Sierksma A, Frenken LG, et al. Inhibition of iron absorption by calcium is modest in an iron-fortified, casein- and whey-based drink in Indian children and is easily compensated for by addition of ascorbic acid. J Nutr. 2014;144(11):1703-9.

18. Abizari AR, Moretti D, Schuth S, Zimmermann MB, Armar-Klemesu M, Brouwer ID. Phytic acid-to-iron molar ratio rather than polyphenol concentration determines iron bioavailability in whole-cowpea meal among young women. J Nutr. 2012;142(11):1950-5.

19. Petry N, Egli I, Zeder C, Walczyk T, Hurrell R. Polyphenols and phytic acid contribute to the low iron bioavailability from common beans in young women. J Nutr. 2010;140(11):1977-82.

20. Crompton DW. Preventive chemotherapy in human helminthiasis: Coordinated use of anthelminthic drugs in control interventions: a manual for health professionals and programme managers. Geneva, Switzerland: World Health Organization; 2006.

21. Hidalgoa M, Castelo-Branco C, Palacios S, Haya-Palazuelos J, Ciria-Recasens M, Manasanch J, et al. Tolerability of different oral iron supplements: a systematic review. Curr Med Res Opin. 2013;29(4):291-303.

22. Peña-Rosas JP, De-Regil LM, Garcia-Casal MN, Dowswell T. Daily oral iron supplementation during pregnancy. Cochrane Database Syst Rev. 2015;(7):CD004736.

23. Lopez A, Cacoub P, MacdougallI C, Biroulet LP. Iron deficiency anemia. Lancet. 2016;387:907-16.

24. Christoph P, Schuller C, Studer H, Irion O, De Tejada BM, Surbek D. Intravenous iron treatment in pregnancy: comparison of high-dose ferric carboxymaltose vs. iron sucrose. J Perinat Med. 2012;40(5):469-74.

25. Kochhar PK, Kaundal A, Ghosh P. Intravenous iron sucrose versus oral iron in treatment of iron deficiency anemia in pregnancy: A randomized control trial. J Obstet Gynaecol Res. 2013;39(2):504-10.

26. Auerbach M, Deloughery T. Single-dose intravenous iron for iron deficiency: a new paradigm. Hematology Am Soc Hematol Educ Program. 2016;2016(1):57-66.

27. World Health Organization. Treatment for iron deficiency anemia in pregnancy. [online] Available from: http://apps.who.int/rhl/pregnancy_childbirth/medical/anaemia/gwguide/en/. [Last accessed June, 2020].

28. Royal College of Obstetricians and Gynaecologists (2015). Blood transfusion in Obstetrics. Green top Guideline No. 47. [online] Available from: https://www.rcog.org.uk/globalassets/documents/guidelines/gtg-47.pdf. [Last accessed June, 2020].

29. Sharma JB, Shankar M. Anemia in pregnancy. JIMSA. 2010;23(4):253-60.

Hypertension: Manage the Risk

Girija Wagh

INTRODUCTION

Hypertensive disorders in pregnancy (HDP) are a spectrum of disorders ranging from already existing chronic hypertension in pregnancy to complex multisystem disorder[1] such as pre-eclampsia leading to the complications such as eclampsia, HELLP (hemolysis, elevated liver enzymes, and low platelet count) syndrome, pulmonary edema, stroke, and left ventricular failure (LVF).

INCIDENCE

World Health Organization (WHO) 2014[2] has attributed 19% of maternal deaths to hypertension in pregnancy. As per the National Eclampsia Registry (NER) of the FOGSI-ICOG, incidence of pre-eclampsia was found to be 10.3% and incidence of eclampsia is 1.9% of all the pregnancies.[3] More than half (50%) of the eclampsia cases are antepartum, and approximately 20% of the cases occurred postpartum. Maternal mortality is 4–6% and the perinatal loss is as high as 30–40%.[4]

CLASSIFICATION AND DIAGNOSIS OF HDP

Blood pressure (BP) of more than or equal to 140 mm Hg systolic blood pressure (SBP) and 90 mm Hg diastolic blood pressure (DBP) before, during, and after pregnancy should be considered as abnormal. This also holds true in women seeking preconceptional counseling. Correct BP assessment is the crux of the diagnosis.[5]

Blood Pressure Measurement

The standard of care is a well-calibrated mercury sphygmomanometer but for the paucity of its availability, automated or aneroid devices can be used. The patient should be rested for 5 minutes prior to the check-up and should be sitting comfortably with feet placed on the ground and the back supported. The hospitalized mother can be checked in a semipropped up position with the arm well-supported at the level of the heart. The cuff should be of appropriate size, i.e., 40% of the arm circumference and should snugly be applied to the upper arm covering 80% of the area. Appropriate

TABLE 1: Basic laboratory tests for hypertensive disorders in pregnancy (HDP).

Laboratory test	Levels	Inference
Hemoglobin	<11 g/dL and >12 g/dL	Anemia/hemoconcentration
PCV	<30 and >40	Hemodilution/hemoconcentration
TLC	Leukocytosis	Infection/SIRS
Platelets	<1.5 lacs	Thrombocytopenia
SGOT and SGPT	>45 U/L	Elevated liver enzymes
SAP	>250 U/L	Elevated
Creatinine	0.9 mg/dL	Renal involvement
LDH	>600 U/L	Hemolysis
SUA	>7.5 U/L	Adverse neonatal outcome and abruption possible

(PCV: packed cell volume; TLC: total leukocyte count; SGOT: serum glutamic oxaloacetic transaminase; SGPT: serum glutamic pyridoxal phosphate-dependent transaminase; SAP: serum alkaline phosphatase; LDH: lactate dehydrogenase; SUA: serum uric acid)

provisions for large women should be made for correct blood pressure reading **(Table 1)**.

MANAGEMENT OF HYPERTENSIVE DISORDERS IN PREGNANCY

Management of Mild-to-Moderate Hypertension

Antihypertensive Medications

The mainstay of mild-to-moderate HDP is pharmacotherapy to control blood pressure and prevention of severe disease. Use of antihypertensives in mothers with mild-to-moderate hypertension needs more clarity. Mothers with associated organ damage and the ones who have not continued the previous treatment should be given antihypertensives. Mild blood pressure rise (<150 mm Hg SBP and <100 mm Hg DBP) in pregnancy does not put the mother or the fetus at risk. Clarity about similar kind of nonthreatening association with moderate hypertension (SBP: 150–159 mm Hg and DBP: 100–109 mm Hg) does not subsist. Randomized controlled trials involving mothers with mild and moderate hypertension have not revealed any advantage with antihypertensives toward reducing the occurrence of pre-eclampsia or placental abruption or any improvement in the maternal or fetal outcome. However, systematic reviews have made it evident that treatment with antihypertensive medications reduces the severe hypertension incidence.[6] It is thus prudent to continue the antihypertensives in following situations **(Table 2)**:

- If the mother's blood pressure has been stabilized from an early severe hypertension.
- If she is already on medications (can be shifted to labetalol or nifedipine if on any other medications).

TABLE 2: Antihypertensive medications overview—doses.

Antihypertensive	Mechanism of action	Dose
Labetalol	α-1 and selective β-2 adrenergic receptor blocker	100 mg BID initially; increased by 100 mg 12 hourly every 2–3 days Usual dosage range: 200–400 mg BID not to exceed 2,400 mg/day
Nifedipine	Calcium channel blocker	10 mg BID may be increased to 120 mg/day. Slow release preparations preferred
α-methyldopa	Centrally acting α_2-adrenergic agonist	500–2,000 mg per day orally in 3–4 divided doses

TABLE 3: Antihypertensives overview: Adverse effects.

Antihypertensive	Adverse effects	Additional advantages
Labetalol	>10%: Bradycardia, nausea, fatigue, and dizziness >1–10%: Dyspnea, bronchospasm, elevated BUN and creatinine, and positional hypotension	Enhances fetal lung maturity and preserves placental perfusion
Nifedipine	Peripheral edema, dizziness, flushing, headache, burning, heartburn, muscle cramps, mood changes	Uterine relaxation and preserved placental perfusion
α-methyldopa	Fetal bradycardia and elevated liver enzymes	Sedation and fetal safety well established

- If associated organ damage is present. If for any reason, the antihypertensives have been stopped then close surveillance of hypertension has to be part of the antenatal care.

The oral antihypertensives may be used for a longer period of time and it is important to be well-versed with the plausible adverse effects as in the **Table 3**.

The starting drug is labetalol or α-methyldopa; the later may not be easily available. If the maximum dosages are ineffective then a second or sometimes third drug may be added. Expectant management only till safety levels for the mother (organ damage) and the fetus (lung maturity or steroid action) should be the practice. Beta-blockers and calcium channel blockers seem to be more effective in preventing severe hypertensive crisis.[6] Drug safety as all are category-C drugs and cross the placenta. Congenital heart disease in the fetuses seems to be associated with antihypertensive drugs; but these are more linked with maternal hypertension. Uncertainty of such association prevails, and it is suggested that antihypertensive medications should be used when indicated to prevent maternal cardiovascular adverse outcomes **(Table 4)**.[7,8]

The overview of maternal antenatal surveillance[9] is shown in **Figure 1**.

TABLE 4: Antenatal care specific questions and warning signs to inform the patient and her family.

Specific symptoms to be asked ideally to all ANCs after 20 weeks	Warning signs to be informed to the patient with HDP and the relatives
• Visual disturbances • Persistent headaches • Epigastric or right upper quadrant pain • Increased edema	• Upper abdominal pain/acute pain in lower abdomen • Headaches • Feeling unwell and, nauseous or like throwing up • Blurring of vision or seeing flashing lights • Swelling on hands and/or face • Reduced fetal movements • Loss of consciousness/seizures

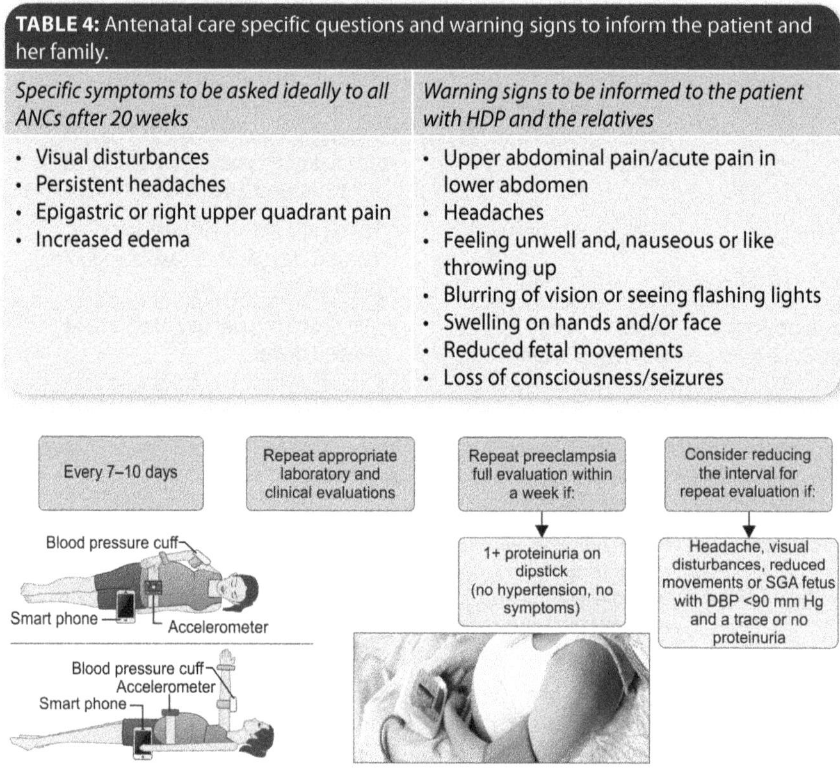

Fig. 1: Antenatal follow-up schedule.

Home blood pressure monitoring by a digital machine or from a nearby healthcare provider should be advised and maintained on a chart and raised BP (^{3}140/90 mm Hg) reading should necessitate visit to the facility.

Supportive Treatment

Strict bed rest is not recommended in mild-to-moderate hypertension. Pre-eclampsia may benefit with rest but immobilization can cause osteopenia and sarcopenia, risk of thrombotic episodes and hypostatic pneumonia. Diet rich in folates and proteins should be advised. Salt restriction is not recommended. Anemia should be corrected and euthyroid levels be achieved. Calcium[10] in the dose of 2,000 mg/day as a dietary source as well as a supplement in divided doses is recommended. Low-dose aspirin[11,12] (100–150 mg) is to be started optimally at 8 weeks of gestation or anytime later preferably before 18 weeks in women high risk for pre-eclampsia. Antiplatelet drugs for prevention of pre-eclampsia and its consequences: systematic review.

Fetal Evaluation

Regular fundal measurement at antenatal visits is optimal surveillance tool for growth restriction. There are no guidelines for ultrasonography schedule

> **BOX 1:** Fetal surveillance with sonography and Dopplers.
>
> - Initial assessment-biometry, AFI and UAD, UmAD, MCA
> - If FGR: Doppler and AFI estimation—1/15 days till delivery
> - UmAD REDF weekly Doppler: AEDF
> - If AEDF: Doppler—2/week—REDF
> - With REDF: >70% of the intervillous circulation is compromised and it is time to deliver by CS
> - Ductus venosus/Umbilical vein: fetal acidemia—poor prognosis
> - Magnesium sulfate to be given for fetal neuroprotection <32 weeks
> - Arterial Doppler significant for fetal prognosis before 32 weeks
> - Venous Doppler later
> - A CPR of >1 gives us time to postpone delivery
>
> (AFI: amniotic fluid index; UAD: uterine artery Doppler; UmAD: umbilical artery Doppler; FGR: fetal growth restriction; AEDF: absent end diastolic flow; REDF: reduced end diastolic flow; CS: cesarean section; CPR: cerebral placental ratio)

especially for HDP.[13] Regular surveillance should be of help to identify FGR earlier in mothers with HDP.[14] After confirmation of fetal developmental normality at 18–20 weeks of gestation, growth scan is scheduled at 28–32 weeks, if clinical fundogram is not satisfactory. It would be ideal to perform a growth scan with Doppler, especially in mothers with pre-eclampsia at a regular basis but evidence does not exist for the same. Typically, it would be ideal to do the uterine artery pulsatility index at 11–13 weeks scan and increased resistance can predict severe pre-eclampsia in high-risk mothers. Likewise at 22–24 weeks, uterine artery diastolic notch can be predictor of severe gestosis (pre-eclampsia) and help in adopting closer stringent surveillance **(Box 1)**. Pre-eclampsia once diagnosed, regular fetal surveillance for FGR would be ideal and once FGR is diagnosed then regular Doppler studies can guide the prognostication and delivery decisions.[15] All these tests, however, may not be easily accessible for all pregnant mothers. In the presence of FGR, Doppler plays a significant role in the timing of delivery for a good neonatal outcome.[16]

Management of Severe Hypertensive Disorders in Pregnancy (Box 2)

Hospitalization

Mothers with severe hypertension and severe features are to be admitted for close supervision and stabilization. Gestational hypertension may be considered for outpatient care after stabilization and evaluation. Inpatient care should include seizure prevention[4] and control, blood pressure control, maternal and fetal evaluation, and supportive care.

Pharmacotherapy

Pharmacotherapy predominantly consists of seizure control and prevention and antihypertensive medications.

> **BOX 2:** Severe features of hypertensive disorders in pregnancy (HDP)*.
>
> - *Clinical features*: Severe hypertension^, epigastric pain, right upper quadrant pain, headache, vomiting, feeling of ill-being, altered sensorium, convulsions^^, unconsciousness, uterine pain, hardened tender gravid uterus (E/O placental abruption), anuria, hyperreflexia (clonus and exaggerated knee jerks), icterus, severe edema, pallor, PO_2 less than 96%, S/O pulmonary edema, hematuria, per vaginal bleeding, fetal bradycardia, or intrauterine death
> - *Laboratory features*: Proteinuria (1+ or more), thrombocytopenia (platelets less than 100,000/mL), raised liver enzymes twice the normal concentrations (75 IU and above), raised creatinine (>0.9 mg/dL), uric acid (>7.5), LDH > 800 IU, schistocytes (fragmented RBCs) on PBS, Se bilirubin more than 1.2 mg/dL
> - *Radiological evidence*: Fetal growth restriction, decelerations on EFM, oligohydramnios AEDF/REDF in the umbilical artery Doppler, abruption or retroplacental hematoma, evidence of pulmonary edema, and embolism.
>
> (AEDF: absent end diastolic flow; PBS: peripheral blood smear; REDF: reduced end diastolic flow)
>
> *Note*: *To be carefully evaluated; ^hypotension or normal BP readings may be transient; ^^every hypertensive mother is at risk of seizures and prevention with magnesium sulfate is effective.

Seizure Prevention and Control

Injection magnesium sulfate to be administered as 4 g (4 ampoules of 50%) in 12 mL of water for injection via a 20 mL syringe or in 100 mL normal saline over a duration of 5–15 min as loading dose. In case of severe disease, full dose consisting of intravenous administration of 5 g magnesium sulfate in 500 mL Ringer's lactate delivered at the drop rate of 25–26 drops per minute is given to ensure the delivery of 1 g of magnesium sulfate over 1 hour. This can also be administered by using infusion pump where the accurate dose is administered. This can effectively prevent seizures and stabilize the mother with the adjuvant use of antihypertensive medications. Intramuscular administration of magnesium sulfate can be considered, if difficult intravenous access encountered and 5 g of magnesium sulfate in addition to the initial intravenous 4 g can be given. In severe thrombocytopenia, intramuscular injections may cause hematoma.

Seizure Control

Injection magnesium sulfate to be administered as 4 g (4 ampoules of 50%) in 12 mL of water for injection via a 20 mL syringe or in 100 mL normal saline over a duration of 5–15 min as loading dose.

Maintenance dose: Intravenous administration of 5 g magnesium sulfate in 500 mL Ringer's lactate delivered at the drop rate of 25–26 drops per minute is given to ensure the delivery of 1 g of magnesium sulfate over 1 hour. This can also be administered by using infusion pump where the accurate dose is administered. The maintenance dose also can be given intramuscularly 5 g in each buttock totaling to 10 g at the onset of therapy and continued as

5 g intramuscularly in alternate buttock. The seizure control regimen has to be continued for 24 hours after the delivery or the last seizure. It is a good practice to use a long 20-gauze needle for intramuscular injection and deliver the drug deeply and strict aseptic precautions used to prevent gluteal abscesses and pain.

Monitoring of magnesium sulfate: Essentially clinical and no serum magnesium levels need to be done for assessment of efficacy and detection of overdosing. Plasma levels of 4–7 mEq/L is enough for effective seizure control. Deep tendon reflexes are obliterated at levels 8–10 mEq/L and this clinical sign can be used to assure adequate magnesium levels. Close monitoring of the respiratory rate should be done and the urine output should be adequate; the urine output, if less than the dose of magnesium sulfate, needs to be adjusted. Magnesium sulfate is not harmful to the kidneys but is excreted by the kidneys, therefore, the levels have to be adjusted in case of impaired renal function to avoid accumulation and overdose. Clinical parameters such as urinary output (30 mL/h), respiratory rate (16 breaths/min), oxygen saturation (98%), and patellar reflexes should be present and be closely monitored.

Monitoring excess dose: Magnesium has a narrow margin of safety. The next dose should be given only if the patellar reflexes are present, respiratory rate is more than 16 breaths/min, patient is alert and UOP is more than 100 mL in the preceding 4 hours.

For reversing magnesium sulfate overdose: 10 mL of a 10% calcium gluconate solution (1 g) IV over 10 minutes is administered. If seizures recur, additional dose of $MgSO_4$ of 2 g IV 20% solution may be given.[15] Thiopentone or diazepam derivatives may be used if seizures persist.

Magnesium sulfate contraindications: Pulmonary edema, renal failure, and myasthenia gravis. Alternative seizure control medicines may be considered in case of patients having recurrence or contraindications to magnesium sulfate. Following anticonvulsant therapy can be used. Lorazepam 2–4 mg IV one dose followed by a repeat dose after 10–15 minutes, phenytoin 15–20 mg/kg IV single dose—10 mg/kg IV may be repeated after 20 minutes if no response and diazepam 5–10 mg IV every 5–10 minutes to maximum dose of 30 mg (fetal hypoxia is associated) are alternative drugs. Phenytoin is avoided in presence of hypotension and cardiac arrhythmias.

Additional Therapy

Mothers with either recurrent convulsions, extreme irritability, severe headache, visual disturbances, or in deep coma can be considered for injection mannitol. Injection mannitol is administered as 100 cc of 20% IV 6 hourly for 48 hours followed with 8 hourly dose for next 24 hours, 12 hourly for next 24 hours and then omitted.

Blood Pressure Control

Urgent but gradual control of blood pressure is necessary in severe hypertension and hypertensive emergency. Antihypertensive therapy is used to prevent stroke, myocardial infarction, and placental abruption.

Sudden lowering of blood pressure may cause shock in the mother and fetal jeopardy and therefore appropriate dosing, route, and method of drugs is essential. Following drugs can be used for acute control of blood pressure[17] **(Fig. 2)**:

- Oral nifedipine 10 mg is given per orally (never sublingually) with close BP monitoring. Repeat dose of 20 mg can be given after 20 minutes, if there is no change in the BP reading. After 20 minutes, if the BP remains unchanged, institute injectable labetalol as per the protocol below. If the BP is lowered then continue the nifedipine regimen with a slow release formulation of 20 mg. Nifedipine 10-20 mg 4-6 hourly can be given with a total dose of 40-60 mg in 24 hours. Nifedipine should never be administered sublingually, as it causes sudden drop in blood pressure and severe maternal tachycardia. After stabilization, other antihypertensives mentioned below can be used for temporization. Nifedipine is contraindicated in presence of maternal tachycardia.
- Labetalol is administered in injectable form for acute control of BP. Initially 20 mg is given IV over 2 minutes and the BP is repeated in 10 minutes. Repeat 40 mg IV over 2 minutes if no change in BP after 10 minutes of the initial dose and if the BP lowers continue BP monitoring. If no change in BP then repeat the third dose of 80 mg labetalol IV over 2 minutes and continue BP monitoring. 10 minutes after the third dose if no change observed with labetalol, hydralazine 10 mg IV over 2 minutes may be considered or labetalol infusion drip may be started. Maximum total cumulative dose of 220 mg in 24 hours can be given. Labetalol is avoided in presence of active asthma, heart disease, or congestive heart failure. It is to be used with caution in mothers with past history of asthma and is avoided in presence of bradycardia (PR < 60 beats/min).

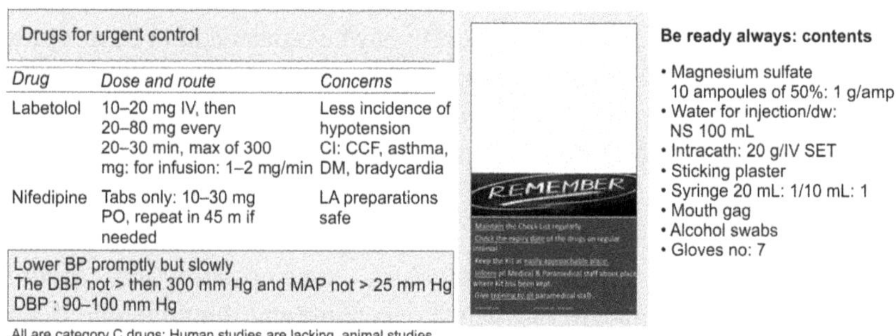

Drugs for urgent control		
Drug	Dose and route	Concerns
Labetolol	10–20 mg IV, then 20–80 mg every 20–30 min, max of 300 mg: for infusion: 1–2 mg/min	Less incidence of hypotension CI: CCF, asthma, DM, bradycardia
Nifedipine	Tabs only: 10–30 mg PO, repeat in 45 m if needed	LA preparations safe

Lower BP promptly but slowly
The DBP not > then 300 mm Hg and MAP not > 25 mm Hg
DBP : 90–100 mm Hg

All are category C drugs: Human studies are lacking, animal studies either positive for fetal risks or lacking, benefits justify the risks to the fetus

Fig. 2: Antihypertensives for urgent blood pressure (BP) control and magnesium sulfate box.

- Hydralazine is administered initially as 5 mg or 10 mg IV injection over 2 minutes and the BP is repeated after 20 minutes. Repeat dose of 10 mg is given, if BP remains the same. After 20 minutes BP check, if no response is noted then labetalol is initiated as per the protocol above. Hydralazine is associated with fetal bradycardia and maternal hypotension.

Additional therapy for blood pressure control: In case of inability of IV access, nifedipine can be instituted or tablet labetalol 200 mg orally repeated in 30 minutes, if BP remains high. Nicardipine can be considered through infusion pump. In extreme emergencies, sodium nitroprusside can be used in the dose for the shortest amount of time, as it is associated with cyanide/thiocyanate toxicity. Initial infusion rate of IV sodium nitroprusside is 0.3–05 µg/kg/min to a maximum rate of 10 µg/kg/min. It is contraindicated in heart diseases and optic atrophy.

Blood Pressure Targets and Monitoring in Hypertensive Emergency

Blood pressure reading of 140 mm Hg SBP and 90 mm Hg DBP is an ideal threshold while 150/100 mm Hg is a reasonable initial target. Antihypertensive medications in an emergency situation have to be administered with frequent blood pressure monitoring as mentioned in the drug protocols above. Once the thresholds are reached then following initial monitoring protocol can be observed—every 10 minutes for 1st hour, every 15 minutes for the 2nd hour, and every 30 minute for the 3rd hour followed by hourly for 4 hours. Additional specific BP monitoring schedule may be individualized.

Fetal Evaluation

Electronic fetal monitoring from 32 weeks for documentation and assessment can be done and mothers receiving alpha-methyldopa may demonstrate reduced baseline variability. Also in the span of 32–34 weeks, accelerations may not be as optimal as a term fetus and this needs considerations. Nonstress testing can help in assessing the FGR babies and delivery decision.

Laboratory Evaluations with Levels

These tests are essential to identify systemic involvement, coagulopathy, and hemolysis. Complete blood count—level of anemia, platelets, leukocytosis, and hemodilution can be depicted. Urinary proteinuria and ketosis can be evaluated from routine urine examination. Systemic involvements and presence of HELLP can be inferred from liver enzyme assessment and renal involvement from creatine and uric acid levels. **Table 5** is the laboratory reference for easy use.

Assessment for occurrence of HELLP and other conditions need to be differentiated. **Table 6** demonstrates the feature of HELLP and other differential diagnoses to be considered.

TABLE 5: Laboratory parameters in severe hypertensive disorders in pregnancy (HDP): Maternal and fetal surveillance.

Maternal condition pregnant/postdelivery mother	Fetus
• CNS (seizure, visual disturbance/headache) • Cyanosis or pulmonary edema • Epigastric or RUQ pain • Impaired liver function • Thrombocytopenia • Hemolysis • Coagulopathy • Oliguria < 30 mL/hour for 2 consecutive hours	• Abnormal fetal tracing • Color Doppler evidence of umbilical artery REDF/AEDF • FGR

TABLE 6: HELLP features and differential diagnosis (D/D) of severe hypertensive disorders in pregnancy (HDP).

Features of HELLP	Differential diagnosis
• Hemolysis (abnormal smear) • Elevated liver enzymes (serum SGOT >70 U/L serum LDH >600 U/L) • Low platelets (<100,000) • *Occurrence*: 20% of pre-eclampsia patients • *Cause*: It is thought to arise because of endothelial and microvascular injury, increased vascular tone and platelet aggregation	• Renal disease • Acute fatty liver • Cholestasis of pregnancy • Hemolytic uremic syndrome • Thrombotic thrombocytopenic purpura • Pheochromocytoma • *Cardiovascular diseases*: Coarctation, subclavian stenosis, aortic dissection, and vasculitis

◾ OBSTETRICAL DECISION MAKING (FIG. 3)

Deliver the severe HDP patient in the following situations after stabilization:

- Eclampsia, HELLP, severe pre-eclampsia, chronic hypertension with superimposed pre-eclampsia and if gestational age is more than or equal to 34 weeks **(Table 7)**.

Vaginal delivery may be considered if attainable in reasonable amount of time. In case of preterm pregnancy, expectant management can be considered with individual assessment and antenatal steroids and rationale use of antihypertensive medications with close supervision to be offered. In presence of these situations, delivery should not be delayed even for the benefit of corticosteroids. Mothers with chronic hypertension can be offered expectant management under close surveillance.

◾ INTRAPARTUM MANAGEMENT

Cesarean section when?

- Severe FGR or REDF in the umbilical artery on color Doppler or any obstetric contraindication for vaginal delivery or failure of induction.

Fluid Management

Inappropriate use of fluids can cause pulmonary edema and maternal death. Fluid restriction is advisable to reduce the risk of fluid overload in the

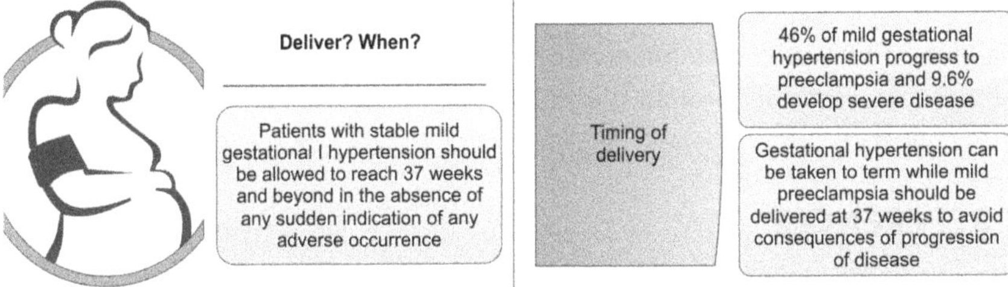

Fig. 3: Delivery decision mild-to-moderate hypertension.

TABLE 7: Delivery decision as per gestational age in severe pre-eclampsia.

23 weeks	24–34 weeks	>34 weeks
Deliver	Expectant management with individualization	If controlled and well-stabilized

intrapartum and postpartum periods. No excessive fluid expansion should be used and total fluid restriction to 80 mL/h or 1 mL/kg/h is beneficial. Additional 700 mL can be used for nonsensical loss.

Intrapartum Monitoring

Intense monitoring for deterioration, progress of labor, and occurrence of placental abruption should be undertaken. Close monitoring of the fetus with continuous or intermittent Doppler device or EFM (electronic monitoring) is preferred. Laboratory investigations may be repeated after 6 hours.

Preventing Postpartum Hemorrhage

Whether a vaginal or a cesarean delivery, active management with oxytocics should be practiced to prevent postpartum hemorrhage (PPH). It is safe to use oxytocin 5 U bolus equally diluted over 2–3 minutes or prostaglandin (PG) intramuscular injections. PG can be used also as misoprostol sublingual, per vaginal, or per rectal. Due to hemoconcentration, even average loss may not be well-tolerated by these patients. Also hypertension, use of magnesium sulfate, and endothelial dysfunction can contribute to more blood loss, which may not be well-compensated for.

> **It is important to diagnose pre-eclampsia early**
> Early identification of pre-eclampsia may allow for interventions, including delivery, that will lessen the risk of progression to severe pre-eclampsia and eclampsia and reduce fetal and maternal morbidity and mortality. It is, therefore, essential for the clinician to look for signs and symptoms of pre-eclampsia.

■ PREDICTION

Uterine artery pulsatility index of more than 2.2 at 12–13 weeks can help to categorize the mother at risk.

SUMMARY

Vigilant and intuitive antenatal care with proper risk assessment and timely therapy can certainly protect the mothers and the babies form disease like pre-eclampsia.

REFERENCES

1. Brown MA, Lindheimer MD, de Swiet M, Van Assche A, Moutquin JM. The classification and diagnosis of the hypertensive disorders of pregnancy: statement from the International Society for the Study of Hypertension in Pregnancy (ISSHP). Hypertens Pregnancy. 2001;20:IX-XIV.
2. Alkema L, Chou D, Hogan D, Zhang S, Moller AB, Gemmill A, et al. Global, regional, and national levels and trends in maternal mortality between 1990 and 2015, with scenario-based projections to 2030: a systematic analysis by the UN Maternal Mortality Estimation Inter-Agency Group. Lancet. 2016;387(10017):462-74.
3. Gupte S, Wagh G. Preeclampsia-eclampsia. J Obstet Gynaecol India. 2014;64(1):4-13.
4. Sibai BM. Diagnosis, prevention, and management of eclampsia. Obstet Gynecol. 2005;105(2):402-10.
5. Working Group on High Blood Pressure in Pregnancy. Report of the National High Blood Pressure Education Program Working Group on High Blood Pressure in Pregnancy. Am J Obstet Gynecol. 2000;183(1):S1-S22.
6. Abalos E, Duley L, Steyn DW, Gialdini C. Antihypertensive drug therapy for mild to moderate hypertension during pregnancy. Cochrane Database Syst Rev. 2018;(10):CD002252.
7. Fitton CA, Steiner MFC, Aucott L, Pell JP, Mackay DF, Fleming M, et al. In-utero exposure to antihypertensive medication and neonatal and child health outcomes: a systematic review. J Hypertens. 2017;35:2123-37.
8. Boesen EI. Consequences of in-utero exposure to antihypertensive medication: the search for definitive answers continues. J Hypertens. 2017;35:2161-4.
9. Heazell A, Norwitz ER, Kenny LC, Baker PN. [2011]. 8 - Identification, diagnosis, and management of suspected preeclampsia. [online] Available from: https://www.cambridge.org/core/books/hypertension-in-pregnancy/identification-diagnosis-and-management-of-suspected-preeclampsia/59BAA086112E364B141A252AC510CBFA. [Last accessed July, 2020]
10. World Health Organization (2018). WHO recommendation: calcium supplementation during pregnancy for prevention of pre-eclampsia and its complications. [online] Available from: https://apps.who.int/iris/handle/10665/277235. [Last accessed July, 2020].
11. Duley L, Henderson-Smart D, Knight M, King J. Aspirin versus placebo in pregnancies at high risk for preterm preeclampsia. BMJ. 2001;322(7282):329-33.
12. Rolnik DL, Wright D, Poon LC, O'Gorman N, Syngelaki A, de PacoMatallana C, et al. ASPRE trial: performance of screening for preterm pre-eclampsia. Ultrasound Obstet Gynecol. 2017;50(4):492-5.
13. Greene MF, Solomon CG. Aspirin to prevent preeclampsia. N Engl J Med. 201717;377(7):613-22.
14. Visintin C, Mugglestone MA, Almerie MQ, Nherera LM, James D, Walkinshaw S, et al. Management of hypertensive disorders during pregnancy: summary of NICE guidance. BMJ. 2010;341:c2207.
15. Sibai BM. Chronic hypertension in pregnancy. Obstet Gynecol. 2002;100:369.
16. Neilson JP, Alfirevic Z. Doppler ultrasound for fetal assessment in high-risk pregnancies. Cochrane Database Syst Rev. 2000;(2):CD000073.
17. Shekhar S, Sharma C, Thakur S, Verma S. Oral nifedipine or intravenous labetalol for hypertensive emergency in pregnancy: a randomized controlled trial. Obstet Gynecol. 2013;122(5):1057-63.

Preterm Labor Pain and Its Prevalence

Tushar Kar

INTRODUCTION

Preterm birth (PTB) refers to a delivery that occurs before 37 weeks of gestation. World Health Organization (WHO) estimated global annual burden of PTB as 15 million. The rate of PTB ranges from 5 to 18% of babies born. India is on the top of the WHO list with maximum number of annual PTBs—3,519,100, whereas Malawi has highest rate of PTBs—18.1 PTBs per 100 births. In India, 13.6% babies born are preterm and that accounts for 18.5% of preterm babies born globally.[1]

Preterm birth is one of the major causes of neonatal morbidity and mortality. The short-term morbidities associated with PTB include respiratory distress syndrome, necrotizing enterocolitis, retinopathy of prematurity, and intraventricular hemorrhage. The prevalence of long-term disability associated with gestational age ranges from 14 to 23% and includes cerebral palsy, neurodevelopmental delay, deafness, visual impairment, and chronic lung disease.

CAUSES OF PRETERM BIRTH

Multiple pregnancies, infections, and chronic illnesses such as diabetes and high blood pressure may lead to PTB, but in most of the cases, no cause is found. It is estimated that 70–80% of PTBs occur spontaneously and rest are due to iatrogenic reasons.

RISK FACTORS FOR PRETERM BIRTH

Certain factors are associated with increased risk of PTB. Identification of these risk factors before conception or in early pregnancy may help in timely interventions and reducing PTBs.

History of previous spontaneous or induced PTB,[2] cervical surgeries,[3] uterine malformations,[4] pregnancies conceived after artificial reproductive techniques, multiple gestation,[5] early pregnancy bleeding, short cervix, infections, genetic factors, adolescent pregnancies, increasing age, pre-existing chronic illness, obesity, short interpregnancy interval of < 6 months, low pre-pregnancy BMI, poor weight gain in pregnancy, longer than 42 hours/week, stood > 6 hours/day, low job satisfaction maternal smoking, and drug abuse are all associated with PTB.

There is an inverse relationship between cervical length (CL) < 25 mm measured at 16–24 weeks and gestational age at delivery.[6] The incidence of PTB < 34 weeks is 19–76% in women with CL < 25 mm as compared to 7–23% with CL > 25 mm.[7] Cervical dilation ≤ 1 cm before 24 weeks of gestation is also associated with an increased risk of preterm.

Predicting the Risk Factors of Preterm Labor

At the first antenatal visit, a PTB risk assessment may be performed in order to triage women into "high risk" so that they can be managed accordingly.

Identify Asymptomatic Women at Risk

At first visit, assessment of clinical risk factors is done by obtaining a detailed medical history, reviewing aspects of all previous pregnancies, and determining their candidacy for prophylactic interventions, such as progesterone supplementation, cervical cerclage, or both.

Biomarkers

Cervicovaginal fetal fibronectin (FFN) can be a useful biomarker for predicting PTB within 7–14 days in women with contractions and mild cervical dilation (symptomatic women). The Preterm Prediction Study evaluated FFN at 24–28 weeks and demonstrated its negative predictive value (NPV) of >96%.[8] However, PPV is <30%. Several studies have evaluated the predictive ability of combined cervical screening and FFN testing. In symptomatic women, with CL < 15 mm and a positive fibronectin test (>50 ng/mL), the sensitivity for predicting of PTB has been shown to be >70% while maintaining NPV > 98%.

A test (PreTRM Test) for two serum proteins, insulin-like growth factor-binding protein 4 (IBP4) and sex hormone-binding globulin (SHBG), became available for clinical use to predict PTB in 2017. In a study to predict spontaneous preterm delivery in asymptomatic pregnant women, the test had sensitivity and specificity of 0.75 and 0.74, respectively.[9]

A 2011 systematic review of other 30 available biomarkers concluded that none of the other biomarkers were clinically useful for predicting PTB in asymptomatic women.

Cervical Screening

Measurement of CL between 14 and 24 weeks of gestation has been shown to be a sensitive predictor of PTB in both low- and high-risk women. Transvaginal cervical ultrasonography has been shown to be a reliable way to assess the length of the cervix. Unlike the transabdominal approach, transvaginal cervical ultrasonography is not affected by maternal obesity, position of the cervix, and shadowing from the fetal presenting part.

■ PREVENTION OF PRETERM LABOR

Cervical Cerclage (Surgical Cerclage)

Indications for cervical cerclage in women with singleton pregnancies are based on either obstetrics history or ultrasound finding of short cervix.

With three or more previous PTB and 2nd trimester losses, cerclage typically are placed at around 12–14 weeks of gestation, obstetric history based or history indicated cerclage. Other indication of surgical cerclage is ultrasound indicated, i.e., patients with previous history of spontaneous PTB and short CL (<25 mm) in present pregnancy. Most of such patients can be safely monitored with serial transvaginal ultrasound examinations only. Surveillance should begin at 16 weeks and is done every fortnightly till end of 24 weeks of gestation. Cerclage is recommended for women who have short CL (<25 mm) with or without the presence of funneling. Cerclage is associated with significant reduction in PTBs, as well as improvements in neonatal morbidity and mortality.[10] In contrast to this, for women in the low-risk population with incidental finding of CL < 25 mm detected between 16 and 24 weeks of gestation, cerclage has not been associated with a significant reduction in PTB and is not recommended.[11]

Progesterone Therapy (Medical Cerclage)

Progesterone is a hormone responsible for maintaining uterine quiescence during pregnancy and may modulate cytokine and contraction associated protein expression and activity. A systematic review and meta-analysis performed in 2012 reported that antenatal vaginal progesterone for women at high risk of PTB with CL < 25 mm was associated with significant reduction in PTB rate (12% vs. 22%).[12] For women with no previous history of PTB (low risk) who develop a short cervix, progesterone supplementation can prolong gestation. A 2018 systematic review and meta-analysis of randomized trials (including OPPTIMUM) found that vaginal progesterone supplementation reduced the risk of PTB and neonatal morbidity and mortality in singleton gestations with midtrimester CL ≤ 25 mm even in low-risk women.[13]

Two trials in which women with a short-CL were randomly assigned to weekly intramuscular hydroxyprogesterone caproate (250 mg or 500 mg) or placebo till 36 weeks reported that treatment with hydroxyprogesterone caproate did not reduce the risk of PTB. Vaginal progesterone clearly inhibits cervical ripening; the effect of hydroxyprogesterone caproate on cervical ripening is less clear.

However, Society of Maternal Fetal Medicine and UpToDate recommend hydroxyprogesterone caproate 250 mg weekly administered intramuscularly for women with a history of spontaneous PTB and natural progesterone 100 mg daily administered vaginally for women with a short cervix (≤20 mm), based on the outcomes reported in the trials.[14]

No evidence exists to support the addition of an alternative form of progesterone to the current progesterone treatment (adding a vaginal form to an intramuscular form).

Maintenance Therapy

The use of progesterone in women who remain undelivered after an episode of threatened preterm labor (PTL) is investigational and it is not routinely recommended.

Other Interventions

A first-trimester urine culture should be performed on all pregnant women, and regular antenatal screening is recommended for women at high risk for asymptomatic bacteriuria. Preconception identification and optimization of chronic medical diseases, such as diabetes and hypertension, can improve maternal health and pregnancy outcome.

■ TERMINOLOGY USED TO DESCRIBE PRETERM LABOR

Suspected preterm labor: A woman with symptoms of PTL with a clinical assessment (including a speculum or digital vaginal examination) of the possibility of PTL but ruled out established labor.

Threatened preterm labor: Frequent uterine contractions without effacement or dilation of the cervix

Diagnosed preterm labor: A woman is in diagnosed PTL, if she has suspected PTL and a positive diagnostic test for PTL. The diagnostic test can either be transvaginal ultrasound of cervical canal length <15 mm or fetal fibronectin positive, >50 ng/mL.

Established preterm labor: A woman with progressive cervical dilatation from 4 cm with regular contractions is in established PTL.

Advanced preterm labor: Cervix dilated more than 3 cm and effaced 80% or more.

Diagnosis of preterm labor pains: Presence of uterine contractions, four or more in 20 minutes or eight or more in 1 hour, each lasts for >40 seconds with progressive dilatation and effacement of cervix (dilatation >1 cm and effacement >80%).

■ EVALUATION OF WOMEN WITH PRETERM LABOR

Assess duration, character, intensity, progressive nature, and interval of pain; it is associated with show or leaking PV; rule out medical and surgical causes of pain; look for risk factor for PTL such as previous history of PTB, polyhydramnios, twin pregnancy, Müllerian anomaly. Also assess for any medical or obstetric indication for termination of pregnancy.

EXAMINATION

Perform general physical examination including vital assessment, orodental hygiene, respiratory and cardiovascular system (r/o heart disease) and rule out any contradictions to tocolysis. On abdominal examination, assess uterine height, presentation, contraction, amount of liquor, and estimated baby weight. Do per speculum examination and bedside test for fetal fibronectin, if available.

Fetal fibronectin (FFN) is a glycoprotein found in the chorioamniotic membranes, decidua and cytotrophoblast are elevated in cervicovaginal secretions of women between 22 and 33 weeks of gestation who are likely to have preterm delivery. If the test is negative, there is no need of tocolysis or corticosteroids administration.

Per vaginam examination is done, if cervical dilatation and effacement cannot be assessed on speculum examination. Unnecessary vaginal examinations should be avoided.

MANAGEMENT OF ESTABLISHED PRETERM LABOR

Woman is admitted to labor room, reassurance, and counseling regarding risk of PTL. Consent regarding prognosis of preterm baby is explained and documented on case records. Monitor pulse, BP, temperature, and uterine contraction; maintain adequate hydration.

Send investigations, routine antenatal investigations, if not already done, complete blood count, urine for routine, microscopy, and culture sensitivity, high-vaginal swab culture, and sensitivity and C-reactive protein (if associated with ruptured membranes).

Ultrasonography is done for assessment of fetal growth, estimated fetal weight, amount of liquor, placental location, and grade. Transvaginal sonography (TVS) is done to assess CL, internal os diameter, and presence of funneling. A sagittal plane of the cervix is obtained in which the entire length of the cervical canal is visualized. After obtaining full view of cervix, the depth is increased so that the image occupies approximately two-thirds of the screen. To obtain the CL, the distance between the internal and external cervical os is measured.

Betamethasone and dexamethasone are preferred over other steroids because they are less extensively metabolized by the placental enzyme 11 beta-hydroxysteroid dehydrogenase type 2. Both are equally effective for accelerating fetal lung maturity and have comparable safety profile; however, use of betamethasone requires fewer injections than dexamethasone.

Dose: Betamethasone—two doses of 12 mg given intramuscularly 24 hours apart or dexamethasone—four doses of 6 mg given intramuscularly 12 hours apart. A nonsulfite-containing preparation of dexamethasone should be used as the sulfite preservative (NNF60211) may be neurotoxic in newborns.

The salt available in India is betamethasone phosphate, which is short acting and requires more frequent administration as compared to the former. Hence, the dosage schedule of betamethasone phosphate available in India is similar to that of the dexamethasone and has no added advantage over dexamethasone.

Following are the recommendations of various international societies:
According to the operational guidelines June 2014, released by Ministry of Health and Family Welfare, Government of India, single course of injection of dexamethasone is to be administered to women with PTL (between 24 and 34 weeks of gestation) at all levels of health facilities in the public as well as the private sector.

According to the Society for Maternal–Fetal Medicine Specialists, women with 34+0 to 36+6 weeks of gestation who are at risk of PTB within 7 days should receive a two-dose course of antenatal betamethasone. For these women with symptoms of PTL, cervical dilation should be ≥3 cm or effacement ≥75% and tocolysis should not be used to delay delivery for completion of the course of steroids. For women with potential medical/obstetric indications for early delivery, steroids should not be administered until a definite plan for delivery has been made.

The American College of Obstetricians and Gynecologists recommends administration of betamethasone for women with a singleton pregnancy at 34+0 to 36+6 weeks of gestation at imminent risk of PTB within 7 days, with the following caveats: antenatal corticosteroid should not be administered to women with chorioamnionitis. Tocolysis should not be used to delay delivery in women with symptoms of PTL to allow completion of corticosteroids course. Medically/obstetrically indicated preterm delivery should not be postponed for steroid administration. Antenatal corticosteroids should not be administered, if the patient has already received a course of corticosteroids. Newborns should be monitored for hypoglycemia.

The NICE guideline (NG25) on PTL and birth suggests considering maternal corticosteroids for women between 34+0 and 35+6 weeks of gestation, who are in suspected, diagnosed, or established PTL, are having a planned PTB, or have preterm prelabor rupture of membranes.

However, some authors have cautioned against universal adoption of antenatal corticosteroids for pregnancies at risk of PTB at 34+0 to 36+6 weeks of gestation because it is unclear whether the short-term benefits (reduction in transient tachypnea of the newborn) clearly outweigh the risks (neonatal hypoglycemia, unknown long-term neurodevelopmental outcome, and metabolic risks).

A 2018 meta-analysis of four randomized trials of antenatal corticosteroids (betamethasone or dexamethasone) administered 48 hours before planned cesarean delivery at ≥37 weeks of gestation found reductions in neonatal respiratory morbidity compared with placebo or no treatment.

What is the harm in administering antenatal corticosteroids after 34+0 weeks of gestation?

Antenatal steroids may have effect on the neurodevelopment outcomes of the fetuses exposed to corticosteroids beyond 34+0 weeks of gestation. This is due to the fact that exponential brain growth occurs after 34 weeks of gestation. The fetus brain grows by 35%, cortical volume increases by 50%, and 25% of cerebellar development occurs after 34 weeks of gestation. Therefore, exposure to exogenous betamethasone or dexamethasone during this time period is likely to have greater adverse consequences on brain development than at any other period of development.

Also, disruption of the normal fetal environment at this critical time may lead to changes in development of the neuroendocrine system, life-long effects on endocrine, behavioral, emotional, and cognitive function, and increased risks for development of a wide range or metabolic, cardiovascular, and brain disorders in later life.

The data on efficacy and safety of antenatal corticosteroid is mainly from the high-income countries. A multifaceted intervention trial (ACT) designed to increase the use of antenatal corticosteroids in low-income and middle-income countries published in the Lancet journal, February 2015, reported increased neonatal and perinatal mortality in the late preterm and early term fetuses exposed to antenatal corticosteroids. The study also observed increased infectious morbidity in steroid-exposed mother and the babies. However, one of the limitations of the study was that instead of gestational age, baby weighing less than 5 percentile were taken as a proxy for PTB.

Tocolysis for 48 hours for delaying delivery for maximum effect of steroids (optimum benefit of steroid begins 24 hours after therapy and lasts for 7 days). Tocolysis is not recommended.

What are contraindications to tocolysis therapy?

Tocolysis is contraindicated when the maternal/fetal risks of prolonging pregnancy or the risks associated with these drugs are greater than the risks associated with PTB. Established contraindications to labor inhibition include—*intrauterine fetal demise, lethal fetal anomaly, nonreassuring fetal status, pre-eclampsia with severe features or eclampsia; maternal hemorrhage with hemodynamic instability; intra-amniotic infection; preterm prelabor rupture of membranes, and medical contraindications to the tocolytic drug.*[15]

What is the aim of giving tocolytic drugs to women in PTL?

There is no evidence exists that tocolytic therapy has any direct favorable effect on neonatal outcomes or that any prolongation of pregnancy afforded by tocolytics actually translates into statistically significant neonatal benefit.[16]

According to the current view, the objectives of tocolysis are:[17]

- Prolongation of the pregnancy by at least 48 hours to ensure completion of induction of lung maturation using corticosteroids

- To enable an in utero transfer of the pregnant woman to a perinatal centre with a neonatal intensive care unit (NICU)
- To complete fetal neuroprotection using magnesium sulfate < 32 weeks of pregnancy.

These measures are evidence-based methods to decrease neonatal morbidity and mortality.

The ACOG also recommends tocolytics to prevent PTL when it is safe to do so and when there are underlying, self-limited conditions that can cause labor, such as pyelonephritis or abdominal surgery, and are unlikely to cause recurrent PTL.[16]

Nifedipine: Initial oral dose is 20 mg, followed by 10–20 mg 3–4 times daily, adjusted according to uterine activity for up to 48 hours. Main adverse effects include flushing, palpitations, nausea and vomiting, and hypotension. Nifedipine is contraindicated in cardiac disease; it should be used with caution in diabetes or multiple pregnancy, owing to risk of pulmonary edema. The oral route of administration, low costs, and a possible efficacy in reducing neonatal morbidity favor the use of CCBs.

Oxytocin antagonist/atosiban: Atosiban is a nonapeptide, desamino-oxytocin analog, and a competitive vasopressin/oxytocin receptor antagonist (VOTra). It inhibits the oxytocin-mediated release of inositol trisphosphate from the myometrial cell membrane. As a result, reduced release of intracellular, stored calcium from the sarcoplasmic reticulum of myometrial cells and reduced influx of Ca^{2+} from the extracellular space through voltage-gated channels occur. In addition, atosiban suppresses oxytocin-mediated release of PGE and PGF from the deciduas.

The onset of uterus relaxation following atosiban is rapid, uterine contractions being significantly reduced within 10 minutes to achieve stable uterine quiescence.

Each vial of 5 mL solution contains 37.5 mg atosiban (as acetate). Each mL of solution contains 7.5 mg atosiban.

Atosiban is administered intravenously in three successive stages—an initial bolus dose (6.75 mg)/0.9 mL solution for injection, immediately followed by a continuous high-dose infusion (loading infusion 300 μg/min) for 3 hours, followed by a lower dose (subsequent infusion 100 μg/min) up to 45 hours.

Indomethacin: Cyclooxygenase (COX, or prostaglandin synthase) is the enzyme responsible for conversion of arachidonic acid to prostaglandins, which are critical in parturition. Nonspecific cyclooxygenase inhibitors reduce prostaglandin production by inhibition of both COX-1 and COX-2. In comparative trials, indomethacin reduced the risk of birth within 48 hours of initiation of treatment compared with any β-agonist and appeared to be as effective as nifedipine.

- *Dosage:* Initial dosage 50–100 mg oral or rectal, followed by 25–50 mg every 4-6 hours for 48 hours. Fetal blood concentrations are 50% of maternal values, but the half-life in the neonate is substantially longer than that in the mother.

To avoid premature closure of the ductus arteriosus, it is recommended to administer COX inhibitors only up to the 32nd week of pregnancy for 48 hours.[16] Prior to 32 weeks of pregnancy, an echocardiographic examination of the fetal ductus arteriosus with assessment of the tricuspid valve (tricuspid regurgitation) is recommended, if treatment lasts >48 hours.[15] According to the recommendations of the European Association of Perinatal Medicine 2017, the amount of amniotic fluid should be checked prior to starting therapy and after 48–72 hours as indomethacin, results in oligohydramnios in 5–15% of cases, and even in up to 70% of cases in the case of use for >72 hours.[15] Indomethacin should only be given if there is a normal amount of amniotic fluid and if oligohydramnios occurs; it should be discontinued or at least the dose should be reduced. Side effects include nausea, vomiting, esophageal reflux, gastritis, constriction of the ductus arteriosus, and oligohydramnios. It is contraindicated in presence of platelet dysfunction or bleeding diathesis, hepatic dysfunction, gastrointestinal ulcerative disease, renal dysfunction, and asthma (in women with hypersensitivity to aspirin.[17]

Beta-agonists: β-agonists, such as isoxsuprine and ritodrine, reduce the sensitivity to calcium, and total intracellular calcium concentrations, thereby causing myometrial relaxation. According to a 2012 network meta-analysis, β-sympathomimetics are indeed effective in prolonging pregnancy for 48 hours, but significantly less effective than calcium channel blockers and indomethacin and also have the highest rate of maternal adverse effects of all tocolytics in comparison to placebo.[18]

The β-2 receptor agonist, terbutaline, is now *not* recommended for use in PTL due to these serious side effects (US Food and Drug Administration, 2011). However, terbutaline is still used for emergency treatment of intrapartum uterine hyperstimulation to aid resuscitation of a fetal bradycardia.[16] *In the current guidelines, β-sympathomimetics are no longer recommended for tocolysis.* However, recently published multicentric studies from India and Korea have reported β-sympathomimetics to be still the most popular tocolysis used as first line. Jaju et al. also found significant improvement in mean latency period, prolongation of delivery beyond 48 hours, and perinatal outcomes among patients on isoxsuprine versus other pharmacological agents.

Less Effective Tocolytic Drugs

Magnesium sulfate: Use of magnesium sulfate as a tocolytic is controversial. In a 2014 systematic review of randomized trials comparing magnesium sulfate with no treatment/placebo control, magnesium sulfate administration did not result in a statistical reduction in birth <48 hours after trial entry (RR: 0.56; 95% CI: 0.27–1.14; three trials, 182 women) or improvement in neonatal and maternal outcomes.[13] Magnesium sulfate causes fewer minor maternal side effects than β-agonists, but the risk of major adverse risk events is comparable. Except in the US, magnesium sulfate is *no longer recommended for tocolysis* in current reviews and guidelines.

Magnesium sulfate reduces the severity and risk of cerebral palsy in surviving infants if administered when birth is anticipated before 32 weeks of gestation. Hence, it has a role in neuroprotection.[15]

Nitrous oxide donor—as transdermal application of nitroglycerin (patches—10 mg/24 h) was considered for some years to be a new and innovative method for tocolysis since it is effective, has few side effects, is easy to apply, and cost-efficient. In a 2014 meta-analysis of randomized trials that compared glyceryl trinitrate by any route with placebo (three trials), β-adrenergic receptor agonists (nine trials), and nifedipine (one trial), use of glyceryl trinitrate did not significantly prolong pregnancy by ≥48 hours, reduce PTB, or result in improved neonatal outcomes compared with any of the comparators.

Magnesium sulfate for fetal neuroprotection: Consider intravenous (IV) magnesium sulfate for neuroprotection of the baby for women between 28 and 32 weeks of pregnancy who are in established PTL or having a planned PTB within 24 hours.

Give a 4-g IV bolus of magnesium sulfate over 15 minutes, followed by an β infusion of 1 g per hour until the birth or for 24 hours (whichever is sooner).

For women on magnesium sulfate, monitor for clinical signs of magnesium toxicity at least every 4 hours by recording pulse, blood pressure, respiratory rate, and deep tendon (e.g., patellar) reflexes. If a woman has or develops oliguria or other signs of renal failure, monitor more frequently for magnesium toxicity and think about reducing the dose of magnesium sulfate.

Long-term in utero exposure to magnesium sulfate is associated with fetal and neonatal bone demineralization and fractures.

Management of Labor

- *First stage*: Avoid repeated digital examination, P/V to be repeated only when indicated. Fetal heart rate (FHR) monitoring is done by cardiotocography (CTG)/intermittent auscultation.
- *Second stage:* Vacuum is contraindicated, if required forceps may be used for instrumental delivery.

If a preterm baby needs to be moved away from the mother for resuscitation, or there is significant maternal bleeding, consider milking the cord and clamp the cord as soon as possible. Otherwise delay cord clamping of preterm babies by 30–60 seconds, if the mother and baby are stable.

Position the baby at or below the level of the placenta before clamping the cord. Neonatologist should be available to attend baby at delivery. Inform pediatrician for making surfactant available, if required.

Management of Threatened Labor

In a subgroup analysis of the APOSTEL-I study, the combination of CL measurement on ultrasound and the determination of fetal fibronectin proved to be cost-effective through the reduction in inpatient admissions, tocolysis, and induction of fetal lung maturation.[4]

It is currently being discussed whether, in addition to CL measurement on ultrasound, the additional determination of a biomarker such as fibronectin significantly improves the prediction of preterm delivery and thus should be included in the clinical management in the event of threatened preterm delivery.[2,3,5]

The NICE guidelines 2016 advised against using combination of transvaginal ultrasound and FFN for diagnosis of PTL.

It is suggested that if a woman is less than 29+6 weeks of gestation and is in suspected PTL, she should receive treatment for PTL (admission, tocolysis, antenatal corticosteroids, and magnesium sulfate if indicated). For women with more than 30+0 weeks of gestation, transvaginal USG should be done and only women who have CL ≤ 15 mm should receive treatment for PTL.

If it is not feasible to do CL measurement, FFN is done and if value is >50 ng/mL, treatment for PTL should be started.

However, *Society of Maternal and Fetal Medicine recommends* that all women between 23+0 and 33+6 weeks of gestation presenting with symptoms of PTL should be evaluated for CL on transvaginal USG, if CL is >30 mm, FFN is not advocated, no treatment is required and woman is kept under observation. If CL is 20–29 mm, FFN is done if positive treatment for PTL is started. In women with CL < 20 mm, treatment for PTL is given without performing FFN.

The sample for FFN should be obtained before TVS to avoid false-positive report.

Are tocolytics indicated and safe to administer in multiple gestations?
The use of tocolytics to inhibit PTL in multiple gestations has been associated with a greater risk of maternal complications, such as pulmonary edema. In addition, prophylactic tocolytics have not been shown to reduce the risk of PTB or improve neonatal outcomes in women with multiple gestations.

Adequate data do not exist to specifically demonstrate benefit from the use of antenatal corticosteroids in multiple gestations. However, because of the clear benefit attributable to the use of antenatal corticosteroids in singleton gestations, most experts recommend their use in preterm multiple gestations.[15]

Is there any role of other pharmacological and nonpharmacological methods in management of PTL?

Antibiotics should not be used to prolong gestation or improve neonatal outcomes in women with PTL and intact membranes, as there is no evidence-based role for antibiotic therapy in the prevention of prematurity in patients with acute PTL.[15]

- *Progesterone supplementation:* Women in acute PTL do not benefit from progesterone supplementation.[16]
- *Bed rest and hydration* have not been shown to be effective for the prevention of PTB and should not be routinely recommended.[15]

SUMMARY

Preconception identification and optimization of chronic medical diseases, such as diabetes and hypertension, can improve maternal health and pregnancy outcome.

A first-trimester urine culture should be performed on all pregnant women, and regular antenatal screening is recommended for women at high risk for asymptomatic bacteriuria.

It is recommended that in women with a previous PTB, progesterones are started in the second trimester (16–20 weeks) and continued till 36 weeks of gestation.

Serial TVS is done to follow their CL once in 2 weeks and more frequently (once a week), if CL is between 25 and 30 mm until 24 weeks of gestation and consider cerclage, if CL is <25 mm.

All women should undergo CL assessment at the time of anomaly scan. In those with incidental finding of short CL < 20 mm before or at 24 weeks of gestation, vaginal progesterone is recommended.

Women between 23+0 and 33+6 weeks of gestation presenting with symptoms of PTL should be evaluated for CL on transvaginal USG, if CL is >30 mm, FFN is not advocated, no treatment is required, and woman is kept under observation. If CL is 20–29 mm, FFN is done if positive treatment for PTL is started, i.e., tocolysis, antenatal corticosteroids, and magnesium sulfate, if <32 weeks. In women with CL < 20 mm, treatment for PTL is given without performing FFN. *The sample for FFN should be obtained before TVS to avoid false-positive report.*

The aim of tocolytic therapy is to allow administration of antenatal corticosteroids and magnesium sulfate and in utero transfer of baby to a tertiary care center.

Nifedipine and atosiban are suitable tocolytics with regard to efficacy, adverse effect profile, and effects on the child. Indomethacin is a potent tocolytic with anti-inflammatory effects and a low rate of maternal adverse effects and should be justified, especially in early preterm delivery.

Beta-sympathomimetics although not recommended by International Society Guidelines due to the high rate of maternal and fetal adverse effects are again gaining popularity in India.

Magnesium sulfate should not be used as a tocolytic due to the controversial study results and the adverse effect profile at a high dose.

Maintenance treatment with tocolytic drugs or repeat tocolytic treatment does not appear to improve perinatal outcome and therefore is not recommended.

Use of multiple tocolytic agents should be avoided due to the risk of increasing adverse effects. Caution should be exercised, if tocolytics are administered in multiple gestations due to the increased risk of adverse effects.

Consider IV magnesium sulfate for neuroprotection of the baby for women between 28 and 32 weeks of pregnancy who are in established PTL or having a planned PTB within 24 hours. Nifedipine in combination with magnesium sulfate should be used with caution.

Antenatal corticosteroids should be administered to women at 23+0 to 33+6 weeks of gestation, who are at high risk of spontaneous or induced preterm delivery within 7 days.

Antenatal corticosteroids in women at gestation 22+0 to 22+6 weeks should be used after consultation with the fetal medicine specialist and neonatologist. This should be done after proper counseling and informed consent from the woman and family.

Although administration of corticosteroids before PTBs between 34 and 37 weeks of gestation has been reported to have potential benefits, till more data on safety of antenatal corticosteroids in Indian population is available, administration of antenatal corticosteroids in women at ≥34+0 weeks of gestation should be done after counseling and informed consent.

■ REFERENCES

1. Chawanpaiboon S, Vogel JP, Moller AB, Lumbiganon P, Petzold M, Hogan D, et al. Global, regional and national estimates of level of preterm birth in 2014: a systematic review and modelling analysis. Lancet. 2019;7(1):PE37-46.
2. Mercer BM, Goldenberg RL, Moawad AH, Meis PJ, Iams JD, Das AF, et al. The preterm prediction study: effect of gestational age and cause of preterm birth on subsequent obstetric outcome. National Institute of Child Health and Human Development Maternal-Fetal Medicine Units Network. Am J Obstet Gynecol. 1999;181(5 Pt 1): 1216-21.
3. Meis PJ, Goldenberg RL, Mercer BM, Iams JD, Moawad AH, Miodovnik M, et al. The preterm prediction study: risk factors for indicated preterm births. Am J Obstet Gynecol. 1998;178(3):562-7.
4. Koike T, Minakami H, Kosuge S, Usui R, Matsubara S, Izumi A, et al. Uterine leiomyoma in pregnancy: its influence on obstetric performance. J Obstet Gynaecol Res. 1999;25(5):309-13.
5. Kiely JL. What is the population-based risk of preterm birth among twins and other multiples? Clin Obstet Gynecol. 1998;41(1):3-11.
6. Newman RB, Goldenberg RL, Iams JD, Meis PJ, Mercer BM, Moawad AH, et al. Preterm prediction study: comparison of the cervical score and Bishop score for prediction of spontaneous preterm delivery. Obstet Gynecol. 2008;112(3):508-15.
7. Guzman E, walters C, Ananth C, O'Reilly-Green C, Benito CW, Palermo A, et al. A comparison of sonographic cervical parameters in predicting spontaneous preterm birth in high-risk singleton gestations. Ultrasound Obstet Gynecol. 2001;18(3):204-10.

8. Goepfert AR, Goldenberg RL, Mercer B, Iams J, Meis P, Moawad A, et al. The preterm Prediction Study: Quantitative fetal fibronectin values and the prediction of spontaneous preterm birth. Am J Obstet Gynecol. 2000;183(6):1480-3.

9. Saade GR, Boggess KA, Sullivan SA, Markenson GR, Iams JD, Coonrod DV, et al. Development and validation of a spontaneous preterm delivery predictor in asymptomatic women. Am J Obstet Gynecol. 2016;214(5):633.e1-633.e24.

10. Brown JA, Pearson AW, Veillon EW, Rust OA, Chauhan SP, Magann EF, et al. History- or ultrasound-based cerclage placement and adverse perinatal outcomes. J Reprod Med. 2011;56(9-10):385-92.

11. Berghella V, Odibo AO, To MS, Rust OA, Althuisius SM. Cerclage for short cervix on ultrasonography: meta-analysis of trials using individual patient-level data. Obstet Gynecol. 2005;106:181-9.

12. Romero R, Nicolaides K, Conde Agudelo A, Tabor A, O'Brien JM, Cetingoz E, et al. Vaginal progesterone in women with an asymptomatic sonographic cervix in the midtrimester decreases preterm delivery and neonatal morbidity: a systematic review and meta-analysis of individual patient data. Am J Obstet Gynecol. 2012;206(2):124. e1-19.

13. Romero R, Conde-Agudelo A, Da Fonseca E, O'Brien JM, Cetingoz E, Creasy GW, et al. Vaginal progesterone for preventing preterm birth and adverse perinatal outcomes in singleton gestations with a short cervix: a meta-analysis of individual patient data. Am J Obstet Gynecol. 2018;218(2):161-80.

14. Norwitz ER, Lockwood CJ; UpToDate (2019). Progesterone supplementation to reduce the risk of spontaneous preterm birth. [online] Available from: https://www.uptodate.com/contents/progesterone-supplementation-to-reduce-the-risk-of-spontaneous-preterm-birth [Last accessed June, 2020].

15. ACOG (2016). Practice Bulletin No. 171: Management of Preterm Labor. [online] Available from: https://journals.lww.com/greenjournal/Fulltext/2016/10000/Practice_Bulletin_No__171__Management_of_Preterm.61.aspx#:~:text=The%20most%20beneficial%20intervention%20for,of%20delivery%20within%207%20days [Last accessed June, 2020].

16. ACOG Committee Opinion (2017). Antenatal Corticosteroid Therapy for Fetal Maturation. [online] Available from: https://www.acog.org/clinical/clinical-guidance/committee-opinion/articles/2017/08/antenatal-corticosteroid-therapy-for-fetal-maturation [Last accessed June, 2020].

17. Tsatsaris V, Carbonne B, Cabrol D. Atosiban for preterm labour. Drugs. 2004;64(4):375-82.

18. Smaill F, Vazquez JC. Antibiotics for asymptomatic bacteriuria in pregnancy. Cochrane Database Syst Rev. 2007;(8):CD000490.

Growth Discrepancy in Fetus

Asis Kumar Mukhopadhyay, Sumitra Bachani

INTRODUCTION

Fetal growth restriction (FGR) is an obstetrical condition with clinical variance in diagnosing, monitoring, and delivering a growth-restricted fetus. There are multiple variables and indices, which have to be assessed to determine the correct time and mode of delivering such a fetus. There is an added risk of prematurity associated with delivering at different gestational ages, which adds to the neonatal morbidity. The first aim in the management of growth-restricted fetus is to distinguish constitutionally small for gestational age (SGA) fetus from "true" FGR as the latter are at a higher risk of stillbirth and adverse perinatal outcomes. The second aim is to identify which growth restricted fetus is at risk of severe fetal hypoxia or death in utero so as to time the delivery. In this chapter, we will discuss the stage-based management approach to FGR, which entails a proper identification of FGR versus SGA, can help reduce clinical variability, and determines the monitoring protocol to decide the decision for termination of pregnancy.

IDENTIFICATION OF "FETAL GROWTH RESTRICTION" VERSUS "(CONSTITUTIONAL) SMALL FOR GESTATIONAL AGE"

A growth-restricted fetus is defined as one which has failed to achieve its biologically established growth potential. It is associated with signs of placental insufficiency manifesting as abnormal Doppler indices and associated maternal comorbidities such as pre-eclampsia. There are various risk factors which are associated with a growth restriction in the fetus **(Table 1)**. The initial history and examination should be followed by relevant investigations to confirm any associated comorbidity like maternal hypertension, antiphospholipid syndrome, maternal infection, renal insufficiency, and, in some cases, genetic syndromes. SGA fetuses have a good perinatal outcome as the any other normal grown fetus. Most guidelines recommended that estimated fetal weight (EFW) < 10th centile and any one of the additional deranged Doppler parameters among the three namely abnormal uterine artery pulsatility index (PI) (>95th centile), abnormal umbilical artery pulsatility index (UAPI) (>95th centile), and abnormal

TABLE 1: Risk factors for fetal growth restriction (FGR).

Odds ratio > 3	Odds ratio > 2
• Previous stillbirth • Antiphospholipid syndrome (APLS) • Diabetes and vascular disease • Unexplained antepartum hemorrhage • Renal impairment • Low maternal weight gain • Paternal SGA • Low maternal weight gain • Cocaine use • Previous SGA baby • Daily vigorous exercise	• Maternal SGA • Chronic hypertension • PIH severe • Pre-eclampsia • Smoking > 10 cigarettes per day • Low pregnancy associated plasma protein A (PAPP-A) < 0.4 MoM • Threatened miscarriage • Elevated AFP > 2.0 MoM and hCG > 2.5 MoM • Echogenic bowel found in the fetus

(AFP: alpha-fetoprotein; SGA: small for gestational age; MoM: multiples of the median)

cerebroplacental ratio (CPR) (<5th centile) to establish the diagnosis of FGR. A recently published Delphi survey, which incorporated opinions of 45 experts, has reached a consensus for defining FGR and differentiating early and late-onset phenotypes.[1]

Late-onset FGR is defined as onset of growth restriction at or after 32 weeks or more.

Presence of two solitary parameters that is AC or EFW < 3rd centile and four contributory parameters AC or EFW < 10th centile, CPR < 5th centile, or UAPI > 95th centile on sonography were designated indices for definition. The algorithm for diagnosis includes one solitary or two contributory parameters that is one each of biometry and Doppler parameters to confirm late FGR.

Early-onset FGR is defined as onset of growth restriction prior to 32 weeks. Presence of three solitary parameters is considered either AC < 3rd centile or EFW < 3rd centile and absent end-diastolic velocity (AEDF) in the umbilical artery (UA). The four contributory parameters of either AC < 10th centile or EFW < 10th centile, uterine artery PI, and/or UAPI > 95th centile were designated indices for definition. The algorithm defines one solitary or two among three contributory parameters including Doppler to confirm early FGR **(Table 2)**.

Early-or-late onset FGR is due to the difference in severity of placental insufficiency and the degree of fetal adaptation to the hypoxia in utero. The deterioration in Doppler indices of both phenotypes is different **(Table 3)**.[2]

INDICES FOR FETAL ASSESSMENT AND ROLE IN MANAGEMENT

Doppler indices, which are used for establishing the diagnosis of FGR and are relevant for the decision as to whether delivery is indicated when term pregnancy is reached, are diagnostic variables. Another set of indices, which are useful to determine whether there is a high risk of short-term deterioration, and hence indicators for delivery prior to term are prognostic variables.

TABLE 2: Delphi consensus for definition of intrauterine growth restriction (IUGR).[1]	
Early FGR: <32 weeks	*Late FGR: ≥ 32 weeks*
Solitary biometric: • AC < 3rd centile • EFW < 3rd centile • *Solitary Doppler:* Absent end-diastolic flow in umbilical artery	*Solitary biometric:* • AC < 3rd centile • EFW < 3rd centile
Contributory biometric: • AC < 10th centile • EFW< 10th centile	*Contributory biometric:* • AC < 10th centile • EFW< 10th centile • *Biometric relative:* AC or EFW crossing centile more than two quartiles
Contributory Doppler: • UtrPI > 95th centile • UAPI > 95th centile	*Contributory Doppler:* • UAPI > 95th centile • Abnormal CPR < 5th centile
Algorithm: One solitary or two contributory one each of biometry and Doppler parameters	One solitary or two among three contributory including Doppler
(CPR: cerebroplacental ratio; EFW: estimated fetal weight; FGR: fetal growth restriction)	

TABLE 3: Early-and late-onset fetal growth restriction (FGR)—Pathophysiology.[2]	
Early onset	*Late onset*
Challenge—management prevalence: 1–2%	Challenge—diagnosis prevalence: 3–5%
Severe placental disease: UA Doppler abnormal, high association with PE	Mild placental disease: UA Doppler normal, low association with PE
Severe hypoxia ++: Systemic CV adaptation	Mild hypoxia: Central CV adaptation
High mortality and morbidity	Lower mortality (but common cause of late stillbirth)

Uterine Artery Doppler

High pulsatility index (>95th centile) is one of the factors included the diagnosis of FGR **(Fig. 1)**.

Umbilical Artery Doppler

The umbilical artery Doppler **(Fig. 2)** is the only index that has both diagnostic and prognostic role in the management of FGR. Worsening of Doppler parameters to absent or reversal of end-diastolic flow have been reported to be present at least a week prior to acute deterioration.[3] Reversed end-diastolic flow in the UA has a sensitivity and specificity of about 60% as a predictor of adverse perinatal outcome, which is likely independent of prematurity.[4] Cosmi E et al. reported a 29% reduction in perinatal mortality on using UA Doppler in high-risk pregnancies.[5] Once the fetus has attained 30 weeks of gestation, the risk of stillbirth in a fetus with isolated reversed

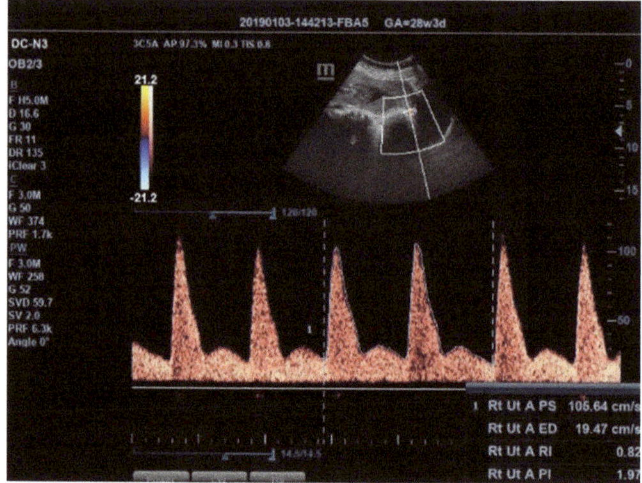

Fig. 1: Uterine artery Doppler.

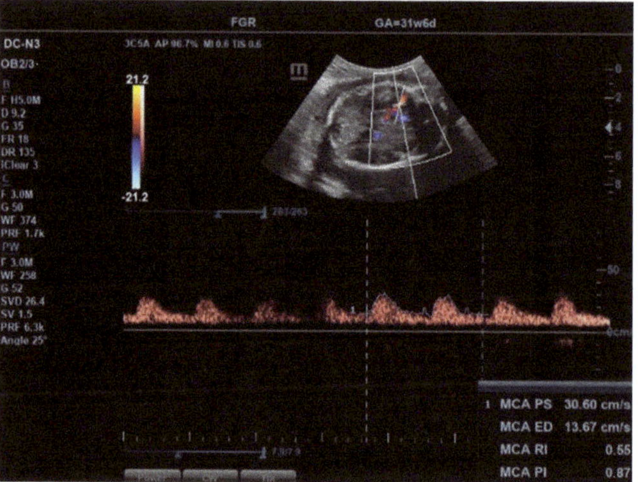

Fig. 2: Umbilical artery Doppler.

end-diastolic velocities in the UA Doppler the risk of stillbirth is higher than that of morbidity of prematurity hence delivery is recommended in such fetuses.[6-8]

Middle Cerebral Artery Doppler/Cerebroplacental Ratio

A hypoxic fetus redistributes the blood flow to the most vital organ—the brain. As more vasodilation marks the fall in resistance of middle cerebral artery (MCA), it is an indicator of redistribution of flow with brain sparing **(Fig. 3)**. It is a surrogate marker to determine the degree of fetal hypoxia. Abnormal MCA-PI can be associated with adverse perinatal and neurological outcome; however, it is not established whether in preterm fetuses, an early delivery before term will be of benefit. In late-onset FGR, the MCA is particularly

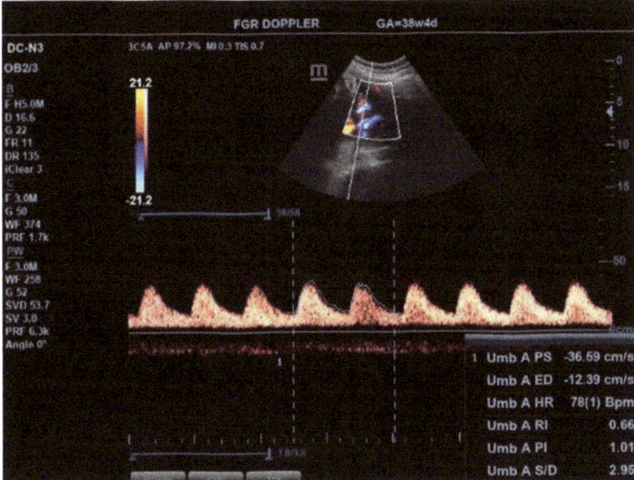

Fig. 3: Middle cerebral artery Doppler flow showing redistribution.

valuable independently of the UA Doppler for the identification and prediction of adverse outcome.[8,9] Few authors have reported that fetuses with abnormal MCA-PI had a sixfold increased risk of emergency cesarean section for fetal distress when compared with SGA fetuses with normal MCA-PI.[10,11] This is particularly relevant because labor induction at term is the current mode of management of late-onset FGR.[12,13] Late FGR with abnormal MCA-PI has poorer neurobehavioral scores at term-corrected age and at 2 years of age.[14] MCA Doppler has a low sensitivity and acceptable specificity for the detection of FGR and it is improved by the use of CPR. The ratio of MCA-PI to UAPI improves upon the individual sensitivity of UA and MCA Doppler. The CPR is already decreased when its individual components show mild changes but are still within normal ranges.[15,16] Abnormal CPR can be present before delivery in 20–25% of the cases of late-onset FGR and is associated with a higher risk of adverse perinatal outcome after labor induction.[11]

Ductus Venosus Doppler

Ductus venosus (DV) flow waveforms **(Fig. 4)** become abnormal only in advanced stages of fetal compromise.[3,5] Absent and reversed velocities (atrial contraction/a wave) are associated with perinatal mortality independent of the gestational age at delivery,[17] with a risk ranging from 40 to 100% in early-onset FGR.[18] Absent "atrial wave" in DV or reversal "a" wave is sufficient to recommend delivery at any gestational age, after completion of steroid cover. DV is the single-most strong Doppler parameter, which predicts the short-term risk of stillbirth in early-onset FGR. In 50% cases, abnormal DV precedes the loss of short-term variability in computerized cardiotocography (cCTG) and in about 90% of cases, it is abnormal 48–72 hours before the biophysical profile (BPP).[18] Therefore, it provides a better window of opportunity for

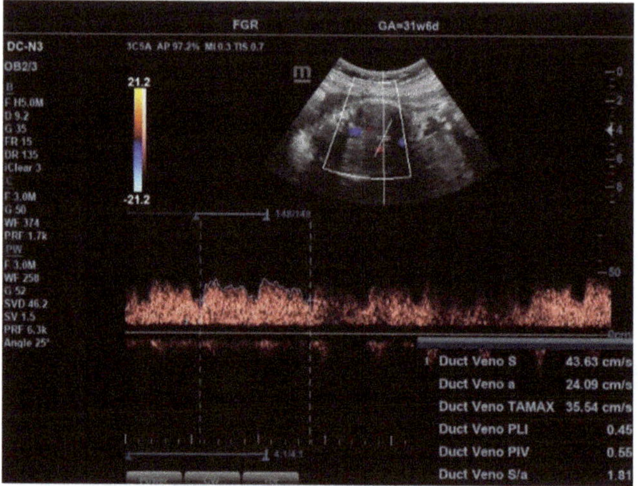

Fig. 4: Ductus venosus Doppler.

delivering fetuses in critical conditions, biding time to complete corticoids administration for fetal lung maturation.

Evidence from the Growth Restriction Intervention Trial (GRIT) study shows that after 30 weeks, the risk of mortality is 5%.[6,7] This risk is overbalanced by the risk of stillbirth secondary to abnormal DV[19] and, therefore, delivery after this gestational age seems reasonable. There is a biological gradient whereby the more severe the abnormalities in the DV, the higher the risk;[19] it would seem also reasonable that in cases of absent/reversed, the threshold for delivery should be even earlier.

Aortic Isthmus Doppler (Fig. 5)

This area shows the balance between the impedance of the brain and systemic vascular system.[20] Reverse aortic isthmus (AoI) flow is a sign of advanced deterioration, and it is further in the sequence of abnormal Doppler after UA and MCA Doppler. Abnormal AoI PI is associated with adverse perinatal outcome and neurological deficit in the infant.[21] However, longitudinal studies show that the AoI Doppler abnormality precedes DV abnormalities by 1 week,[22,23] and thus, it is not as good as to predict the short-term risk of stillbirth.[11] In contrast, AoI seems to improve the prediction of neurodevelopmental outcome at 2–5 years of age.[21] The interpretation of CTG is challenging in very preterm fetuses with a physiologically reduced variability due to subjective interpretation. The cCTG has provided new insights into the pathophysiology and management of FGR. cCTG evaluates short-term variability of the FHR, using a computer-based software and thus, it is not prone to error due to subjective analysis. Current evidence suggests that cCTG is sensitive to detect advanced fetal deterioration, and it provides a prediction risk for short-term fetal death, which is similar to DV reverse atrial flow.[24] However, cCTG is yet to be incorporated in the labor room protocols in India.

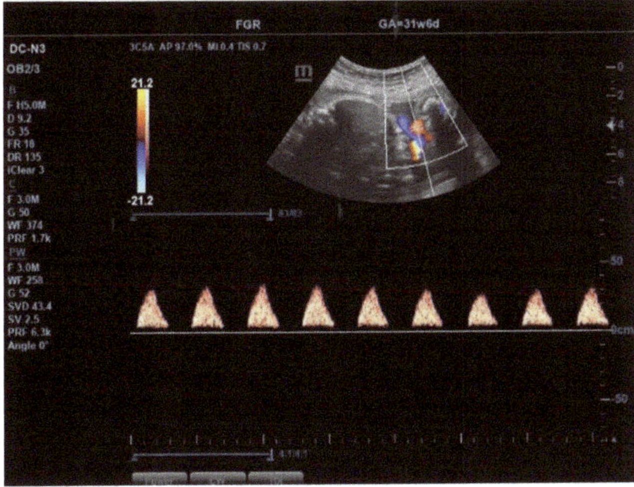

Fig. 5: Site of aortic isthmus.

EVIDENCES ABOUT TIMING OF DELIVERY IN FETAL GROWTH RESTRICTION

The main management strategy is to monitor the fetus for signs of deterioration and deliver it timely to improve perinatal outcome.[25] No specific treatment has been established to be of benefit in growth restriction.[26-29] The GRIT study[7] was a multicentre randomized controlled trial (RCT) including 548 pregnancies between 24 and 36 weeks with FGR, aimed to compare the effect of delivering early with delaying birth for as long as possible. The study observed that when obstetricians were uncertain about timing of delivery based on UA Doppler, the timing of delivery varied up to 4 days. However, the results of early delivery or delayed birth were almost similar terms of perinatal outcome.

The Trial of Randomized Umbilical and Fetal Flow in Europe (TRUFFLE) of management of preterm FGR between 26 and 32 weeks[30] was a study of early FGR (<32 weeks) where mothers were allocated to 1 of 3 monitoring strategies to indicate timing of delivery: (1) reduced fetal heart rate short-term variability on CTG; (2) early changes in fetal DV waveform; or (3) late changes in fetal DV waveform. Many infants were delivered because of safety-net criteria that is abnormal cCTG and STV or for maternal and other fetal indications, or at >32 weeks of gestation when the protocol was no longer applied. TRUFFLE study proved that delaying delivery until late changes occur in the DV or the CTG shows abnormal trace is associated with improved fetal and neonatal outcomes at 2 years of age.

Timing of Delivery in Late-onset Fetal Growth Restriction

In fetuses with FGR who show abnormal Doppler indices (raised UAPI, raised UtAPI, or reduced cerebral Doppler indices) or isolated severe FGR (EFW < 3rd centile), the majority of guidelines (83%) recommend delivery

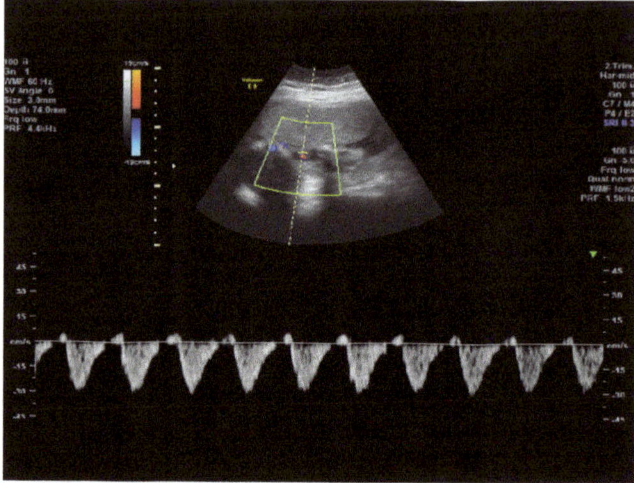

Fig. 6: Umbilical artery Doppler showing absent end-diastolic flow.

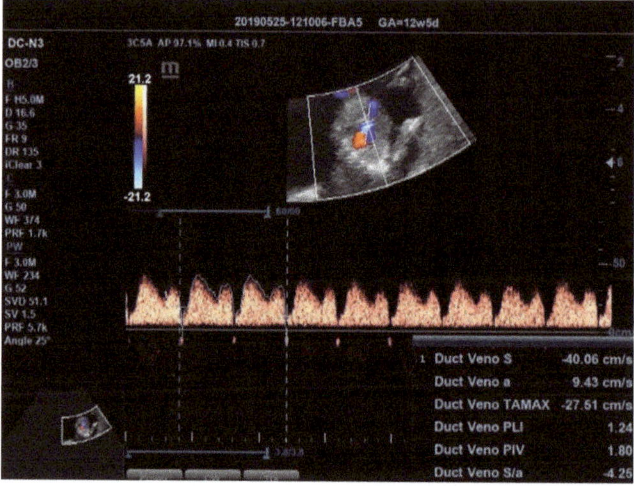

Fig. 7: Umbilical artery Doppler showing reversed end-diastolic flow.

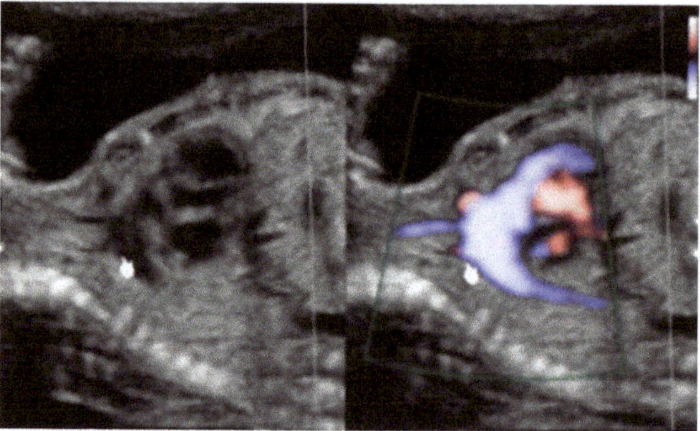

Fig. 8: Ductus venosus showing absent a wave (atrial flow).

at 37–38 weeks.[31,32] Another 33% recommend a more conservative approach when Doppler studies are normal and the FGR is not severe (i.e., EFW not <3rd centile).[31,32] These recommendations are based on the findings of the Disproportionate Intrauterine Growth Intervention Trial at Term study[13] in which 650 women with suspected FGR > 36 weeks were randomized to induction or expectant management with Doppler surveillance carried out biweekly. There was no difference in the primary outcome of severe neonatal morbidity or in cesarean delivery. Women who were offered conservative/ expectant management had a twofold increased risk of developing pre-eclampsia (7.9% vs. 3.7%; $p < 0.05$) and were more likely to have a baby with birth weight < 3rd centile (30% vs. 13%; $p < 0.001$). The recommendation was that "it is rational to choose induction to prevent possible neonatal morbidity and stillbirth." Additional data were published on outcomes in the children. There was no difference overall in neonatal morbidity between induction of labor and expectant management groups, but induction at <38 weeks was associated with increased admission in neonatal unit. It was recommended to continue pregnancy up to 38 weeks with close monitoring. On follow-up at 2 years, one of the "Ages and Stages" questionnaires was administered. Severe FGR (birth weight < 2.3 centile positively correlated with abnormal "Ages and Stages" scores).[33] A health economics analysis demonstrated that costs were lower with induction at 38 weeks compared to earlier gestations.[34] These findings suggest that delivery at 38 weeks in the fetus with suspected FGR may be optimum, unless there are earlier concerns about fetal well-being, and are consistent with findings from population-based studies that show a marked increase in stillbirth from 38 weeks in the SGA baby.

Timing the Delivery in Early-onset Fetal Growth Restriction

Most guidelines (83%) recommend undertaking cerebral Doppler studies[35-37] and using the information to influence management. There is no established consensus in terms of frequency for ongoing growth scans after diagnosis of SGA/FGR (2–4 weekly) and fetal surveillance methods such as undertaking cardiotocography (CTG) and timing of delivery.[35-37] When Doppler studies are normal, the recommendation varies between delivery at 37 and 40 weeks.[35] There is universal agreement about use of corticosteroids before birth that is likely to occur at <34 weeks 0 days; however, the RCOG alone recommends corticosteroids up to 35 weeks 6 days.[38] Four of six (67%) recommend use of magnesium sulfate for neuroprotection before very preterm delivery,[35-37] with gestation of administration varying from <30[35] to 32–33 weeks.[37] Regarding timing of delivery for preterm FGR with absent or reversed end-diastolic velocity, the recommendations for timing of delivery vary from 32 to 34 weeks[35-37] and 30 to 34 weeks,[37] respectively, with the majority (67%)[35-38] specifying that cesarean delivery should be undertaken with this severe Doppler abnormality. The most common criterion for deciding timing of delivery for fetal indication/deterioration was a computerized antenatal CTG (50%) or cCTG.[36-39]

A STAGE-BASED PROTOCOL FOR MANAGING FETAL GROWTH RESTRICTION

Due to lack of firm recommendations and clinical variance regarding monitoring and delivery, the best approach is to follow an integrated protocol, which incorporates the best available evidence. One approach (Barcelona protocol)[40] is to group in stages those indices that are associated with similar risks to the fetus, as they indicate similar follow-up intervals and timing of delivery.

- *SGA*: Doppler and growth assessment very fortnightly constitutes standard practice. Labor induction should be recommended at 40 weeks.[40]

- *Stage I FGR (severe smallness or mild placental insufficiency)*: Uterine artery, UA or MCA Doppler, and the CPR are abnormal. Fetus is at low risk of deterioration before term. Delivery mode by labor induction beyond 37 weeks, however, the risk of intrapartum fetal distress is increased and needs close monitoring in labour.[17]

- *Stage II FGR (severe placental insufficiency)*: This stage is defined by absent end-diastolic flow in umbilical artery (UA-AEDF). Reverse AoI may also be present, however, it is not considered for timing of the termination of pregnancy. Delivery is recommended at or after 34 weeks. The risk of emergency cesarean section at labor induction exceeds 50%, and elective cesarean section can be a reasonable option. Until then biweekly monitoring should be done.

- *Stage III FGR (advanced fetal deterioration, low incidence of fetal acidosis)*: The stage is characterized by reversed end-diastolic flow in the umbilical artery (UA-REDV) or DV-PI > 95th centile. This fetus is at higher risk of stillbirth and poorer neurological outcome. However, elective delivery can be delayed till signs suggesting a very high risk of stillbirth within days are not present yet like absent atrial wave in DV or abnormal CTG/BPP. This will decrease the effects of severe prematurity. Elective delivery should be done by cesarean section at or after 30 weeks. Monitoring has to be done every 24–48 hours meanwhile.

- *Stage IV FGR (high incidence of fetal acidosis and stillbirth)*: There are spontaneous FHR decelerations, reduced short-term variability (<3 ms) in the cCTG, or reverse atrial flow in the DV Doppler. Elective delivery after 26 weeks by cesarean section at a tertiary care center should be planned after steroid treatment for lung maturation and magnesium sulfate to improve neurodevelopment outcome. Parents need to be counseled by multidisciplinary teams regarding only 50% intact survival after 26–28 weeks, and before this threshold. Until delivery monitoring should be carried out every 12–24 hours **(Table 4)**.

TABLE 4: Stage-based management of early-onset fetal growth restriction (FGR).

Stage	Pathophysiological correlate	Criteria (any of)	Monitoring	GA/mode of delivery
I	Severe smallness or mild placental insufficiency	EFW < 3rd centile MC-PI < 5th centile CPR < p5 UAPI > 95th centile UtAPI > 95th centile	Weekly	37 weeks Labor induction
II	Severe placental insufficiency	UA-AEDF Reversed AoI	Biweekly	34 weeks CS
III	Low suspicion fetal acidosis	UA-REDF DV-PI > P95	1–2 days	30 weeks CS
IV	High suspicion fetal acidosis	DV reversal in a wave cCTG < 3 ms FHR decelerations	12 hourly	26 weeks CS

KEY MESSAGES

- Fetal growth is a complex process controlled by many factors including genetic factors so management of this category is essentially empirical.
- Fetal growth restriction can be correctly diagnosed and differentiated from SGA based on the solitary and contributory parameters on biometry and Doppler indices.
- Certain Doppler indices have diagnostic while some indices predict the prognosis and neonatal outcomes.
- A universal stage-based management protocol can be applied to reduce variability in treatment protocols of FGR.

REFERENCES

1. Gordijn SJ, Beune IM, Thilaganathan B, Papageorghiou A, Baschat AA, Baker PN, et al. Consensus definition of fetal growth restriction: a DELPHI procedure. Ultrasound Obstet Gynecol. 2016;48(3):333-9.
2. Savchev S, Figueras F, Sanz-Cortes M, Cruz-Lemini M, Triunfo S, Botet F, et al. Evaluation of an optimal gestational age cut-off for the definition of early- and late-onset fetal growth restriction. Fetal Diagn Ther. 2014;36(2):99-105.
3. Ferrazzi E, Bozzo M, Rigano S, Bellotti M, Morabito A, Pardi G, et al. Temporal sequence of abnormal Doppler changes in the peripheral and central circulatory systems of the severely growth restricted fetus. Ultrasound Obstet Gynecol. 2002;19(2):140-6.
4. Alfirevic Z, Stampalija T, Gyte GM. Fetal and umbilical Doppler ultrasound in high-risk pregnancies. Cochrane Database Syst Rev. 2010;(1):CD007529.
5. Cosmi E, Ambrosini G, D'Antona D, Saccardi C, Mari G. Doppler, cardiotocography, and biophysical profile changes in growth-restricted fetuses. Obstet Gynecol. 2005;106(6):1240-5.
6. Thornton JG, J Hornbuckle, A Vail, D J Spiegelhalter, M Levene; GRIT study group. Infant wellbeing at 2 years of age in the Growth Restriction Intervention Trial (GRIT): multicentred randomised controlled trial. Lancet. 2004;364(9433):513-20.

7. GRIT Study Group. A randomised trial of timed delivery for the compromised preterm fetus: short-term outcomes and Bayesian interpretation. BJOG. 2003;110(1):27-32.

8. Cruz-Lemini M, Crispi F, Van Mieghem T, Pedraza D, Cruz-Martínez R, Acosta-Rojas R, et al. Risk of perinatal death in early-onset intrauterine growth restriction according to gestational age and cardiovascular Doppler indices: a multicenter study. Fetal Diagn Ther. 2012;32(1-2):116-22.

9. Eixarch E, Meler E, Iraola A, Illa M, Crispi F, Hernandez-Andrade E, et al. Neurodevelopmental outcome in 2-year-old infants who were small-for gestational age term fetuses with cerebral blood flow redistribution. Ultrasound Obstet Gynecol. 2008;32(7):894-9.

10. Hershkovitz R, Kingdom JC, Geary M, Rodeck CH. Fetal cerebral blood flow redistribution in late gestation: identification of compromise in small fetuses with normal umbilical artery Doppler. Ultrasound Obstet Gynecol. 2000;15(3):209-12.

11. Cruz-Martinez R, Figueras F, Hernandez-Andrade E, Oros D, Gratacos E. Fetal brain Doppler to predict cesarean delivery for nonreassuring fetal status in term small-for-gestational-age fetuses. Obstet Gynecol. 2011;117(3):618-26.

12. Boers KE, van Wyk L, van der Post JAM, Kwee A, van Pampus MG, Spaanderdam MEA, et al. Neonatal morbidity after induction vs expectant monitoring in intrauterine growth restriction at term: a subanalysis of the DIGITAT RCT. Am J Obstet Gynecol. 2012;206(4):344e1-e7.

13. Boers KE, Vijgen SMC, Bijlenga D, van der Post JAM, Bekedam DJ, Kwee A, et al. Induction versus expectant monitoring for intrauterine growth restriction at term: randomised equivalence trial (DIGITAT). BMJ. 2010;341:c7087.

14. Oros D, Figueras F, Cruz-Martinez R, Padilla N, Meler E, Hernandez-Andrade E, et al. Middle versus anterior cerebral artery Doppler for the prediction of perinatal outcome and neonatal neurobehavior in term small-for-gestational-age fetuses with normal umbilical artery Doppler. Ultrasound Obstet Gynecol. 2010;35(4):456-61.

15. Arbeille P, Maulik D, Fignon A, Stale H, Berson M, Bodard S, et al. Assessment of the fetal PO2 changes by cerebral and umbilical Doppler on lamb fetuses during acute hypoxia. Ultrasound Med Biol. 1995;21(7):861-70.

16. Gramellini D, Folli MC, Raboni S, Vadora E, Merialdi A. Cerebral-umbilical Doppler ratio as a predictor of adverse perinatal outcome. Obstet Gynecol. 1992;79(3):416-20.

17. Schwarze A, Gembruch U, Krapp M, Katalinic A, Germer U, Axt-Fliedner R. Qualitative venous Doppler flow waveform analysis in preterm intrauterine growth-restricted fetuses with ARED flow in the umbilical artery—correlation with short-term outcome. Ultrasound Obstet Gynecol. 2005;25(6):573-9.

18. Baschat AA, Gembruch U, Weiner CP, Harman CR. Qualitative venous Doppler waveform analysis improves prediction of critical perinatal outcomes in premature growth-restricted fetuses. Ultrasound Obstet Gynecol. 2003;22(3):240-5.

19. Bilardo CM, Wolf H, Stigter RH, Ville Y, Baez E, Visser GHA, Hecher K. Relationship between monitoring parameters and perinatal outcome in severe, early intrauterine growth restriction. Ultrasound Obstet Gynecol. 2004;23(2):19-25.

20. Fouron JC, Skoll A, Sonesson SE, Pfizenmaier M, Jaeggi E, Lessard M. Relationship between flow through the fetal aortic isthmus and cerebral oxygenation during acute placental circulatory insufficiency in ovine fetuses. Am J Obstet Gynecol. 1999;181(5 Pt 1):1102-7.

21. Fouron JC, Gosselin J, Raboisson MJ, Lamoureux J, Tison CA, Fouron C, et al. The relationship between an aortic isthmus blood flow velocity index and the postnatal neurodevelopmental status of fetuses with placental circulatory insufficiency. Am J Obstet Gynecol. 2005;192(2):497-503.

22. Cruz-Martinez R, Figueras F, Hernandez-Andrade E, Oros D, Gratacos E. Changes in myocardial performance index and aortic isthmus and ductus venosus Doppler in term, small-forgestational age fetuses with normal umbilical artery pulsatility index. Ultrasound Obstet Gynecol. 2011;38(4):400-5.

23. Figueras F, Benavides A, Del Rio M, Crispi F, Eixarch E, Martinez JM, et al. Monitoring of fetuses with intrauterine growth restriction: longitudinal changes in ductus venosus and aortic isthmus flow. Ultrasound Obstet Gynecol. 2009;33(1):39-43.

24. Hecher K, Bilardo CM, Stigter RH, Ville Y, Hackelöer BJ, Kok HJ, et al. Monitoring of fetuses with intrauterine growth restriction: a longitudinal study. Ultrasound Obstet Gynecol. 2001;18(6):564-70.

25. Gulmezoglu AM, Hofmeyr GJ. Plasma volume expansion for suspected impaired fetal growth. Cochrane Database Syst Rev. 2000;(2):CD000167.

26. Gulmezoglu AM, Hofmeyr GJ. Betamimetics for suspected impaired fetal growth. Cochrane Database Syst Rev. 2001;(4):CD000036.

27. Laurin J, Persson PH. The effect of bedrest in hospital on fetal outcome in pregnancies complicated by intra-uterine growth retardation. Acta Obstet Gynecol Scand. 1987;66(5):407-11.

28. Say L, Gulmezoglu AM, Hofmeyr GJ. Maternal nutrient supplementation for suspected impaired fetal growth. Cochrane Database Syst Rev. 2003;(1):CD000148.

29. Say L, Gulmezoglu AM, Hofmeyr GJ. Maternal oxygen administration for suspected impaired fetal growth. Cochrane Database Syst Rev. 2003;(1):CD000137.

30. Lees CC, Marlow N, van Wassenaer-Leemhuis A, Arabin B, Bilardo CM, Brezinka C, et al. 2 year Neurodevelopmental and intermediate perinatal outcomes in infants with very preterm fetal growth restriction (TRUFFLE): a randomized trial. Lancet. 2015;385(9983):2162-72.

31. American College of Obstetricians and Gynecologists. Fetal growth restriction. Practice bulletin no. 134. Obstet Gynecol. 2013;121:1122-33.

32. Society for Maternal-Fetal Medicine Publications Committee, Berkley E, Chauhan SP, Abuhamad A. Doppler assessment of the fetus with intrauterine growth restriction. Am J Obstet Gynecol. 2012;206(4):300-8.

33. van Wyk L, Boers KE, van der Post JA, van Pampus MG, van Wassenaer AG, van Baar AL, et al. Effects on (neuro)developmental and behavioral outcome at 2 years of age of induced labor compared with expectant management in intrauterine growth-restricted infants: long-term outcomes of the DIGITAT trial. Am J Obstet Gynecol. 2012;206(5):406.e401-7.

34. Vijgen SM, van der Ham DP, Bijlenga D, van Beek JJ, Bloemenkamp KWM, Kwee A, et al. Economic analysis comparing induction of labor and expectant management in women with preterm prelabor rupture of membranes between 34 and 37 weeks (PPROMEXIL trial). Acta Obstet Gynecol Scand. 2014;93(4):374-81.

35. New Zealand Maternal Fetal Medicine Network. Guideline for the management of suspected small for gestational age singleton pregnancies and infants after 34 weeks' gestation. New Zealand Maternal Fetal Medicine Network; 2014.

36. Institute of Obstetricians and Gynecologists Royal College of Physicians of Ireland (2017). Fetal growth restriction—recognition, diagnosis management. Clinical practice guideline no. 28. [online] Available from: https://www.hse.ie/eng/services/publications/clinical-strategy-and-programmes/fetal-growth-restriction.pdf [Last accessed June, 2020].

37. Vayssiere C, Sentilhes L, Ego A, Bernard C, Cambourieu D, Flamant C, et al. Fetal growth restriction and intra-uterine growth restriction: guidelines for clinical practice from the French College of Gynecologists and Obstetricians. Eur J Obstet Gynecol Reprod Biol. 2015;193:10-8.

38. Royal College of Obstetricians and Gynecologists (2013). The investigation and management of the small-for-gestational-age fetus (Green-top guideline no. 31), 2nd edition. [online] Available from: https://www.rcog.org.uk/globalassets/documents/guidelines/gtg_31.pdf [Last accessed June, 2019].

39. McCowan LM, Figueras F, Anderson NH. Evidence-based national guidelines for the management of suspected fetal growth restriction: comparison, consensus, and controversy. Am J Obstet Gynecol. 2018;218(2S):S855-68.

40. www.fetalmedicinebarcelona.org. [Last accessed June, 2020].

Care of Breasts during Breastfeeding: Gynecologist's Perspective

Kawita Bapat, Sneha Bhuriyar

BEST POSITIONS FOR BREASTFEEDING

The best position is where mother and baby both are comfortable and relaxed and do not have to strain to hold the position or keep nursing. Here are some common positions for breastfeeding baby **(Figs. 2 and 3)**:

- *Cradle position*: Rest the side of baby's head in the crook of elbow with his whole body facing you. Position your baby's belly against your body so he feels fully supported. Your other, "free" arm can wrap around to support your baby's head and neck, or reach through your baby's legs to support the lower back.
- *Football position*: Line your baby's back along your forearm to hold your baby like a football, supporting his head and neck in your palm. This works best with newborns and small babies. It is also a good position, if you are recovering from a cesarean birth and need to protect your belly from the pressure or weight of your baby.
- *Side-lying position*: This position is good for night feedings in bed. Side lying also works well if you are recovering from an episiotomy, an incision to widen the vaginal opening during delivery. Use pillows under your head to get comfortable. Then snuggle close to your baby and use your free hand to lift your breast and nipple into your baby's mouth. Once your baby is correctly "latched on," support your baby's head and neck with your free hand so there is no twisting or straining to keep nursing **(Fig. 4)**.

ABCs OF BREASTFEEDING

- *A (Awareness):* Watch for baby's signs of hunger, and breastfeed whenever baby is hungry. This is called "on demand" feeding. The first few weeks, nursing is required 8 to 12 times every 24 hours. Hungry infants move their hands toward their mouths, make sucking noises or mouth movements, or move toward your breast. Do not wait for baby to cry. That is a sign he is too hungry.
- *B (Be patient):* Breastfeed as long as baby wants to nurse each time. Do not hurry your infant through feedings. Infants typically breastfeed for 10–20 minutes on each breast.

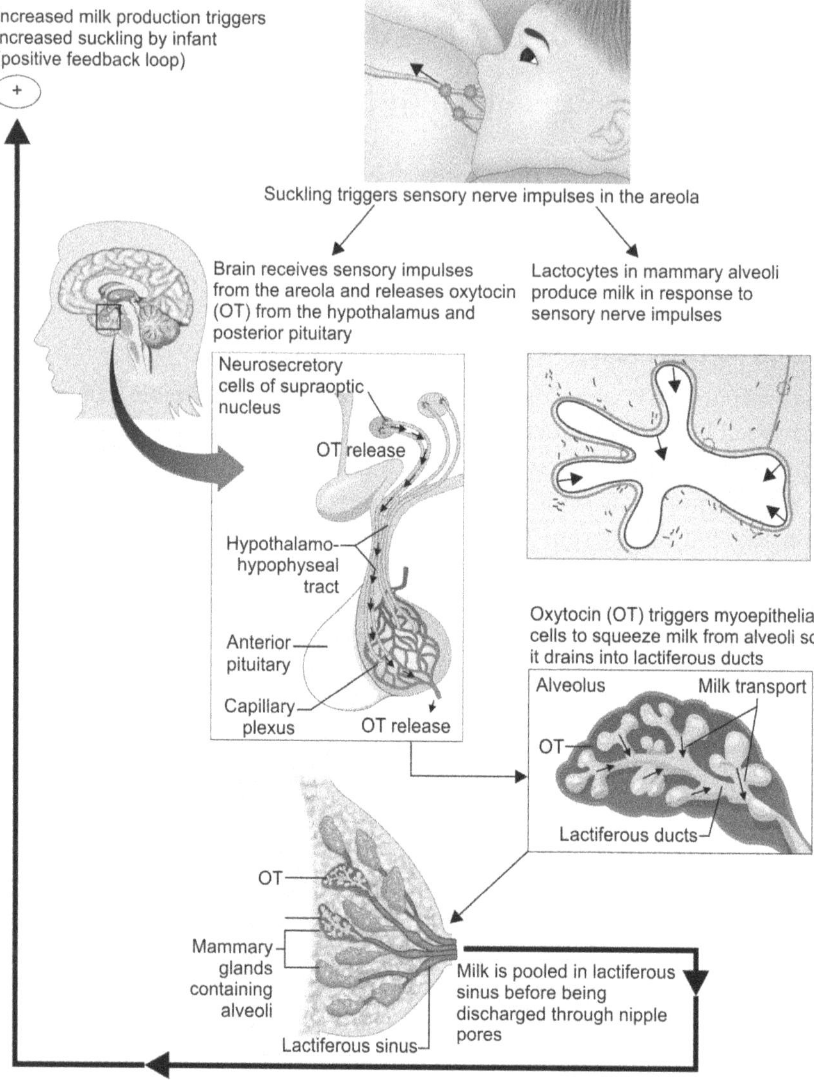

Fig. 1: Hormonal control of breastfeeding.

- *C (Comfort):* This is the key. Relax while breastfeeding, and milk from breast is more likely to "let down" and flow. Positions should be comfortable with pillows as needed to support arms, head, and neck, and a footrest to support feet and legs before one begins to breastfeed.

CONTRAINDICATIONS OF BREASTFEEDING

In a few situations, breastfeeding could cause harm to your baby. You should not breastfeed if:
- HIV positive
- Active and untreated tuberculosis

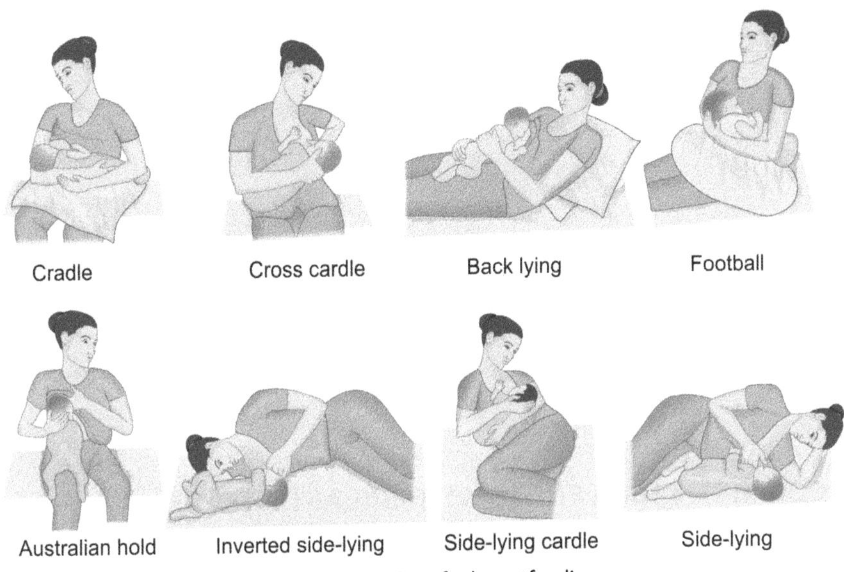

Fig. 2: Best positions for breastfeeding.

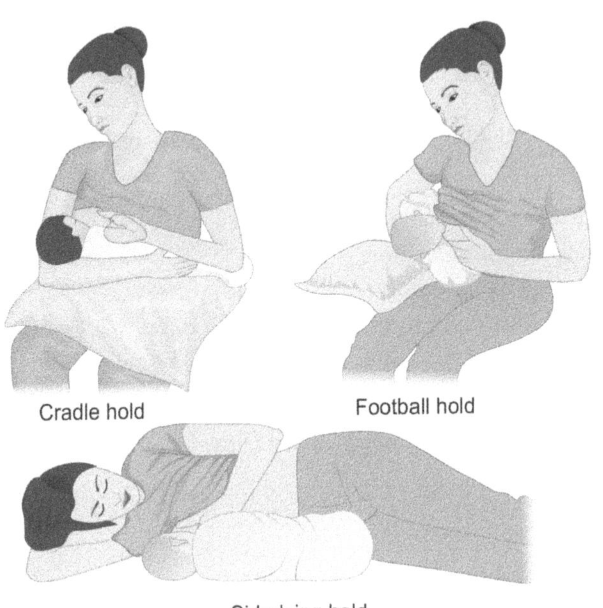

Fig. 3: Right breastfeeding positions.

- On chemotherapy for cancer
- Drug addictions, such as cocaine or marijuana
- Baby has a rare condition called galactosemia and cannot tolerate the natural sugar, called galactose, in breast milk
- Mother on prescription medications, such as some drugs for migraine headaches, Parkinson's disease, or arthritis.

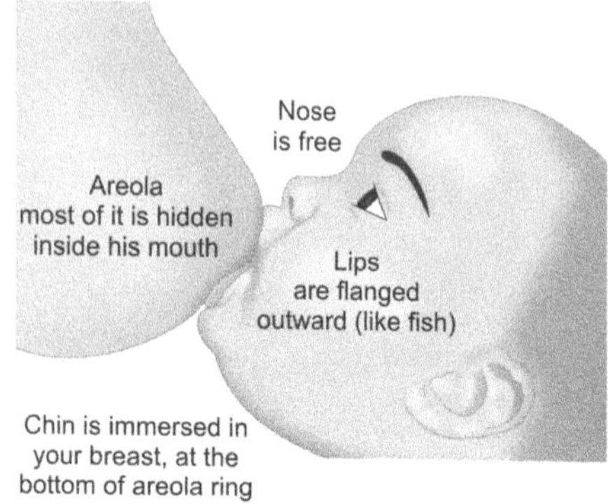

Fig. 4: Signs of correct latch.

■ COMMON CHALLENGES WITH BREASTFEEDING

Cracked/Sore/Damaged Nipples (Fig. 5)

You can expect some soreness in the 1st weeks of breastfeeding. Causes are:
- Improper latch on
- Fungal infection
- Tight frenulum
- Improper position
- Frequent washing of nipple and areola with soap and water.

Management:
- Good latching technique
- Proper breastfeeding position
- Routine, once a day, cleaning of breast with water
- Treat fungal infection in mother as well as in baby.

Surgical correction of tongue-tie:
- Use one finger to break the suction of babies' mouth after each feeding to prevent sore nipples. Keep nipples dry between feedings
- Cold compression
- Using cotton bra pads.

Worries about Producing Enough Milk

A general rule of thumb is that a baby who is wetting six to eight diapers a day is most likely getting enough milk. Avoid supplementing breast milk with formula, and never give infant plain water. Body needs the frequent and regular demand of baby's nursing to keep producing milk. Some women mistakenly think that they cannot breastfeed, if they have small breasts. But small-breasted women can make milk just as well as large-breasted women. Good nutrition, plenty of rest, and staying well hydrated all help too:
- *Pumping and storing milk*: You can get breast milk by hand or pump it with a breast pump. It may take a few days or weeks for baby to get used

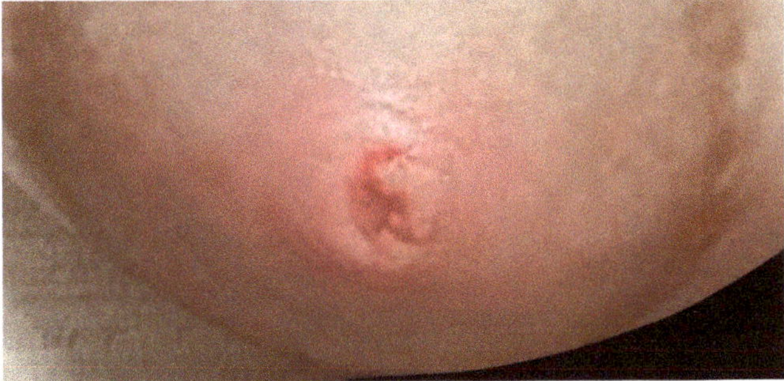

Fig. 5: Cracked nipple.

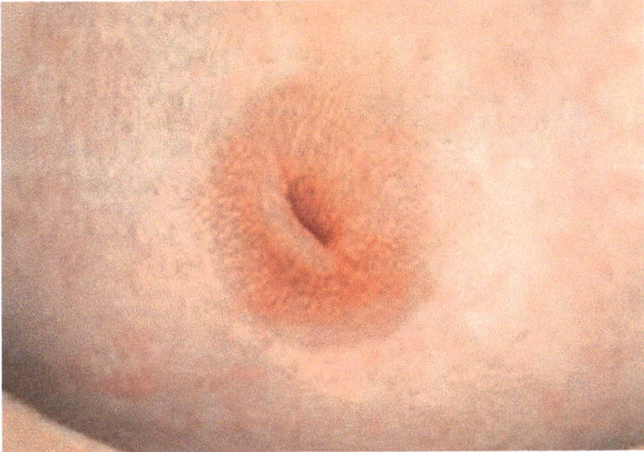

Fig. 6: Retracted and inverted nipple.

to breast milk in a bottle. So begin practicing early if going back to work. Breast milk can be safely used within 2 days if it is stored in a refrigerator. You can freeze breast milk for up to 6 months. Do not warm up or thaw frozen breast milk in a microwave. That will destroy some of its immune-boosting qualities, and it can cause fatty portions of the breast milk to become super hot. Thaw breast milk in the refrigerator or in a bowl of warm water instead.

- *Retracted and inverted nipples (Fig. 6)*: The pulling back of the nipple may be harmless (majority) or malignant (breast cancer). The retracted nipple appears flat and broad and cannot be pulled outward. It does not protrude or becomes erect when stimulated or hold. An inverted nipple can be pulled out and mother should be taught during antenatal care visits about inverted nipple. Syringe method can be tried in few mothers.
- *Breast engorgement (Fig. 7)*: Breast fullness is natural and healthy. It happens as breasts become full of milk, staying soft and pliable. But, breast engorgement means the blood vessels in breast have become congested. This traps fluid in your breasts and makes them feel hard, painful, and swollen. Alternate heat and cold, for instance using ice packs and hot

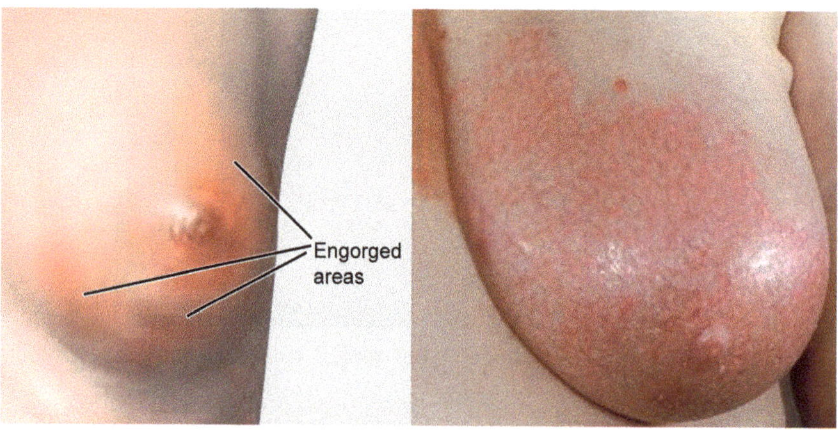

Fig. 7: Breast engorgement and infection.

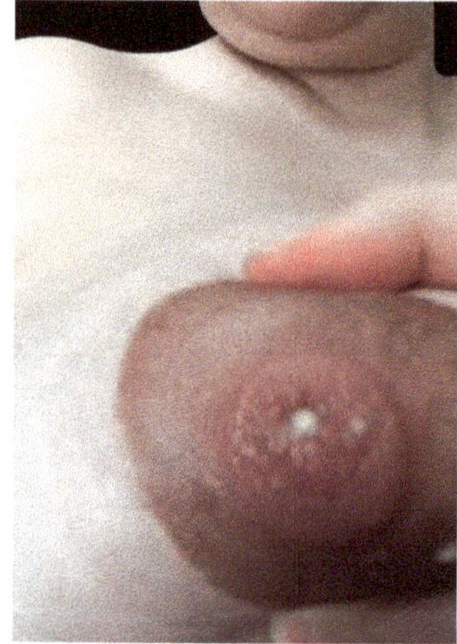

Fig. 8: A single sore spot on breast.

showers, to relieve mild symptoms. It can also help to release your milk by hand or use a breast pump.

- *Blocked ducts*: A single sore spot on breast **(Fig. 8)**, which may be red and hot, can signal a plugged milk duct. This can often be relieved by warm compresses and gentle massage over the area to release the blockage. More frequent nursing can also help.
- *Breast infection (mastitis)* **(Fig. 9)**: It is preventable but common problem and occurs due to:
  - Milk stasis
  - Hyperlactation
  - Cracked nipple
  - Insufficient milk removal
  - Maternal stress
  - Use of nipple creams.

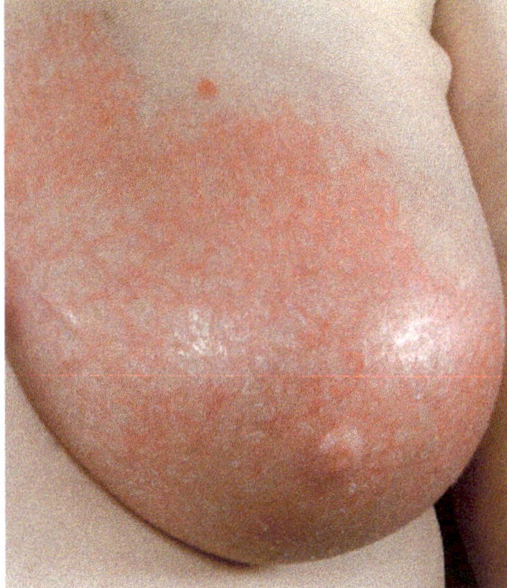

Fig. 9: Mastitis.

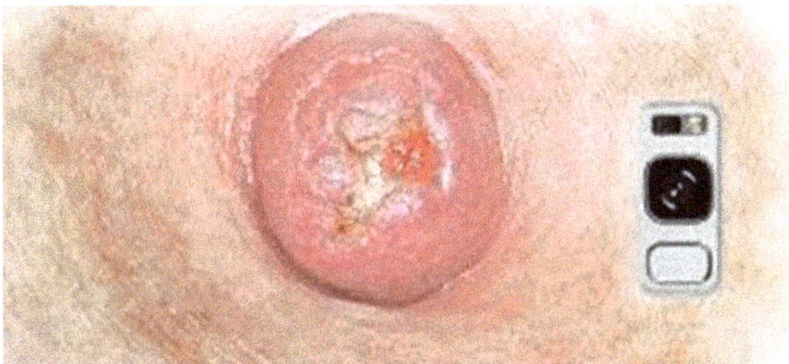

Fig. 10: Herpes simplex with active oozing nipple and areola.

Prevention and Treatment

- Breastfeeding information and education, adequate rest, good nutrition, psychological support, proper handwashing, warm moist packs, or cold. Cabbage compresses between feeds. Proper antibiotic therapy.
- *Breast abscess*: If mastitis is not treated, it may progress to breast abscess. The baby should be allowed to continue breastfeed and abscess can be treated with aspiration technique.
- *Galactocele*: It is a benign cyst, which should not interrupt feeding breast.
- Duct ectasia, also called as granulomatous mastitis, can be aggravated by lactation.
- *Dermatitis involving breast nipple and areola*: Herpes simplex with active oozing nipple and areola **(Fig. 10)** are contraindications for the breastfeeding till the lesions heal.
- *Vasospasm of nipple (Raynaud's phenomenon like condition)* **(Fig. 11)**: It causes burning and pain in the nipple. Management includes—
  - Feeding on the less tender side first
  - Correct positioning

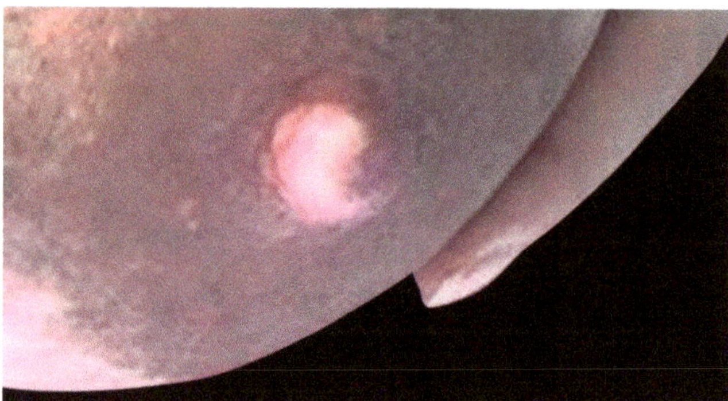

Fig. 11: Vasospasm of nipple.

- Warm compress
- Avoid cold air
- Initiate the milk ejection reflux
- Express the drops of colostrums before putting baby to the breast
- Reduction of the caffeine and nicotine intake
- Use of safe analgesics
- Supplementation of vitamin B6, calcium, and magnesium
- Nifedipine.

Insufficient Milk Supply

Mother should be taught about normal physiological breastfeeding about 8–12 or more times in 24 hours, feeding at night, and not to decrease the frequency of breastfeeding to let the breast fill. One breast should be fully drained before offering the second one. Mother should constantly be supported and encouraged by teaching different positions of breastfeeding.

Pathophysiological lactation failure: The reasons of failure are:
- Delayed lactogenesis II
- Maternal nipple anomalies
- Insufficient glandular tissue
- Chronic illness of mother, anemia, and infection.

How to care for breasts while breastfeeding?

Here are some tips to help care for nursing mothers and prevent some of the common problems of breastfeeding.

- *Practice good hygiene*: Wash hands before touching breasts. Keep breasts and nipples clean by washing them each day with warm water in the shower or bath. Avoid using soap on breasts since it can cause dry, cracked, and irritated skin. It can also remove the natural oils produced by the Montgomery glands located on the dark area surrounding nipples. These oils help to keep the nipples and areola clean and moisturized.
- *Wear a supportive bra*: Nursing mothers should choose a nursing bra or a regular bra that fits well, but is not too tight. Cotton is an excellent choice of fabric since it allows skin to breathe.

- *Good latching technique and nursing very often*—at least every 2–3 hours—can help to prevent the development of painful breast problems such as sore nipples, breast engorgement, plugged milk ducts, and mastitis.
- Proper position of breastfeeding as shown in **Figure 2**.
- *Changing breast pads often*: If mother is using breast pads or cotton squares inside bra to soak up the breast milk from leaking breasts, she should change them when they become wet. Clean, dry nursing pads can help to prevent sore nipples, thrush, or mastitis from occurring.
- *Moisturize nipples with breast milk*: After nursing baby, rub some of breast milk on nipples and areola then let them air dry.
- *Remove child from breast correctly*: When mother is ready to take baby off of the breast, avoid pulling the baby. Instead, place one finger in the corner of her mouth to break the suction between baby's mouth and breast.
- *Discuss sore nipples with doctor*: If mother has sore nipples, she should talk to a lactation consultant about using purified lanolin or hydrogel pads to help soothe breasts.
- *Treat breast engorgement*: If the breasts become painful overfull, hard, and swollen, cold cabbage leaves or cold compresses to reduce inflammation and relieve pain can be used.
- *Feeding the baby before he/she becomes too hungry.*
- *Continue to perform monthly breast self-examination*: In nursing mothers also, it is important to check breasts each month. While it is normal for breasts to feel lumpy when they are full of milk, the lumps should go away with breastfeeding, pumping, or massaging the breasts.

Caring for Your Breasts to Suppress Lactation

It could take a few weeks or months to dry up the breast milk in breasts. Here are some tips for caring for breasts, if in case breastfeeding has to be stopped. *The followings have to be taught to mothers*:

- Wear a bra that is supportive but not tight.
- Use breast pads or a cotton cloth to soak up leaks.
- Place a cold compress or cold cabbage leaves on your breasts to help relieve swelling and discomfort.
- If breasts are painfully full, pump or hand express a little bit of breast milk to relieve some of the pressure. Pumps are better avoided.
- Try not to touch nipples or breasts. Regular stimulation of the breasts and nipples tells body to keep producing milk.
- Medicines for pain relief can be given.

Useful Nipple Care Products (Figs. 12 to 17)

- *Nipple cream* made from ultra-pure lanolin—a natural product obtained from sheep's wool. This moisturizes and supports healing. It is harmless for baby, so there is no need to wash off lanolin before breastfeeding.
- *Hydrogel pads* can be placed on sore nipples to offer instant breastfeeding pain relief, as well as creating ideal conditions for healing.

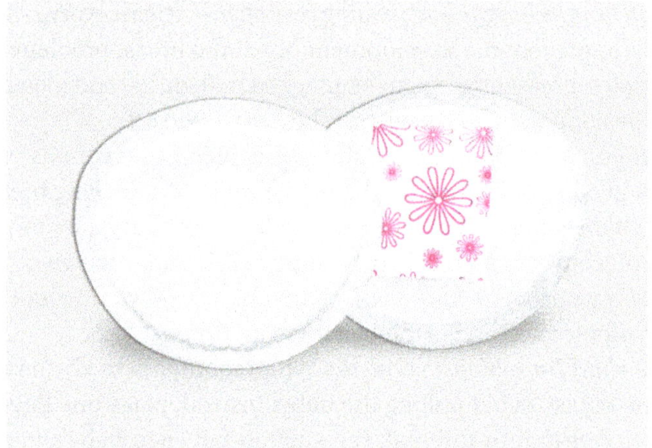

Fig. 12: Safe and Dry™ ultra thin nursing pads.

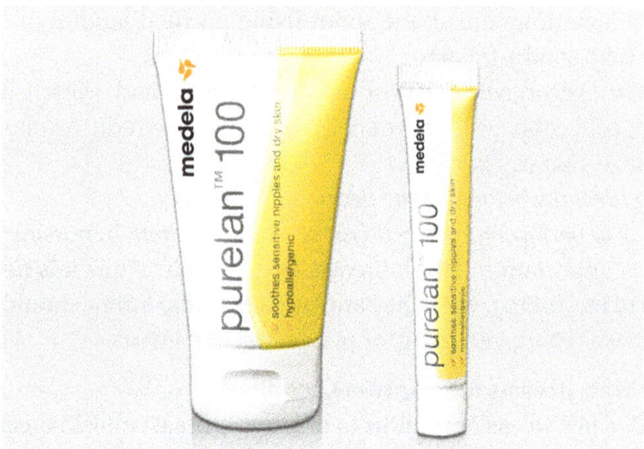

Fig. 13: Purelan™ 100 lanolin cream.

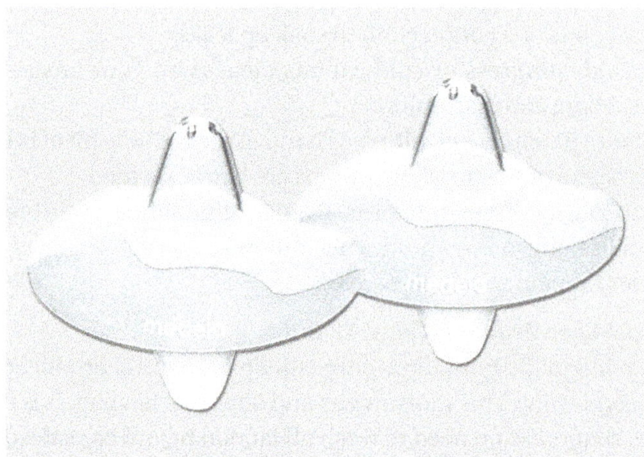

Fig. 14: Contact™ nipple shields.

Fig. 15: Safe and Dry™ washable bra pads.

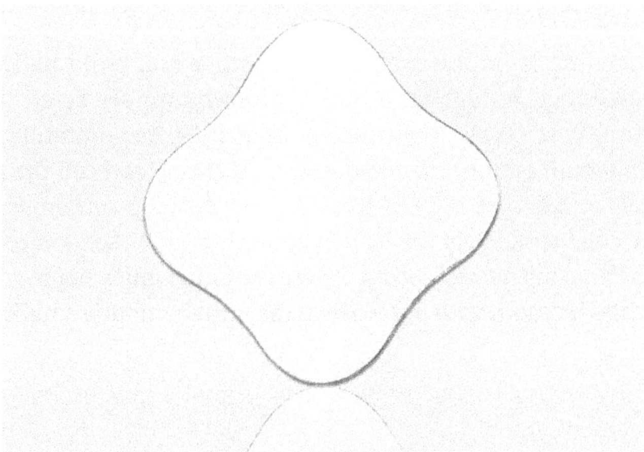

Fig. 16: Hydrogel pads.

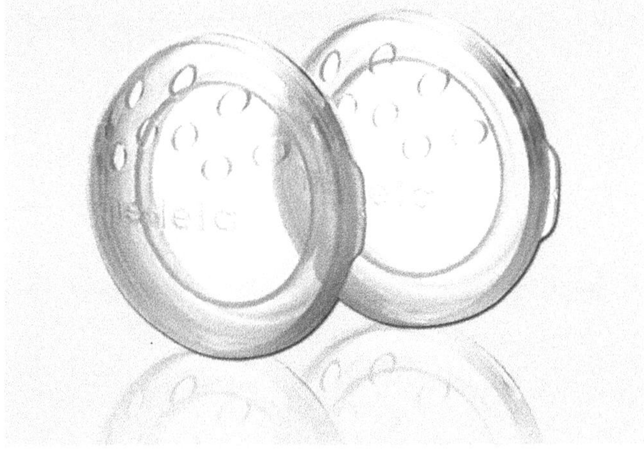

Fig. 17: Breast shells.

- *Breast shells* fit inside bra. They are good for stopping clothing rubbing against sore nipples, and have holes in so air can still get to nipples to help them heal.
- *Nursing bras* made from either a breathable material like cotton, or a fabric that dries quickly and wicks excess moisture away from damaged nipples.
- *Nipple shields* are silicone covers that fit over nipples, with small holes for breast milk to flow through as you breastfeed. They protect the skin underneath and can give a baby with a poor latch something firmer to attach to. In general, nipple shields should be considered a short-term solution. If problems or pain occur, consult lactation consultant or breastfeeding specialist.

If you are breastfeeding and have sore or cracked nipples, Medela hydrogel pads support.

CONCLUSION

The breastfeeding is important for both mother and child and it needs proper counseling, guidance, education, and support at all levels to overcome troubles, which occur during pregnancy, lactation till weaning. As gynecologists, it is our first and foremost duty to teach all the mothers about proper techniques of breastfeeding and develop self-confidence in them. Every child should get the benefit of mother's milk so as to reduce the complications during infancy. So let the every mother enjoy her motherhood and every child blossom with pure love in the form of mother's milk.

Birth Preparedness: It Matters

Arup Kumar Majhi, Semanti Bose

■ INTRODUCTION

India has made great strive in reducing its maternal mortality ratio (MMR) by 77%, from 556 per 100,000 live births in 1990 to 130 per 100,000 live births in 2016.[1] Even then India did not manage to meet the Millennium Development Goal of MMR of 109 per 100,000 live births. Hence, greater efforts are necessary, if we are to meet the target of 70 per 100,000 by 2030 as per the Sustainable Development Goals. Besides, World Health Organization (WHO) estimates that 300 million women in the developing world suffer from short-term to long-term illness brought about by pregnancy and childbirth.

It is estimated that most of the maternal deaths occur either during delivery or within 24 hours of delivery[2] and near one-third of neonatal deaths occur on 1st day of life.[3]

Seeking in care is delayed due to delay in:
- Identifying the complications
- Deciding to seek care
- Delay in reaching health facility, and
- Delay in adequate and appropriate treatment in the facility.[4]

Inadequacy or lack of birth and emergency preparedness[5] is the reason for delay, resulting these morbidity and mortality.

Birth preparedness and complication readiness is the important strategy to reduce the maternal and perinatal morbidity and mortality and important component of safe motherhood program.

■ BIRTH PREPAREDNESS AND COMPLICATION READINESS

Birth preparedness is the prior planning and advance preparation for delivery. Birth preparedness and complication readiness (BPCR/BPACR) ensures that the pregnant mother can reach the appropriate place for delivery when labor begins and/or complication arises and helps to reduce the delays to get the appropriate care by the skilled care providers.

Complications occurring during birthing in an unprepared family may lead to catastrophic consequences due to delay in identifying the problem, in getting money, in finding transport, and reaching the appropriate referral facility. This delay in the decision-making process can be solved by proper use of birth preparedness and complication readiness plan.[6-8] BPACR is one intervention that addresses the delays by encouraging and increasing awareness among pregnant women, their families, and communities to do prior planning for births and to tackle the emergencies, if they occur. Hence, BPCR is not only of advanced planning and preparation for delivery but also anticipation of steps to be taken in case of any complications during the birth process. It has been an essential element of antenatal care (ANC) package as per WHO. For implementation of BPCR, not only the pregnant mother but also her family, community, and health personnel are involved. The active involvement of those persons is critical in ensuring to adequately prepare for delivery and to carry out a birth plan and to combat complications, if they arise.

Components of BPCR:
- Early registration of pregnancy
- Antenatal care
- Knowledge of danger signs and seeking for care
- Plan for where to give birth
- Plan for presence of a skilled birth attendant
- Plan for transportation
- Picking a birth companion
- Identification of compatible blood donors in case of emergency
- Saving money for delivery, and
- Feedback from the pregnant woman.

Registration of Pregnancy

Early registration to ANC is imperative for the timely diagnosis and treatment of pregnancy-related morbidities.[9] This may require community health workers to visit a family and motivate pregnant women for seeking ANC.

The ideal gestational age for booking is within the first 10 weeks of pregnancy. The first visit or registration of a pregnant woman for ANC should take place as soon as the pregnancy is suspected. Ideally, the first visit should take place in the first trimester, before or at the 12th week of pregnancy.[10,11]

Antenatal Care

Antenatal care is defined as the care provided by skilled healthcare professionals to pregnant women and adolescent girls in order to ensure the best health conditions for both mother and baby during pregnancy. Birth preparedness is an essential part of ANC counseling:
- ANC includes identification of risk factors, prevention and management of pregnancy-related or concurrent complications, and health education and health promotion. ANC ensures referral of at-risk pregnancies to an appropriate level of care. And thus, ANC reduces maternal and perinatal morbidity and mortality.

- *Number and timings of antenatal visit*: The WHO 2016 ANC model[12] recommends a minimum of *eight ANC contacts*, with the first contact scheduled to take place in the first trimester (up to 12 weeks of gestation), two contacts scheduled in the second trimester (at 20 and 26 weeks of gestation), and five contacts scheduled in the third trimester (at 30, 34, 36, 38, and 40 weeks). Thereafter, women are advised to return for delivery at 41 weeks of gestation, if not given birth or sooner if they experience danger signs.
- Previous four-visit focused ANC (FANC) model is no longer recommended by World Health Organization (WHO), as it does not offer women adequate contact with healthcare practitioners.
- In this model, the word "contact" has been used instead of "visit", as it implies an active connection between a pregnant woman and a healthcare provider. In the new model, an additional contact is recommended at 20 weeks of gestation, and an additional three contacts are recommended in the third trimester since this period represents the period of greatest antenatal risk for both mother and baby.
- In every visit, patient's history taking and examination are mandatory. BP measurement is essential component. During the contact/visit, mother is advised regarding rest, diet, immunization, and birth preparedness. Minimum investigations such as hemoglobin estimation, urine, and other tests are detailed in the respective chapter.
- As per "Anemia Mukt Bharat Operational Guideline, 2018"[13] by Government of India, daily 1 iron and folic acid tablet (each tablet containing 60 mg elemental iron + 500 µg folic acid) starting from 4th month of pregnancy (that is from the second trimester) is continued throughout pregnancy (minimum 180 days during pregnancy) and to be continued for 180 days, postpartum.
- Deworming of pregnant woman in the second trimester by administration of one dose of 400 mg albendazole is advocated by Government of India.
- Most pregnant and lactating women in India have low dietary calcium intake, hence calcium supplementation is a routine. All pregnant and lactating women to be counseled about intake of calcium-rich foods.
- Government of India (2014 guideline) suggests calcium tablets (500 mg) to be swallowed twice daily (total 1 g calcium/day, but not at a time) starting from 14 weeks of pregnancy up to 6 months postpartum. Calcium and iron folic acid (IFA) tablets should not be taken together since calcium inhibits iron absorption. IFA tablets should be taken preferably 2 hours after a meal. One calcium tablet should contain 500 mg elemental calcium and 250 IU vitamin D3. Vitamin D increases calcium absorption.
- Two doses of injection tetanus toxoid 0.5 mL are given intramuscularly at interval of 6 weeks between 16 and 24 weeks. Recently, Tdap vaccine (tetanus, diphtheria, and acellular pertussis) are suggested instead of only

tetanus toxoid preferably between 27 and 36 weeks to maximize passive antibody transfer to fetus.

Knowledge of Danger Signs (Table 1)

Pregnant women and their family members should be made aware of the danger signs, which should prompt their immediate reporting to a knowledgeable healthcare provider.

Plan for where to give Birth

Birth plan should identify the nearest healthcare center where delivery shall take place. Pregnancy should ideally be registered in the same center as well.

Plan for Skilled Birth Attendant

Deliveries in rural areas are often conducted by untrained dais without any aseptic precautions. Secondly, the disparaging doctor to patient ratio in a developing nation as India does not always allow for access to a skilled birth attendant (doctor and nurse). Training of TBAs (trained birth attendants) has been shown to increase the utilization of prenatal, antenatal, and postnatal healthcare of women who otherwise are unable to seek treatment from a skilled birth attendant.[14] Without formal training, TBAs are unable to identify the signs of a critical pregnancy or labor and delivery danger signs, which can significantly put a mother's life at risk.[15]

Training of TBAs is recommended in addition to an increase of hospital births and informing women who utilize TBAs to request that they refer them to a health facility, if they are unable to care for them properly.

Plan for Transportation

An analysis of the causes of maternal deaths in India found that more than half of the maternal deaths occurred in instances where institutional care had not been availed at the time of delivery.[16] The distance from home to health facility was less than 5 km in 49% of institutional deliveries, and as the distance increased, number of women having institutional delivery decreased. Among

TABLE 1: Danger signs during pregnancy and labor.

Danger signs during pregnancy	Danger sign in labor
• Severe bleeding • Plain abdomen • Swelling of hands and face • Reduced fetal movement • Leakage per vagina • Headache • Blurring of vision • Excessive vomiting • Fever for more than 24 hours	• Severe vaginal bleeding • Prolonged labor • Convulsions • Retained placenta

the reasons for not delivering in health facility, insufficient transport facilities (10.4%) are featured as a significant cause.[17]

During BPCR counseling, the pregnant woman should ascertain the mode of transportation available from her home to the health center system where she plans to deliver. It is important for the local health officials to familiarize women regarding the transport facility services provided by the Government that they can avail.

At present, India has over eighteen different models of transportation for emergency, pregnant women, children, and other categories of patients. These can be broadly categorized as follows:

- *Statewide models*: This is the "108 Emergency Transport Facility", where the ambulance comes with equipment and trained staff to manage emergencies during transit.
- *Decentralized district or block-level public–private partnership (PPP) models*: The fleet includes government and contracted private vehicles, such as the Janani Express Yojana in Madhya Pradesh, and the District Health Society manages the services.
- *Decentralized community-based models*: These are managed by community-based organizations and there is significant involvement of communities and private vehicle owners. Typically, the vehicles are not dedicated for RT*. Examples are Cheeranjeevi Yojana in Gujarat, Ayushmati Scheme in West Bengal, in Khunti district of Jharkhand, and in Dhaulpur district of Rajasthan.[18,19]
- *Picking a birth companion*: An elderly woman of the house or a neighbor should be available to the woman during her labor to provide emotional support.
- *Identification of compatible blood donors in case of emergency*: Blood grouping of the pregnant woman should be done during her booking visit and at least two family members or acquaintances should be identified and undergo counseling for voluntary blood donation in case the woman faces any obstetric emergency.

Obstetric complications that may require blood transfusion:
- Anemia
- Abruptio placentae
- Recurrent bleeding from placenta previa
- Ruptured ectopic pregnancy
- Postpartum hemorrhage
- Disseminated intravascular coagulation (DIC)
- Rupture uterus.

Saving Money for Delivery

Even though the Indian Government has made arrangements to provide most services for free to pregnant mothers under Janani Sishu Suraksha Karyakram

(JSSK) such as free transport to hospital, free delivery services, free drugs, and free blood and blood products;[20] woman and her family members should set aside funds for unavoidable out of pocket expenses that may arise in the event of any complications.

Feedback from the Pregnant Woman

Healthcare provider after each session must ask the woman whether she understands the messages correctly and if the pregnant woman cannot recall most of the messages, healthcare provider should make them understand by explaining one more time.

BPCR Providers

- Treating doctors at maternity hospitals
- Accredited Social Health Activist (ASHA), Auxiliary Nurse Midwife (ANM), and Anganwadi workers
- Home visits by community health workers.

Information to be provided:
- Signs of onset of labor
- Danger signs during pregnancy
- Danger signs during postpartum
- Newborn care.

Implementation

Government Level

- Janani Sishu Suraksha Karyakram launched by Government of India in 2011 is aimed at increasing institutional deliveries across India in a bid to reduce maternal and neonatal mortality. *ASHA workers* who are a key component of JSSK form an important link between the community and health workers and should be utilized to improve knowledge about BPCR.
- Government-sponsored *mass media campaigns* (radio, television, etc.) to educate public about services available for pregnant mothers.
- Initiatives to promote *private-public partnerships* in the health sector to increase ANC visits among women and optimize BPCR practices.
- Increase number of skilled birth attendants (SBAs) in rural areas.

Hospital Level

- Skilled birth attendants should provide BPCR information during antenatal visit to all women.
- Pamphlets and posters regarding BPCR to be made available.
- Questionnaires in local languages to gauge preparedness level of pregnant women and to ascertain aspects in which knowledge is lacking.

Community Level

Trained birth attendants such as ANM in rural areas to provide information regarding BPCR by home visits, birth preparedness, determine the blood group of pregnant women and identify a donor, and advise regarding emergency transportation. They should also explain the danger signs and guide pregnant women to visit an appropriate healthcare facility, if there are any risk factors.[21]

Impact of BPCR: Evidences

Promotion of BPACR has several positive impacts on maternal and child healthcare by improving preventive behaviors, increasing knowledge of mothers about danger signs, and overall improving in care seeking during antenatal period and obstetric emergency. There is evidence from India,[22,23] rural Nepal,[24] Ethiopia,[25]and Burkino Faso.[26]

A systematic review and meta-analysis (2014) of randomized trials of BPCR interventions in populations of pregnant women living in developing countries consisting of fourteen randomized studies (292,256 live births) concluded that BPCR interventions with adequate population coverage are effective in reducing maternal and neonatal mortality in low-resources settings.[21]

The published studies showed that BPACR is inadequate and low proportions of pregnant are full prepared for childbirth and complications in many developing countries.[27] Improving socioeconomic status and strengthening community-based education and awareness regarding full attendance of ANC concept of BPACR will improve the maternal and neonatal outcome. Involvement of health administrators and healthcare providers from central to grass root level is needed to improve birth preparedness and complication readiness. On the other hand, more research assessing BPACR is needed involving not only the pregnant woman but the family, community, and health facility level to explore for evidences to prevent maternal and perinatal death and disabilities.

◼ REFERENCES

1. World Health Organization. (2018). India has achieved groundbreaking success in reducing maternal mortality. [online] Available from: https://www.who.int/southeastasia/news/detail/10-06-2018-india-has-achieved-groundbreaking-success-in-reducing-maternal-mortality#:~:text=WHO%20commends%20India%20for%20its,000%20live%20births%20in%202016.&text=Women%20in%20India%20are%20more,able%20to%20read%20and%20write. [Last accessed June, 2020].
2. Ronsmans C, Graham WJ; Lancet Maternal SurvivalSeries Steering Group. Maternal mortality: Who, When, Where, and Why. Lancet. 2006;368(9542):1189-200.
3. International Institute for Population Sciences. (2007). National family health survey (NFHS-3), 2005-06, Volume I.. [online] Available from: https://dhsprogram.com/pubs/pdf/FRIND3/FRIND3-Vol1AndVol2.pdf. [Last accessed June, 2020].
4. Thaddeus S, Maine D. Too far to walk: maternal mortality in context. Soc Sci Med. 1994;38(8):1091-110.

5. UNPF; WHO (2005). Millennium Development Goals (MDGs): "Fact sheets on maternal mortality Geneva, Switzerland." [online] Available from: http://www.who.int/mediacentre/factsheets/fs290/en/index.html. [Last accessed June, 2020].

6. Acharya AS, Kaur R, Prasuna JG, Rasheed N. Making pregnancy safer—birth preparedness and complication readiness study among antenatal women attendees of a primary health center, Delhi. Indian J Community Med. 2015;40(2):127-34.

7. Khanna J, Bergsjo P, Lashley K, Peters C, Sherrat D, Villar J (2002). WHO antenatal care randomized trial: manual for the implementation of the new model. [online] Available from: https://apps.who.int/iris/handle/10665/42513. [Last accessed June, 2020].

8. Bankole A, Sedgh G, Okonofua F, Imarhiagbe C, Hussain R, Wulf D, et al. Birth preparedness and complication readiness: a matrix of shared responsibility. Revised. J Clin Med Res. 2010;2(4):55-60.

9. Begashaw B, Tesfaye Y, Zelalem E, Ubong U, Kumalo A. Assessment of Birth Preparedness and Complication Readiness among Pregnant Mothers Attending Ante Natal Care Service in Mizan-Tepi University Teaching Hospital, South West Ethiopia. Clin Mother Child Health. 2017;14:257.

10. American Academy of Pediatrics; American College of Obstetricians and Gynecologists. Guidelines for perinatal care, 5th edition. Elk Grove Village, (IL): American Academy of Pediatrics and American College of Obstetricians and Gynecologists; 2002.

11. Maternal Health Division, Department of Family Welfare Ministry of Family Health & Family Welfare, Government of India. (2005). Guidelines for Pregnancy Care and Management of Common Obstetric Complications by Medical Officers. [online] Available from: http://www.nrhmorissa.gov.in/writereaddata/upload/documents/normal_delivery_and_management_of_obstetric_complications_.pdf. [Last accessed June, 2020].

12. World Health Organization (2016). WHO recommendations on antenatal care for a positive pregnancy experience. [online] Available from: who.int/reproductivehealth/publications/maternal_perinatal_health/anc-positive-pregnancy-experience/en/. [Last accessed June, 2020].

13. Ministry of Health and Family Welfare, Government of India. (2018). "Anemia Mukt Bharat operational guideline, 2018". [online] Available from: https://www.fitterfly.com/site/pdf/anemia-mukt-bharat.pdf. [Last accessed June, 2020].

14. Sibley LM, Sipe TA. Transition to skilled birth attendance: is there a future role for traditional birth attendants? J Health Popul Nutr. 2006;24(4):472-8.

15. Doctor HV, Findley SE, Cometto G, Afrenyadu GY. Awareness of critical danger signs of pregnancy and delivery preparations for delivery and utilization of skilled birth attendants in Nigeria. J Health Care Poor Underserved. 2013;24(1):152-70.

16. Dikid T, Gupta M, Kaur M, Goel S, Aggarwal AK, Caravotta J. Maternal and perinatal death inquiry and response project implementation review in India. J Obstet Gynecol India. 2013;63(2):101-7.

17. UNICEF. (2009). Coverage evaluation survey. [online] Available from: http://www.indiaenvironmentportal.org.in/files/National_Factsheet_30_August_no_logo.pdf. [Last accessed June, 2020].

18. United Nations Environment Programme. Transport for a Changing World. Position paper prepared by the Division of Technology, Industry and Economics, Nairobi: Transport Unit, UNEP (2014).

19. Raj AX (2014). Saving lives through rural ambulance services: Experiences from Karnataka and Tamil Nadu states, India. Transport and Communication Bulletin for Asia and Pacific: No 84. [online] Available from: https://www.unescap.org/sites/default/files/Bulletin%2084_Article5.pdf. [Last accessed June, 2020].

20. Center for Health Informatics; National Health Portal New Delhi (2013). Janani Sishu Suraksha Karyakram (JSSK). [online] Available from: https://www.nhp.gov.in/janani-shishu-suraksha-karyakaram-jssk_pg. [Last accessed June, 2020].

21. Soubeiga D, Gauvin L, Hatem MA, Johri M. Birth preparedness and complication readiness (BPCR) interventions to reduce maternal and neonatal mortality in developing countries: systematic review and meta-analysis. BMC Pregnancy Childbirth. 2014;14:129.
22. Kumar V, Mohanty S, Kumar A, Mishra RP, Santosham M, Baqui AH, et al. Effect of community-based behavior change management on neonatal mortality: a cluster-randomized controlled trial in Shivgarh, Uttar Pradesh, India. Lancet. 2008;372(9644):1151-62.
23. Agarwa S, Sethi V, Srivastava K, Jha PK, Baqui AH. Birth Preparedness and Complication Readiness among Slum Women in Indore City, India. J Health Popul Nutr. 2010;28(4):383-91.
24. McPherson RA, Khadka N, Moore JM, Sharma M. Are birth-preparedness programmes effective? Results from a field trial in Siraha district, Nepal. J Health Popul Nutr. 2006;24(4):479-88.
25. Fullerton JT, Killian R, Gass PM. Outcomes of a community- and home-based intervention for safe motherhood and newborn care. Health Care Women Int. 2005;26(7):561-76.
26. Moran AC, Sangli G, Dineed R, Rawlins B, Yameogo M, Baya B. Birth-preparedness for maternal health: findings from Koupela district, Burkina Faso. J Health Pop Nutr. 2006;24(4):489-97.
27. Bank TW; WHO, United Nations Population Fund; UNICEF (2009). Pregnancy, childbirth, postpartum and newborn care. A guide for essential practice, 3rd edition. [online] Available from: https://www.who.int/maternal_child_adolescent/documents/imca-essential-practice-guide/en/. [Last accessed June, 2020].

Contraception Advice during Antenatal Care: Is It the Right Time?

Shobha N Gudi

▦ INTRODUCTION

It is commonly asserted that maternal and child outcomes are negatively affected when pregnancies are "too early, too late, too many, and too close".

Advice on contraception during pregnancy is a value addition to the plan of antenatal care. The right messages for spacing between births and family planning should be integrated into the counseling.

What is the need?

The need for such a step is mandatory to meet the unmet need for contraception.

We are now 1.36 billion people of the 7.7 billion in the world.[1] The unmet need for contraception is higher in India than anywhere else in the world. Unmet need of course is defined as the couples or women who are considered fecund and do not wish for pregnancy in near future, but have no awareness, information, or accessibility of contraceptive methods.

Approximately 13% of currently married females between the ages 15 and 49 years in India have an unmet need for contraception.[2] This translates to millions of women. The FP 2020 vision document of the Government of India states clearly that for the mean couple protection rate to increase from 53.9 to 54.3%, an additional 48 million women should be covered annually. Therefore, every opportunity should be taken to make an effort to reduce the number of unintended pregnancies.

In fact, in a planned pregnancy, preconceptionally there is a strong role of introducing the concept of reproductive planning, where in the couple can make a conscious decision of how many children they want and what should be the interval between them.

Public health initiatives to be implemented have more complexity as they involve procedures, medications, and clinic visits for preventive care in essentially well women.

Is pregnancy the right time?

The best time for the obstetrician to speak about contraceptive choices may be during pregnancy for several reasons.

Firstly, the rate of institutional deliveries and care has increased in our country to almost 85%. The hospitals in public sector are better equipped now to take on the care of more deliveries. Though women may not come to hospital only for contraceptive services, it is certain that they will visit the hospital for pregnancy care.

Secondly, during pregnancy, they are in a positive mindset in expectation of a new life and more receptive to ideas of spacing and limiting the number of pregnancies.

Thirdly, counseling for contraception during antenatal care can be streamlined as part of an integrated service wherein the woman is informed about the choices by the Obstetrician and is then directed to a dedicated contraception clinic. This room will have a special ambience, which emphasizes on availability of choice, safety of methods, benefits of spacing, and limiting family size. A trained medical staff and a paramedical personnel can offer the woman the basket of choice after the consultant obstetrician has identified the basket to be offered.

Fourthly, as compared to the postnatal period when they are overwhelmed by the tasks of breastfeeding and other care for the newborn, during pregnancy, the opportunity of offering postpartum intrauterine contraceptive device (PPIUCD) and inserting it postpartum should not be lost on any count as large number of women can be provided for in this way.[3]

An important step is to check the options after offering the basket and using a seal on the patient's antenatal card and document her choice. This choice can be confirmed after childbirth **(Fig. 1)**.

The possibility of initiation in the immediate postpartum period is particularly advantageous for women unlikely to return for a postpartum care visit **(Fig. 2)**.

THE IMPORTANCE OF MEDICAL ELIGIBILITY CRITERIA

The medical eligibility criteria (MEC) for contraceptive methods utilized to judge the safety of the method for a particular situation are as follows:

- *Category 1*: No restrictions to use
- *Category 2*: Benefits outweigh the risks; generally use
- *Category 3*: Risks generally outweigh benefits; generally do not use
- *Category 4*: Too risky to use; do not use.

FP OPTIONS

☐ OCPs	☐ PPIUCD
☐ Injectable	☐ Tubal ligation
☐ Condom	☐ Vasectomy
☐ Interval IUCD	☐ LAM

Fig. 1: Seal on antenatal card (IUCD: intrauterine contraceptive device; LAM: lactational amenorrhea method; PPIUCD: postpartum intrauterine contraceptive device).

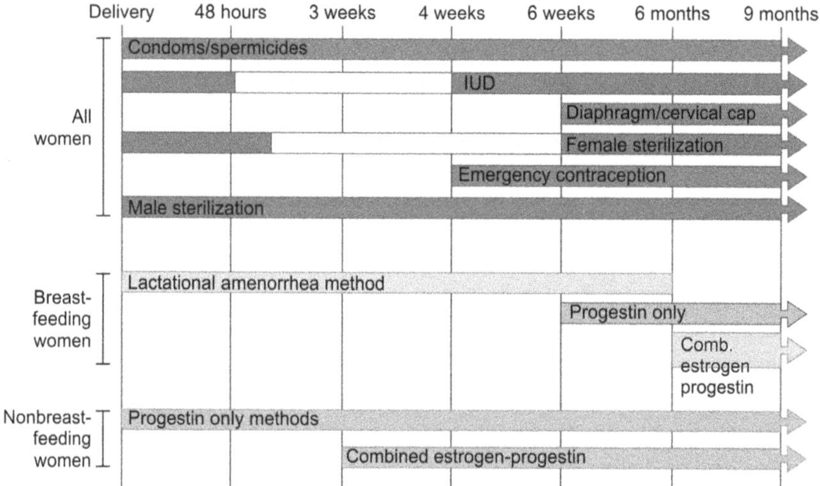

Fig. 2: Options postpartum to be discussed antepartum.

This classification is best depicted on a WHO MEC wheel, a tool to be kept handy in our clinics. It shows the life situation, MEC category for method and special information on important methods to be checked while prescribing.

IDENTIFYING THE METHOD EFFICACY IN THE BASKET[4]

The other tool used while offering the basket of choice is a chart showing different methods with their effectiveness and guidance of how best to increase efficacy of a particular method **(Fig. 3)**.

So, we need to be reasonably convinced that discussing postpartum contraception prenatally lays the groundwork for decisions about postpartum contraception and increases the possibility of initiation in the immediate postpartum period. This is particularly advantageous for women unlikely to return for a postpartum care visit and is especially true for high-risk pregnancy.

During antenatal period, depending on the situation, we can constitute the basket for the woman and send her for counseling to a special room identified for the purpose.

To consider a few situations:
- In low-risk gravida who have completed family-limiting methods of tubal sterilization and vasectomy and long-acting reversible contraceptives (LARC) methods including PPIUCD are good options.
- For women who need spacing and are breastfeeding can be given hormonal contraceptives with progesterone only pills and implants within 6 weeks, but injectable progestogens such as Depot injection medroxyprogesterone intramuscular or subcutaneous are suitable only after 6 weeks; whereas, combined hormonal contraception can be given only after 6 months. The important methods always to be included in the basket are the intrauterine devices (IUDs), both the Cu IUDs and

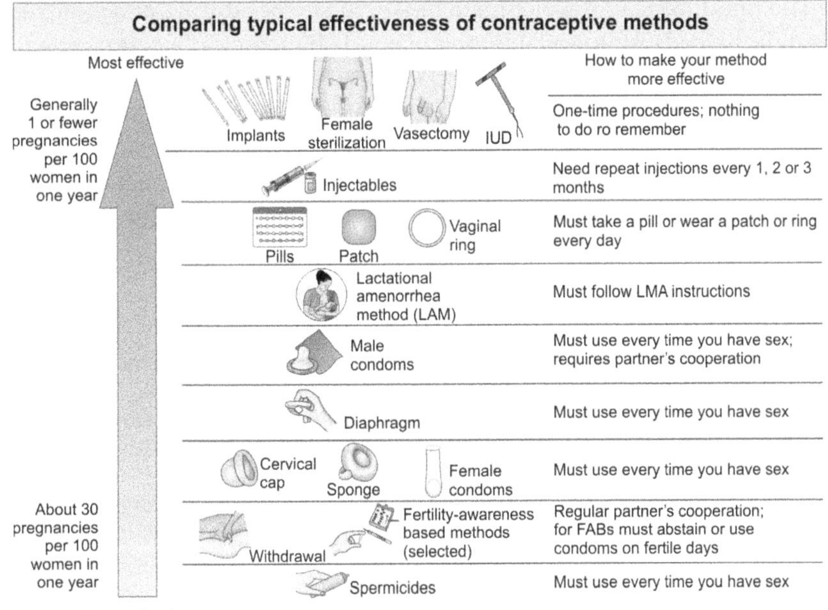

Fig. 3: Method efficacy.
(FAB: fertility awareness-based; IUD: intrauterine devices)

the levonorgestrel-releasing intrauterine system (LNG-IUS) are suitable for postpartum insertion anytime before 48 hours and then again after 4 weeks onward.

- Women who are not breastfeeding can be prescribed combined hormonal contraception after 3 weeks and all other hormonal contraceptives as stated above. As we outline the method as part of antenatal care, the woman is sensitized and develops familiarity with the structure and form of the methods.

- Let us consider the situation of an HIV-positive woman with her first pregnancy. She will require a sure method of spacing apart from barrier contraception. Those with mid disease of stage 1 or 2 can use hormonal method as other women postpartum. The category for initiating LNG-IUD remains.[2] Women who have stage 3 and 4 and have delivered, and are also on antiretroviral therapy can be prescribed hormonal contraception as in other postpartum women, but initiation of IUDs to be avoided (Category 3).

- Women with well-controlled diabetes and no vascular complications can be prescribed almost all methods even if they are on insulin; those with vascular problems cannot be prescribed combined hormonal methods and progesterone only injections (Category 3).

- Women with well-controlled hypertension and pre-eclampsia can be prescribed all methods except combined hormonal methods. Those women who are at high risk for arterial thrombosis can be prescribed all methods except combined hormonal methods and injectable progestogens.

The fine-tuning of developing a basket of choices during pregnancy is greatly facilitated by the available tools of WHO MEC criteria for contraceptive methods.

As Indian obstetricians, we shoulder a tremendous responsibility for contributing substantially toward population stabilization. Introducing the concept of contraception and family planning to women at first contact during antenatal care will go a long way for achieving both short-term objectives and long-term goals.

REFERENCES

1. Office of the Registrar General & Census Commissioner, India. 2011 census. [online] Available from: https://censusindia.gov.in/. [Last accessed June, 2020].
2. Ministry of Health and Family Welfare, India. National family Health Survey (NFHS-4) 2015-16. [online] Available from: http://rchiips.org/nfhs/NFHS-4Reports/India.pdf. [Last accessed June, 2020].
3. World Health Organization [2012]. Statement for collective action for postpartum family planning. [online] Available from: http://www.who.int/reproductivehealth/topics/family_planning/Statement_Collective_Action.pdf. [Last accessed June, 2020]
4. Stoddard A, Mcnicholas C, Peipert JF. Efficacy and safety of long-acting reversible contraception: literature review. Drugs. 2011;71(8):969-80.

21st Century Antenatal Care: Special Issues in Special Times

- **Respectful Care in Labor**
  Nandita Palshetkar, Ameya Purandare, Rohan Palshetkar, Ruchika Garg

- **Management of IVF Pregnancy**
  Sadhana Gupta, Mousumi Das Ghosh

- **Surgical Intervention in Antenatal Period**
  Parul Kotdawala, Nidhi Nagar

- **E-Technology for Antenatal Care**
  Aswath Kumar, Reshma Joy

- **Antenatal Screening: Quiz**
  Sebanti Goswami, Abha Rani Sinha, Seema Hakim

Respectful Care in Labor

Nandita Palshetkar, Ameya Purandare, Rohan Palshetkar, Ruchika Garg

INTRODUCTION

In September 2014, a statement was released by the World Health Organization on preventing disrespect and abuse during institutional childbirth. In addition, respectful and dignified care is also needed for the newborns. Awareness of childbirth as a natural process is required for the provision of respectful care in labor. The duty is to provide access to clinical interventions as required, along with need for woman-centered humanistic care. Avoidance of overmedicalization and inappropriate interventions contributes to respectful care. Good working relationships among staffs are also very important, as staffs functioning at their best can improve the experience of women. Institutionalizing respectful care alongside evidence-based clinical practice represents the goal of "mother–baby friendly birthing facilities" as advocated by International Federation of Obstetrics and Gynecology (FIGO).

RESPECTFUL CARE FOR MOTHER AND NEONATES

Documented examples of disrespectful care are neglect, painful, and unnecessary examinations, refusals to provide analgesics, breaches of confidentiality, and the lack of informed consent including in the context of sterilization. The use of abusive, harsh, or rude language threats to withhold treatment or of poor outcomes, accusatory remarks are very common. Women are vulnerable to mistreatment during childbirth due to their socioeconomic status, health status, viral infections, and/or location. WHO, in 2014, released a statement which rightfully states that while "disrespectful and abusive treatment of women may occur throughout pregnancy, childbirth, and the postpartum period, women are particularly vulnerable during childbirth". The WHO statement argues that "every woman has the right to the highest attainable standard of health, which includes the right to dignified and respectful health care".

World Health Organizations' statement calls for:

- Greater support from governments and enhancement of research
- Programs to improve the quality of maternal health care

- Greater emphasis on women rights
- Involvement of stakeholders in effort to improve quality of care and elimination of disrespect.

In a 2010 landscape analysis, Bowser and Hill described seven categories of disrespectful and abusive care during childbirth—physical abuse, nonconsented clinical care, nonconfidential care, nondignified care, discrimination, abandonment, and detention in health facilities.

Freedman and colleagues built on the Bowser and Hill categories to propose a definition of disrespectful and abusive care during childbirth as "interactions or facility conditions that local consensus deems to be humiliating or undignified, and those interactions or conditions that are experienced as or intended to be humiliating or undignified".

Mistreatment to which women are subjected during childbirth includes physical, verbal, and sexual abuse and denials of privacy, confidentiality, and high-quality care. Women sometimes reported lack of informed consent and confidentiality, conduction of vaginal examinations without consent, and neglect or abandonment. The overall goal for respectful care during normal birth was to achieve a healthy mother and child using the least possible interventions.

MATERNAL HEALTH

World Health Organization estimates that 536,000 maternal deaths occur globally each year and 136,000 of them take place in India. According to the Family Welfare Statistics in India, the maternal mortality ratio (MMR) was estimated to 301 maternal deaths per 100,000 live births in 2003. Even though there has been big decrease in the maternal mortality nationwide, Uttar Pradesh still reports MMR of 450 per 100,000. In the southern states though, Kerala and Tamil Nadu have reported MMR of 66 and 88 respectively, which is comparable with MMR in middle-income countries.

BOLOGNA SCORE

The Bologna Score tool is constructed to measure both attitudes and practices in care in labor and is based on the WHO's guidelines for how care in normal birth should be managed. The Bologna Score consists of three indicators:

1. *Indicator A*: It investigates the requirements for a safe delivery and is defined as the percentage of women attended by a skilled attendant in labor.
2. *Indicator B*: It is used to estimate the number of women falling outside the scope by measuring the percentage of women with induced labor or undergoing elective cesarean section.
3. *Indicator C*: It strives to measure the management of normal labor and consists of five key measures—presence of a companion at birth, use of a partograph, absence of augmentation as for example external pressure on

the fundus or emergency cesarean section, use of nonsupine position for birth, and skin-to-skin contact of mother and baby for at least 30 minutes within the 1st hour.

CARE IN LABOR

The practices used throughout labor where classified depending on whether they were considered useful, harmful, used inappropriately, and practices for which insufficient evidence exists.

Useful practices include use of the partograph for monitoring progress of labor, nonsupine position in labor, and early skin-to-skin contact between mother and child. Harmful practices include routine intravenous infusion in labor and use of supine position during labor. Inappropriate practice is liberal or routine use of episiotomy and electronic fetal monitoring. The practices for which insufficient evidence exists include fundal pressure and early clamping of the umbilical cord and these practices should be used with caution until there is further research done.

In WHO's definition of normal birth, it is made clear that, for example, cesarean section and preterm labor is not considered normal. On the other hand, it is not clear if a delivery where epidural anesthesia or oxytocin infusion is used still can be considered as a normal birth.

SKILLED BIRTH ATTENDANT

World Health Organization defines a skilled attendant as "an accredited health professional—such as a midwife, doctor, or nurse—who has been educated and trained in the skills needed to manage normal uncomplicated pregnancies, childbirth and the immediate postnatal period, and in the identification, management, and referral of complications in women and newborns". Studies had found that the use of skilled attendants was more common among younger women with higher levels of education and those belonging to higher economic groups.

PARTOGRAPH

A review of five studies from 2008, assessing the effect on perinatal and maternal outcome while using a partograph and it inferred that there was no significant difference in rate of cesarean section, instrumental vaginal delivery or Apgar score was less than seven at 5 minutes between the group with and without partograph. An exception was the one study carried out in a low-resource setting (Mexico) that showed a lower cesarean section rate when using the partograph.

SUPPORT DURING LABOR

Throughout labor, physical and emotional well-being of a woman should be assessed. It includes attention to privacy, respecting her choice of companions in the labor room. Support during labor can be given by the partner, family members, friends, or hospital staff. In a review with 16 trials, women who had continuous support during labor were more likely to have shorter duration of labor and also are less likely to use analgesics or report dissatisfaction with their childbirth experience.

BIRTH POSITION

World Health Organization states that women in both first and second stage of labor can adopt any position they like. A review with the objective to assess the benefits and risks of the use of different positions during second stage of labor showed that supine position was unfavorable for both mother and baby while incidence of perineal tear was high when birth occurred in nonsupine position.

INTERVENTIONS

Operative Deliveries

Cesarean section is a major operation with great benefits, but also with risks for both mother and baby. When there is an indication for hasten the delivery of the baby, instrumental vaginal delivery may be an option instead of cesarean section. There is evidence that instrumental deliveries increase the maternal morbidity, including perineal lacerations, hematomas, blood loss and anemia, urinary retention, and long-term problems with urinary and fecal incontinence. An American review including over 50,000 vaginal deliveries, third- and fourth-degree perineal lacerations were higher in the vacuum-assisted (10%) and forceps deliveries (20%) compared to the spontaneous vaginal deliveries (2%).

Episiotomy

Episiotomy was earlier considered to lower the risk of third-degree perineal tearing. Recent studies have shown that the risk of third-degree perineal tear is not reduced when episiotomy is performed routinely. A review including eight studies compared the effects of routine episiotomy to restrictive episiotomy and found that restrictive episiotomy resulted in less severe perineal trauma, less suturing, and fewer healing complications.

Artificial Rupture of Membranes

Artificial rupture of membranes (ARMs) can be used to induce labor, if the cervix status is favorable and the presenting part is fixed in the pelvis. It is common practice to start oxytocin infusion within a few hours after ARM, if labor is not established.

Skin-to-skin Care

A review including thirty studies compared early skin-to-skin contact with traditional hospital care with the objective to assess the effects of early skin-to-skin contact (STSC) on breastfeeding, behavior, and physiological adaptation in healthy mothers and newborns. The result indicated that babies placed skin-to-skin after delivery interacted more with their mothers, stayed warmer, and cried less.

■ INDIAN SCENARIO

Despite concerted global efforts to reduce mortality of women during childbirth, maternal mortality continues to be a significant cause of death among women worldwide. One of the important components of the efforts to decrease maternal mortality is to improve the quality of care received by women during delivery. Quality of care during delivery comprises a number of clinical protocols; respectful care during delivery is also a major determinant of quality and has been found to be associated with critical maternal and child health outcomes.

There are concerted global efforts to reduce complications and mortality of women during childbirth, particularly in low-resource countries, maternal mortality continues to be a significant cause of death among women worldwide. A component of quality care that is receiving attention is the issue of mistreatment of women by healthcare providers during childbirth. A growing body of literature suggests that fear of such mistreatment is a key impediment to timely acquisition of care and use of institutional facilities for childbirth, particularly among less educated and poor women, and is associated with poor birth outcomes for both mother and child. Such mistreatment can include a broad array of behaviors, from neglectful or nonconsensual care to verbal or physical abuse against a woman during childbirth.

A recent comprehensive systematic review of 65 qualitative and quantitative studies on the topic documents the following major types of mistreatment by providers—direct abuse (physical, sexual, or verbal), discrimination, failure to meet professional standards of care (nonconsensual or nonconfidential care, neglect or abandonment, and inadequate or poor-quality medical resources), and nonsupportive care. More insight into the limitations and strengths of different ways to measure mistreatment is important, both from the perspective of collecting evidence that adds to understanding of the scale of the problem, and from the perspective of defining mistreatment during childbirth.

In one study done by Arnab et al. on women delivering in public health clinics in Uttar Pradesh, India, provider mistreatment during childbirth has been found to be prevalent and may be under-reported by women, particularly when providers were younger or when they were older or less trained.

FOGSI'S MANYATA INITIATIVE: PROVIDING AND PRIORITIZING QUALITY AND RESPECTFUL MATERNAL CARE ALL OVER INDIA

Manyata is FOGSI's flagship initiative with the private sector providers, which was rolled out in 2017 wherein FOGSI has customized WHO standards for private maternity care providers in India. Led by FOGSI, the program aims to establish synergies between societies of professional healthcare providers and private healthcare. In a span of 3 years, close to 400 private maternity providers across Uttar Pradesh, Maharashtra, and Jharkhand have been approached.

The processes followed under Manyata are facility engagement, quality improvement, and quality assessment. Facility engagement includes orientation and baseline assessment. Quality improvement includes training and mentoring. Quality assessment includes an external assessment, which is carried out by FOGSI-trained lead assessors. On passing the assessment, the hospital is awarded the Manyata certificate. The enrolled hospitals are recognized for their excellence in maternity care. In case they do not match the expected score of 85%, a period of 3 months is generally given for course corrections and then, the center is reassessed. The FOGSI leadership consisting FOGSI office bearers and FOGSI-NPMU along with MSD for Mothers and Jhpiego have worked on developing and validating a viable and investable business model for the quality assurance (QA) mechanism while laying the groundwork for sustainable quality improvement (QI) efforts in the private maternal healthcare sector in India.

Government of Maharashtra and FOGSI have jointly finalized the launch of "LaQshya-Manyata" quality standards for the private maternal services sector in the state of Maharashtra. The registered facilities will be trained on essential patient care, safety, and facility improvement components based on set of 26 standards of quality of care. These standards have been carefully identified by renowned private sector OBGYN specialists, covering components that are vital for delivering quality maternal care. While safety of women and newborn is at the core of the program, LaQshya-Manyata is also valuable for other stakeholders in the maternal care ecosystem such as the private maternity providers. It enables them to build capable teams, with improved ability to manage life-threatening complications during deliveries. Furthermore, the program, with flexible training sessions and simplified standards, is designed to meet private providers' diverse needs, making it particularly suitable for small private sector maternity hospitals.

CONCLUSION

To eliminate the preventable maternal and newborn deaths and stillbirths, we should look beyond survival and basic healthcare, and we must strive for respectful care for women and their babies together and there should be systematic effort to measure and identify quality gaps and childbirth particularly in high-burden settings in India and elsewhere.

Manyata-LaQshya has indeed been a landmark event internationally, focused on providing quality care during childbirth via Manyata and Lakshya to the private and public health facilities, respectively. FOGSI and the Government of India are the FIRST to launch this unique initiative in the world. Indeed, we should be proud of this achievement and certainly it will benefit the millions of women in India and motivate other nations to follow our footsteps to provide quality and respectful maternal care to each and every pregnant woman across the world.

■ SUGGESTED READING

1. Angioli R, G'omez-Marin O, Cantuaria G, O'sullivan MJ. Severe perineal lacerations during vaginal delivery: the university of Miami experience. Am J Obstet Gynecol. 2000;182(5):1083-5.
2. Bc Moore ER, Anderson GC, Bergman N. Early skin-to-skin contact for mothers and their healthy newborn infants. Cochrane Database Syst Rev. 2007;(3):CD003519.
3. Bowser D, Hill K. Exploring evidence for disrespect and abuse in facility-based childbirth: report of a landscape analysis. Washington (District of Columbia): United States Agency for International Development; 2010.
4. Carolli G, Mignini L. Episiotomy for vaginal birth. Cochrane Database Syst Rev. 2009;21(1):CD000081.
5. Chalmers B, Porter R. Assessing effective care in normal labour: the Bologna score. Birth. 2001;28(2):79-83.
6. Dangal G. Preventing prolonged labour by using partograph. Int J Gynecol Obstet. 2007;7(1):1-9.
7. Dystoci AM, Hagberg H, Marsal K, Westgren M. Obstetrik. Lund: Studentlitteratur; 2008.
8. Fraser DM, Cooper MA. Myles Textbook for Midwives, 15th edition. New York: Churchill Livingstone Elsevier; 2009.
9. Freedman LP, Kruk ME. Disrespect and abuse of women in childbirth: challenging the global quality and accountability agendas. Lancet. 2014;384:e42-4.
10. Gupta JK, Hofemeyr GJ. Position for women during second stage of labour. Cochrane Database Syst Rev. 2004;(1):CD002006.
11. Hazarika I. Factors that determine the use of skilled care during delivery in India: implications for achievement of MDG-5 targets. Matern Child Health J. 2011;15(8):1381-8.
12. Hodnett ED, Gates S, Hofmeyr GJ, Sakala C. Continuous support for women during childbirth. Cochrane Database Syst Rev. 2003;(3):CD003766.
13. Lavender T, Hart A, Smyth RM. Effect of partogram use on outcomes for women in spontaneous labour at term. Cochrane Database Syst Rev. 2008;8(4):CD005461.
14. Lundgren I. Professionelltförhållingssätt. In: Kaplan A, Hogg B, Hildingsson I, Lundgren I (Eds). Lärobokförbarnmorskor, 3rd edition. Lund: Studentlitteratur; 2009.
15. Nordström L, Wiklund I. Förlossningensfysiologiochhandläggning. In: Hagberg H, Marsal K, Westgren M (Eds). Obstetrik. Lund: Studentlitteratur; 2008.
16. Svantesson L, Kaplan A. Operationslära. In: Kaplan A, Hogg B, Hildingsson I, Lundgren I, editors. Lärobokförbarnmorskor, 3rd edition. Lund: Studentlitteratur; 2009.
17. Technical Working Group, WHO. Care in normal birth: a practical guide. Birth. 1997;24(2):121-3.

18. Vora KS, Mavalankar DV, Ramani KV, Upadhyaya M, Sharma B, Lyengar S, et al. Maternal health situation in India: a case study. J Health Popul Nutr. 2009;27(2):184-201.
19. Waiswa P, Nyanzi S, Namusoko-Kalungi S, Peterson S, Tomson G, Pariyo GW. I never thought that this baby would survive; I thought that it would die any time: perceptions and care for preterm babies in eastern Uganda. Trop Med Int Health. 2010;15(10):1140-7.
20. Wall SN, Lee AC, Carlo W, Goldenberg R, Niermeyer S, Darmstadt GL, et al. Reducing intrapartum-related neonatal deaths in low- and middle-income countries-what works? Semin Perinatol. 2010;34(6):395-407.
21. World Health Organization (2004). Making pregnancy safer: The critical role of the skilled attendant. [online] Available from: https://www.who.int/maternal_child_adolescent/documents/9241591692/en/. [Last accessed June, 2020].
22. World Health Organization. The prevention and elimination of disrespect and abuse during facility-based childbirth. Geneva: World Health Organization; 2014.

Management of IVF Pregnancy

Sadhana Gupta, Mousumi Das Ghosh

INTRODUCTION

In vitro fertilization (IVF) involves ovarian stimulation with gonadotropin hormones, followed by retrieval of oocytes under sedation with subsequent fertilization by sperm in the laboratory and development of embryos in culture prior to transfer into the uterus.[1]

The technique of IVF has evolved over last four decades and more than five million babies have been born. Managing an IVF pregnancy is challenging; however, the ideal method is not well established. These patients are elderly with comorbid conditions and have undue concern and worry about outcome. IVF is an independent risk factor for antenatal and perinatal complications. This is a high-risk pregnancy and the aim is to optimize a favorable outcome, both for mother and baby.

PRE-PREGNANCY

Pre-pregnancy counseling and evaluation optimizes risks to the mother. A thorough medical evaluation is done and health condition optimized. Those with cardiovascular diseases and Turner syndrome should have specific evaluation and risk counseling. Medical disorders such as diabetes, hypertension, and epilepsy should have prepregnancy assessment and counseling regarding risk reduction strategies.[2] Optimum body weight should be targeted in case of obesity.

Folic acid is started prior to planned pregnancy and advised regarding cessation of smoking and alcohol. Medications are reviewed and switched over to safer alternatives, which are safe periconceptionally and in pregnancy. The couple should understand the risks of IVF such as multiple pregnancy, hypertensive disorders in pregnancy, and preterm labor.

Communication

Clear communication between the healthcare professionals and the couple about the monitoring and treatment plan goes a long way. The woman feels comfortable and a continuity of care is assured. Risk assessment is an integral step with appropriate referrals.[3] Clear referral paths should be outlined so that concerned specialist teams can treat when needed.[4]

The care plan should be tailored according to woman needs, keeping in mind that medical problems and obstetric complications are more common in these women.

EARLY PREGNANCY

Pregnancy is confirmed 14 days after embryo transfer by quantitative β-human chorionic gonadotropin (β-hCG) test. Few centers advise urine pregnancy test for confirmation of pregnancy.[5] Transvaginal ultrasound is usually done, soon after to confirm the site of pregnancy and to rule out ectopic pregnancy. This scan also confirms viability and chorionicity. Multiple gestations will have very high levels of β-hCG.

Biochemical pregnancy loss varies from 11 to 35%. The incidence of ectopic pregnancy, especially heterotopic, is higher in IVF pregnancies.[6]

Antenatal care is sometimes taken care of by the IVF unit or a different maternity center. The first appointment provides the opportunity to evaluate the maternal–fetal risks, revisit the medications of the patient, and to devise and agree an antenatal schedule. Once a viable pregnancy is confirmed, low-dose aspirin is recommended and continued at least 36 weeks of gestation. This reduces the chances of severe pre-eclampsia. Although National Institute of Clinical Excellence (NICE) recommends aspirin from 12 weeks, various studies show that aspirin in first trimester is beneficial and safe.

FIRST TRIMESTER

There is increased risk of spontaneous miscarriage and vaginal bleeding during pregnancy. This can be due to aneuploidy resulting in implantation failure as well as advancing age of mother. Implantation failure can occur for various reasons—patient selection, type of protocol, uterine receptivity, gamete and embryo quality, and transfer efficiency. It is known that the depth of placement of embryos in the uterine cavity, embryo quality, the embryo transfer technique, the use of ultrasound, the type of catheter used, and the presence of blood on the catheter are all important factors in the success of pregnancy and implantation.[7]

Miscarriage increases with lower number of retrieved oocytes (poor responders) where embryo selection is difficult.[8] This can be minimized by selecting chromosomally normal embryos through preimplantation genetic diagnosis. Array comparative genomic hybridization along with morphology screening results in higher pregnancy rates.[9]

The IVF mothers receive progesterone supplementation, which may be discontinued after first trimester.

Some IVF units start low-molecular-weight heparin (LMWH) as an adjuvant therapy, particularly those with history of recurrent miscarriage or poor response to IVF. Risk assessment for venous thromboembolism is advised early in pregnancy. This will decide the antenatal and postnatal thromboprophylaxis. In the absence of indication for thromboprophylaxis, LMWH should be discontinued at the end of first trimester.

Baseline blood tests can be performed. Women with Turner syndrome or structural heart disease are advised baseline echocardiogram.

Conditions, which may be life-threatening in IVF pregnancies, are: ovarian hyperstimulation syndrome, ectopic and heterotopic pregnancy, and ovarian torsion.[10] With rising IVF worldwide, emergency physicians should be aware of the possible risks. Ovarian hyperstimulation syndrome predisposes to unfavorable obstetric outcomes such as miscarriages, pregnancy-induced hypertension, diabetes mellitus, and low birth weight.[11]

Combined Screening

Prenatal screening is an essential part of antenatal care. IVF patients are more likely to have fetuses of chromosomal disorders. This risk is further increased after intracytoplasmic sperm injection (ICSI), mainly autosomal structural aberrations passed on by the father or de novo. This explains genetic assessment of couples, especially fathers with oligospermia before IVF.[12]

Aneuploidy screening provides a background risk for trisomy 21, 13, and 18. The multiple risk factor model includes nuchal translucency (NT), additional markers (nasal bone, ductus venosus flow, and tricuspid regurgitation), maternal serum β-hCG and placental associated plasma protein-A (PAPP-A). Age of the mother, ethnicity, smoking, and diabetes are taken into account. Other details such as donor age in case of egg donation and the day of transfer are also incorporated for risk assessment.

The combined test is offered between 11 weeks 0 days and 13 weeks 6 days in singleton and twin pregnancies. In higher order gestations, along with NT, nasal bone and flow in ductus venosus are used for screening.[4] PAPP-A levels are lower (approximately 0.8 MoM) and thereby increased risk of false positive result compared to those who conceived spontaneously.[13] The false-positive rate for combined screening in IVF pregnancies is increased from 4.7 to 15.9%.[14] There is increased need of invasive procedures such as chorionic villous sampling or amniocentesis for confirmation.[12] This has associated risk of miscarriage. These patients are less likely to opt for invasive procedures because of the risk of spontaneous abortion.[13] The reason for reduction in PAPP-A levels is not known; however, placental problem could be a cause.[15]

Twin pregnancies after IVF is mostly the result of transfer of two embryos, hence dizygotic and dichorionic. Monochorionic twinning is also high, usually after advanced assisted reproduction technologies, such as ICSI, assisted hatching, and blastocyst culture with a 10–15% risk of twin-to-twin transfusion syndrome.[13] Prenatal screening of IVF twin pregnancies faces two problems:

1. First, biochemical tests in dizygotic twins are limited by the masking effect of the normal co-twin and the difficulty in identifying the abnormal twin.

2. The second obstacle is that biochemical marker levels differ between IVF and pregnancies conceived naturally.[14] Hence a "pseudo-risk" for each twin in a dizygotic twin-pair and a combined risk in monozygous twins can be calculated. Visual identification of the affected fetus with the help of the NT is essential to perform this estimation.

■ SECOND TRIMESTER

In the second trimester, cervical length is assessed from 14 weeks of pregnancy by ultrasound. The risk factors such as previous mid trimester losses, multiple pregnancy, and congenital malformations of uterus need special attention. Those at risk of preterm labor are offered prophylactic tocolysis.[4]

Selective fetal reduction is a safe option to reduce the risks of prematurity in triplets and higher order pregnancies. However, the risk of fetal loss is 1%.[15]

Anomaly Scan (18–20 Weeks)

There is increased risk of congenital malformations in IVF pregnancies (3–4%) compared to normal population (2–3%).[9] The risk is further increased in multiple pregnancy. This association could be due to advanced age of the couple, prior treatment and duration for infertility, and chronic diseases such as obesity and diabetes. The composition of culture media and length of time in culture and altered hormonal environment at the time of implantation as well as manipulation of gametes and embryos play a role.[16]

A detailed structural anomaly scan is recommended in all pregnancies. The malformations include neural tube defects, cardiovascular defects, gastrointestinal defects, and musculoskeletal defects.

In addition, uterine artery Doppler studies add value. If the uterine artery pulsatility index is >95th centile (high-resistance uteroplacental circulation), additional surveillance for pre-eclampsia and growth restriction should be done.

Fetal echocardiography is advised in the patients with personal or family history of cardiac abnormality, use of antiepileptic drugs, or monochorionic twin pregnancies. Some IVF units recommend fetal echocardiography in all IVF cases. This must be balanced against available resources.

Alterations in methylation, epigenetics, and imprinting are reported in IVF pregnancies. Abnormalities in imprinting are associated with Beckwith–Wiedemann syndrome, Angelman syndrome, and Prader–Willi syndrome.[2]

■ THIRD TRIMESTER

There is a higher incidence of placenta previa and abruptio placentae in IVF pregnancies. Metabolic changes during embryo culture could be a cause. The other theory is increased tendency of lower segment implantation due to uterine stimulation and contraction during embryo transfer. This risk is lower in frozen cycles compared to fresh ones.

Frequency of antenatal check-ups and growth scan should be individualized. If the patient is at risk of pre-eclampsia or growth retardation based on biophysical (abnormal uteroplacental blood flow at anomaly scan) or biochemical markers (maternal serum PAPP-A below the 5th centile at combined screening), antenatal visits are advised 2 weekly and growth scans 4 weekly till 32–34 weeks, then more frequently. Frequent clinical and sonographic monitoring is also advised in medical disorders such as chronic hypertension, pre-eclampsia, diabetes, antiphospholipid syndrome, multiple pregnancies, and more so in monochorionic ones.

Medical disorders of pregnancy are high due to the age factor. There is increased risk of gestational diabetes in both singleton and twin pregnancies. This may be attributed to insulin resistance and polycystic ovary syndrome (PCOS).

Preterm labor is seen in both singleton and multiple pregnancies conceived by IVF. Efforts to prevent the morbidity and mortality associated with preterm birth may be categorized as tertiary (initiated after the process of parturition has begun, with a goal of preventing delivery or improving outcomes for preterm infants) or secondary (aimed at eliminating or reducing risk in women with known risk factors). Multiple pregnancy increases the risk of prematurity by sixfold. This is a leading cause of infant mortality and long-term physical and mental problems.[17] To reduce the morbidity of prematurity-related illness, antenatal glucocorticoids, antibiotics, and neuroprotectants are used.[14] Antenatal magnesium sulfate reduces intraventricular hemorrhage, cerebral palsy, and perinatal mortality in early premature babies.

The adverse outcome of IVF can be explained by elevated levels of estradiol and vascular endothelial growth factor (VEGF). Hormonal stimulation and embryo culture cause epigenetic alterations in imprinted genes. This along with multiple pregnancies contributes to the adversities.[1]

Timing and Mode of Delivery

Delivery is planned based on maternal and fetal condition and pregnancy risk factors/complications. Singleton pregnancies also have higher induction of labor and cesarean section rates.[6] Cesarean delivery on maternal request is high due to anxiety and apprehension of the mother.

Higher rates of fetal macrosomia, emergency cesarean section, and postpartum hemorrhage are seen in IVF pregnancies. There is an elevated risk of blood transfusion.[2] The risk of stillbirth is high (16.2/1,000 compared with a rate of 2.3/1,000) in naturally occurring pregnancies. Hence, elective induction is offered at 38–39 weeks of pregnancy. In the presence of Turner syndrome with cardiovascular problems such as coarctation of aorta or aortic root dilatation, elective cesarean section is the preferred option.

The newborns are premature and of low birth weight or very low birth weight.[6] It is seen that the risks of prematurity and low birth weight is more significant in female factor infertility. IVF babies have fifteen times more risk of neonatal intensive care unit (NICU) admissions. The main reasons are supportive care for feeding, neonatal jaundice, neonatal sepsis, and respiratory difficulties. The neonatal outcomes are reassuring; however, neonatal death is higher in IVF pregnancies compared to women who conceive naturally.

Frozen transfer cycles had better perinatal outcomes compared to fresh embryo transfer. There is reduced risk of low birth weight, preterm labor, and small for gestation age fetuses.[18] This may be due to self-selection effect of freezing, which filters out compromised embryos that are less likely to survive. Also, this provides more natural uterine environment and synchrony between embryonic development and endometrial receptivity. The effects of elevated estradiol and VEGF levels on placentation are avoided.[1]

POSTNATAL

Parenting stress is an important concern in IVF patients. Those with medical disorders such as chronic hypertension and diabetes are taken care by the physician. Postnatal thromboprophylaxis is advised based on mode of delivery and the ongoing risk factors for venous thromboembolism. Multiple risk factors need to be dealt individually.

Contraception is also discussed. Progesterone-based preparations are preferred.

SPECIAL INDICATIONS FOR IVF

IVF—Egg Donation

Pregnancy following IVF with egg donation is a technique of choice in women with premature ovarian failure, gonadal dysgenesis, poor oocyte quality, or diminished ovarian reserve. This is also used by women with autosomal-dominant conditions or a carrier of an X-linked disorder. The oocyte is obtained from a screened donor in a fresh IVF cycle and fertilized with the recipient's partner's sperm. This is an immune paradox as the fetus is of different genetic composition.

This group of patients is of advanced age and usually suffers from chronic conditions such as chronic hypertension, type 2 diabetes, and cardiovascular disease. They suffer from significant anxiety and need time-to-time assurance from the healthcare providers. Pregnant women with Turner syndrome are at increased risk of deterioration of congenital heart disease, cardiac failure, aortic dilatation, dissection, or rupture. Involving a cardiologist helps in monitoring during pregnancy.

Miscarriage rate is lower than IVF with autologous eggs, as implantation is better. There is minimal risk of ovarian hyperstimulation, as they have no superovulation.

First- and second-trimester bleeding is higher in this group of patients; the probable cause would be abnormal placentation. Multiple pregnancy is common. These pregnancies are associated with higher incidence of pre-eclampsia due to altered immunological processes.[18] Frequent follow-up is advised for surveillance and timely diagnosis. Preterm delivery and lower mean infant birth weights are seen in this group of patients. Operative delivery and cesarean section rates are higher.[19]

Maternal and fetal risks are higher in the presence of medical conditions. Multidisciplinary approach improves perinatal outcome. Obstetricians should be aware about the need for closer surveillance for the development of gestational hypertension and pre-eclampsia.

Male Factor Infertility

There is a reduced complication rate in this group compared to non-male factor infertility. The incidence of preterm premature rupture of the membranes (PPROM) and preterm delivery is low due to lack of medical problems in the mother.[20]

KEY MESSAGES

- In vitro fertilization pregnancy is a high-risk pregnancy.
- Multidisciplinary and tertiary level of antenatal care reduces adverse outcome. Every case should be individualized and clear communication with the patient and family is advisable from time-to-time.
- Risks of miscarriage, ectopic pregnancy, congenital anomalies, gestational hypertension, and gestational diabetes are higher and the obstetrician should be careful in this group of patients. Antenatal visits and ultrasound monitoring are more frequent and should be individualized.
- With rising IVF worldwide, emergency physicians should be aware of the possible life-threatening situations in IVF pregnancies such as ovarian hyperstimulation syndrome, ectopic and heterotopic pregnancy, and ovarian torsion.
- The neonate has more chances of NICU admissions due to prematurity and low birth weight.

REFERENCES

1. Sullivan-Pyke CS, Senapati S, Mainigi MS, Barthart KT. In vitro fertilization and adverse obstetric and perinatal outcomes. Semin Perinatol. 2017;41(6):345-53.
2. The American college of Obstetricians and Gynaecologists (2016). Committee opinion, Number 671: Perinatal Risks Associated with Assisted Reproductive Technology. [online] Available from: https://www.acog.org/clinical/clinical-guidance/committee-opinion/articles/2016/09/perinatal-risks-associated-with-assisted-reproductive-technology [Last accessed June, 2020].
3. British Fertility Society; Royal College of Obstetricians and Gynaecologists (2012). In vitro fertilization: perinatal risks and early childhood outcomes. Scientific Impact paper no 8. [online] Available from: https://www.rcog.org.uk/globalassets/documents/guidelines/scientific-impact-papers/sip_8.pdf [Last accessed June, 2020].

4. Gada D, Tomar G (2011). Monitoring of an IVF pregnancy. FOGSI Focus: Advanced Infertility Management. [online] Available from: https://www.fogsi.org/wp-content/uploads/fogsi-focus/advances_infertility.pdf [Last accessed June, 2020].

5. Chirumamilla L, Raja A, Kini S, Menezes Q, Thong J; Assisted Conception Unit, Royal Infirmary of Edinburgh, Edinburgh, United Kingdom, et al. (2008). Confirmation of pregnancy after assisted conception treatment: a summary of practice in United Kingdom: Abstracts, Volume 90, Supplement 1. [online] Available from: https://www.fertstert.org/article/S0015-0282(08)02848-3/pdf [Last accessed June, 2020].

6. Kathpalia SK, Kapoor K, Sharma A. Complications in pregnancies after in vitro fertilization and embryo transfer. Med J Armed Forces India. 2016;72(3):211-4.

7. Cetin MT, Kumtepe Y, Kiran H, Seydaoglu G. Factors affecting pregnancy in IVF: age and duration of embryo transfer. Reprod Biomed Online. 2010;20(3)380-6.

8. Maaike L, Groen H, Mooij TM, Burger CW, Broekmans FJ, Lambalk CB, et al. Miscarriage risk for IVF pregnancies in poor responders to ovarian hyperstimulation. Reprod Biomed Online. 2010;20(2):191-200.

9. Choi J, Lobo RA. In vitro fertilization. Reprod Endocrinol Infertility. 924-36.

10. Hilbert SM, Gunderson S. Complications of assisted reproductive technology. Emerg Med Clin N Am. 2019;37(2):239-49.

11. Courbiere B, Oborski V, Braunstein D, Desparoir A, Noizet A, Gamerre M. Obstetric outcome of women with in vitro fertilization pregnancies hospitalized for ovarian hyperstimulation syndrome: a case-control. Fertil Steril. 2011;95(5):1629-32.

12. Gjerris AC, Loft A, Pinborg A, Christiansen M, Tabor A. First-trimester screening markers are altered in pregnancies conceived after IVF/ICSI. Ultrasound Obstet Gynecol. 2009;33(1):8-17.

13. Gjerris AC, Tabor A, Loft A, Christiansen M, Pinborg A. First trimester prenatal screening among women pregnant after IVF/ICSI. Hum Reprod Update. 2012;18(4):350-9.

14. Simhan HN. Prevention and management of preterm parturition. Disorders at the maternal–foetal interface. 679-711.

15. Gungor ND. The alteration of first trimester screening markers in fresh and frozen-thawed blastocyst transfers. Eur Res J. 2018;1-5.

16. Zheng Z, Chen L, Yang T, Yu H, Wang H, Qin J. Multiple pregnancies achieved with IVF/ICSI and risk of specific congenital malformations: a meta-analysis of cohort studies. Reprod Biomed Online. 2018;36::472-82.

17. El-Toukhy T, Bhattacharya S, Akande VA; The Royal College of Obstetricians and Gynaecologists. Multiple pregnancies following assisted conception. Scientific Impact Paper No. 22. BJOG. 2018;125(5):e12-8.

18. Palomba S, Homburg R, Santagni S, La Sala GB, Orvieto R. Risk of adverse pregnancy and perinatal outcomes after high technology infertility treatment: a comprehensive systematic review. Reprod Biol Endocrinol. 2016;14:76.

19. Sekhon LH, Gerber RS, Rebarber A, Saltzman Dh, Klauser CK, Gupta S, et al. Effect of oocyte donation on pregnancy outcomes in vitro fertilization twin gestations. Fertil Steril. 2014;101(5):1326-30.

20. Lavie A. Obstetrical outcomes of IVF pregnancies in patients with male factor infertility. Am J Obstet Gynaecol. 2018;218(1):S462-3.

Surgical Intervention in Antenatal Period

Parul Kotdawala, Nidhi Nagar

INTRODUCTION

A surgery during pregnancy, especially one that required anesthesia, was considered a "high-risk" zone for many decades, and was reserved for only desperate cases. The two big worries were the detrimental effect anesthetic agents and the surgical procedure on the growing fetus, and a possible stimulus to the uterus inducing contractions and resulting abortion/PT delivery. Over last 2–3 decades, our trepidation has eased with advent of better anesthetic agents as well as positive team experience and now we do undertake surgeries when needed with more confidence. Surgical procedures unrelated to pregnancy are very occasionally necessary. An incidence of 0.75% was noted in a large series of 720,000 pregnancies, where 5,405 women required an operation unrelated to pregnancy. The most common operations performed during pregnancy are appendicectomy and cholecystectomy. Upon checking published papers, we notice that almost all types of surgeries are reported to have been performed at some time.

Whenever a surgery needs to be performed in a pregnant woman, a consultation among her obstetric team, surgeon, anesthesiologist, and neonatologist becomes vital to coordinate best management plan. Mode and type of anesthesia and surgical procedure may be altered according to the anatomical and physiological changes related to pregnancy and the concerns about the fetus.

As these surgeries are very infrequent and as there is a wide personal variation in the procedure adopted among surgeons, it is almost impossible to conduct a randomized trial to evaluate management protocols of nonobstetric surgery in pregnant women. We have tried to review the current status of this, based upon data from observational studies, expert opinion, and extrapolation from trials during cesarean delivery.

COMMON INDICATIONS

The most common nonobstetric conditions reported as requiring a surgery during pregnancy are appendicitis, cholecystitis ovarian disorders (torsion and neoplasm), trauma, breast or cervical disease, and bowel obstruction.

▇ PHYSIOLOGICAL CHANGES RELATED TO PREGNANCY

Physiological changes related to pregnancy occur in virtually all systems and are caused by both hormonal and mechanical factors. Pertinent changes in major organ systems are summarized here.

Cardiovascular

Cardiac output (CO) increases by 20% at 8 weeks. It continues to rise until 30–32 weeks, when it plateaus and remains approximately 50% above the pre-pregnancy state. After 32 weeks, CO remains stable and is maintained until the beginning of labor. The rise in CO is due to:

- Increased preload from a rise in blood volume
- Decreased afterload from declining vascular resistance
- Increased maternal heart rate by 15–20 beats/min (bpm)
- Supine position at term may lower CO by 25–30% compared with left lateral position, due to compression of the inferior vena cava by a gravid uterus.

Pulmonary Effects

A state of hyperventilation leads to chronic respiratory alkalosis (pH 7.42–7.44) and a drop in the partial pressure of carbon dioxide ($PaCO_2$ 28–32 mm Hg vs. nonpregnant normal range of 34–36 mm Hg). This is a result of the increase in tidal volume and respiratory drive due to the stimulatory effects of progesterone right from the first trimester. As a compensatory response, the plasma bicarbonate concentration decreases to 20 mEq/L and diminishes plasma-buffering capacity.

- PaO_2 may be slightly elevated during pregnancy (104–108 mm Hg) as a result of the increase in CO and minimization of the ventilation/perfusion mismatch in the lung.
- An upward displacement of diaphragm from 20 weeks onward leads to a 20% reduction in functional residual capacity.
- Oxygen consumption increases by almost 20% during pregnancy.

Hematologic

Plasma volume increases by 50% by 32 weeks of gestation; total red blood cell mass increases only by 20–30%, resulting in hemodilution ("physiologic anemia of pregnancy"), with normal hemoglobin levels as low as 11 g/dL in the first and third trimesters, and 10.5 g/dL in the second trimester.

Pregnancy creates a relatively hypercoagulable state caused by an increase in circulating concentrations of the majority of coagulation factors, reduced levels of the endogenous anticoagulant cofactor protein S, and reduced fibrinolysis due to increases in circulating type 1 and 2 plasminogen activator inhibitor. The risk of deep vein thrombosis (DVT) is highest in the first 4–6 weeks postpartum. There is also a mild leukocytosis during pregnancy.

Gastrointestinal

Gastroesophageal reflux occurs in 30–50% of pregnancies, most likely related to increases in intra-abdominal pressure and to decreased lower esophageal sphincter tone during all trimesters. Gastric emptying is not affected by pregnancy, though it is slowed by labor and opioid analgesics.

Renal

Glomerular filtration rate and renal blood flow rise markedly during pregnancy, resulting in a physiologic fall in the serum creatinine concentration.

■ LABORATORY CHANGES (TABLE 1)

Pregnancy-induced physiological changes can alter the range of normal laboratory values in pregnant women.

■ PREOPERATIVE EVALUATION

Pregnant patients who require surgery should be evaluated preoperatively in the same manner as nonpregnant patients. Additional testing is not indicated in an uncomplicated pregnancy. A thorough history should document underlying medical and obstetrical conditions, and physical examination should include detailed assessment of the airway. Laboratory and other testing should be performed as indicated by the patient's medical problems and the proposed surgery.

Timing

Nonurgent surgery that cannot wait until delivery is generally performed during the second trimester. Urgently needed surgery should be performed regardless of the trimester; whereas, completely elective surgery should be postponed until after delivery.

There is no strong evidence of increased risk of miscarriage or teratogenesis from anesthetic agents used during early pregnancy. Because common first-trimester adverse outcomes (e.g., miscarriage, vaginal bleeding, and fetal structural anomalies) may be attributed to surgery and anesthesia in the absence of other obvious causes, it is prudent to minimize exposure of the fetus to surgery and medication during pregnancy, especially during organogenesis. Furthermore, the safety of drug use in pregnancy cannot be conclusively evaluated.

The first trimester background miscarriage rate is approximately 8–16% of clinically recognized pregnancies under 13 weeks of gestation, and it is 2–4% of pregnancies between 13 and 20 weeks. A literature review of studies of pregnancy outcome after nonobstetric surgical intervention reported an incidence of miscarriage within this range, 10.5% of patients in the first

TABLE 1: Physiological changes in pregnancy.

System	Physiological change	Anesthetic implications
Cardiovascular	• ↑ CO up to 50% • ↑ Uterine perfusion to 10% of CO • ↓ SVR, ↓ PVR, ↓ AP • Aortocaval compression from 13 weeks	 • Uterine perfusion not autoregulated • Hypotension common under regional and general anesthesia • Supine hypotensive syndrome requires left lateral tilt
Respiratory	• ↑ Minute ventilation • Respiratory alkalosis ($PaCO_2$, 3.7–4.2 kPa) • ↓ ERV, ↓ RV, ↓ FRC • ↑ V/Q mismatch • ↑ Oxygen consumption • Upward displacement of diaphragm • ↑ Thoracic diameter • Mucosal edema	• Faster inhalation induction • Maintain $PaCO_2$ at normal pregnancy levels • Potential hypoxemia in the supine and Trendelenburg positions • Breathing more diaphragmatic than thoracic • Difficult laryngoscopy and intubation; bleeding during attempts
CNS	• ↑ Epidural vein engorgement • ↓ Epidural space volume • ↑ Sensitivity to opioids and sedatives	• Bloody tap more common • More extensive local anesthetic spread
Hematological	• ↑ Red cell volume 30%, ↑ WCC • ↑ Plasma volume 50% • ↑ Coagulation factors • ↓ Albumin and colloid osmotic pressure	 • Dilutional anemia • Thromboembolic complications (DVT prophylaxis) • Edema, decreased protein binding of drugs
Gastrointestinal	• ↑ Intragastric pressure • ↓ Barrier pressure	• ↑ Aspiration risk • Antacid prophylaxis, RSI after 18 weeks gestation
Renal	• ↑ Renal plasma flow, ↑ GFR • ↓ Reabsorptive capacity	• Normal urea and creatinine may mask impaired renal function • Glycosuria and proteinuria

(CO: cardiac output; SVR: systemic vascular resistance; PVR: pulmonary vascular resistance; AP: arterial pressure; ERV: expiratory reserve volume; RV: residual volume; FRC: functional residual capacity; V/Q: ventilation/perfusion; MAC: minimum alveolar concentration; WCC: white cell count; GFR: glomerular filtration rate; CNS: central nervous system: RSI: rapid sequence intubation)

trimester. Some studies have reported higher rates of miscarriage in women who undergo first trimester abdominal surgery. However, it is not clear whether these higher rates were due to the surgery itself, the underlying maternal condition prompting the surgery (e.g., infection and high fever), maternal characteristics (e.g., smoking and older age), or other factors, such as damage to the corpus luteum early in gestation.

The recommendation to perform surgery during the second rather than the third trimester is primarily mechanical—the early-second-trimester uterus is still small enough to not obliterate an abdominal operative field, and the risk of preterm labor may be lower when surgery is performed during the second trimester as compared with third trimester.

Patient Preparation

In addition to standard preoperative procedures, preparation of pregnant women takes into account risks of aspiration, difficult intubation, thromboembolism, and the well-being of the fetus. Pregnant patients also have a greater risk of carotid puncture during central venous catheterization due to the tendency of the internal jugular vein to overlie the carotid artery in pregnancy.

Fetal Heart Rate Monitoring

The fetal heart rate (FHR) should be documented pre- and postoperatively, regardless of gestational age. The American College of Obstetricians and Gynecologist (ACOG) states that the decision to use intraoperative fetal monitoring should be individualized based on factors such as gestational age, type of surgery, and available resources. If technically possible, continuous monitoring of all viable fetuses (>26–28 weeks' gestation) should be employed throughout the surgery. Although continuous FHR monitoring has not shown improved fetal outcome conclusively in women under general anesthesia, such cases should be performed in hospitals with good quality neonatal ICU backup. An obstetrician should be readily available in case an emergency cesarean delivery is indicated.

Fasting Guidelines

Standard adult fasting guidelines are applicable to nonobstetric surgery in pregnant patients. The American Society of Anesthesiologists (ASA) recommends that patients abstain from solid food for at least 6 hours prior to surgery (8 hours for fried or fatty foods); clear liquids, which have a more rapid gastric transit time, may be ingested until 2 hours prior to surgery.

Aspiration Avoidance

The actual risk of aspiration appears to be quite small. Preoperative medication to minimize risk from aspiration in pregnant women is a reasonable precaution, although no specific intervention has shown improved clinical outcome. In a retrospective review of 51,000 + first trimester and 11,000 + second trimester pregnant patients undergoing deep sedation with propofol, there were no cases of perioperative pulmonary aspiration even though preoperative antacids or cricoid pressure were not routinely utilized. Pregnant patients with a BMI > 40 kg/m^2 were not suitable candidates for deep sedation.

Thromboprophylaxis

Pregnancy is a hypercoagulable state due to an increase in majority of coagulation factors and a decrease in protein S levels. This effect protects against excessive blood loss at delivery, but also increases the risk of a thromboembolic event in the postsurgical period.

Mechanical or pneumatic compression should be placed on all pregnant women undergoing surgery. The need for pharmacologic thromboprophylaxis should be determined on a case-to-case basis keeping in mind the expected scope and length of the procedure, and whether the woman has risk factors for venous thrombosis in addition to the pregnancy (e.g., thrombophilia, prolonged immobilization, past history of venous thrombosis, malignancy, diabetes mellitus, varicose veins, paralysis, or obesity).

American College of Chest Physicians (ACCP) "clinical practice guideline (2012)" on prevention and treatment of thrombosis recommends mechanical or pharmacologic thromboprophylaxis for all pregnant patients undergoing a surgery. For laparoscopic procedures (gynecologic or general surgical), which are likely to last 45+ minutes, a use of low-molecular weight heparin is suggested. For a shorter procedure, a mechanical thromboprophylaxis is a reasonable alternative. After surgery, thromboprophylaxis is continued until the patient is fully mobile. Early mobilization is encouraged to minimize the risk of DVT.

Antibiotic Prophylaxis

The need for antibiotic prophylaxis depends on the specific procedure. Following antibiotics have a good safety profile in pregnant women—the cephalosporins, penicillins, erythromycin (except estolate), azithromycin, and clindamycin. Aminoglycosides are relatively safe, but carry a risk of fetal (and maternal) ototoxicity and nephrotoxicity.

Prophylactic Corticosteroids

A course of antenatal glucocorticoids 24–48 hours prior to surgery between 24 and 34 weeks of pregnancy can reduce perinatal morbidity/mortality, if a preterm birth occurs. This decision depends upon the urgency of the surgery and the obstetrician's estimate of whether the patient is at increased risk of preterm birth because of the underlying disease or the planned procedure. Although antenatal glucocorticoids have the potential benefits for the fetus, they are best avoided in the setting of systemic infection (e.g., sepsis or a ruptured appendix), because they may impair the ability of the maternal immune system to contain the infection.

Prophylactic Tocolytics

There is no proven benefit to routine administration of prophylactic perioperative tocolytic therapy. Tocolytics are indicated for treatment of preterm labor until resolution of the underlying, self-limited condition that may have caused the contractions. Minimizing uterine manipulation may reduce the risk of development of uterine contractions and preterm labor.

ANESTHESIA MANAGEMENT

Positioning

Although the value of left displacement of the uterus is being questioned, a supine patient beyond 18–20 weeks of gestation should be positioned with a 15° left lateral tilt, to reduce aortocaval compression and cardiovascular compromise. Left uterine displacement can be accomplished by either tilting the operating table, or by placing a wedge under the patient's right hip.

Intraoperative Fetal Heart Rate Monitoring

Intraoperative FHR monitoring can be achieved either by using an electronic FHR monitor or by Doppler ultrasound. For abdominal operations, some centers use transvaginal ultrasound to monitor FHR. If adequate maternal oxygenation and uterine perfusion are maintained, the fetus usually tolerates surgery and anesthesia well.

With induction of general anesthesia, the FHR typically displays reduced variability, probably by anesthetizing the brainstem center that modulates intrinsic cardiac automaticity. Baseline FHR usually remains within the normal range. Ephedrine crosses the placenta and can produce changes in the FHR in accordance with their vasoactive effects.

One should optimize uteroplacental oxygen delivery and blood flow by minimizing aortocaval compression, whenever fetal bradycardia, tachycardia, or repetitive decelerations are observed and also to correct maternal hypovolemia and hypotension. To maintain maternal hyperoxia and normocarbia, an adjustment of the fraction of inspired oxygen (FiO_2) and appropriate ventilation are necessary. These measures are recommended and may be of benefit.

Type of Anesthetic

Anesthesia plan for a pregnant patient must take into account:
- Type of surgery
- Underlying medical conditions (including changes of pregnancy)
- Effects of anesthesia and surgery on both the patient and the fetus
- Preferences of the patient, anesthesiologist, and surgeon.

There are no studies showing differences in neonatal outcome (teratogenicity or preterm delivery) based on type of anesthetic; however, concerns regarding fetal drug exposure, maternal intubation, and maternal aspiration lead to a preference for regional anesthesia when possible. However, as most nonobstetric surgery in pregnancy is suprapelvic (laparotomy or laparoscopy), a general anesthesia is employed most often.

Sedation (Light Anesthesia)

Often called "monitored anesthesia", this involves monitoring of patient by an anesthesia provider, possible administration of analgesic and/or anxiolytic medication, and further intervention and support as needed during a procedure; the surgeon usually provides local anesthetic infiltration for analgesia to minimize the need for excessive sedation.

The most common medications used during monitored anesthesia care are propofol for sedation, fentanyl as an analgesic, and midazolam as an anxiolytic. Each of these, when used, is administered in small incremental doses.

Sedation is generally minimized due to concerns related to the administration of sedative drugs during pregnancy:

- Sedation-induced hypoventilation may cause respiratory acidosis, with deleterious effects on placental circulation.
- Aspiration may occur during deep sedation, due to decreased gastroesophageal sphincter tone in pregnancy.
- Patients often request that drugs, which may affect the fetus, be avoided.

Regional Anesthesia

Regional anesthesia, which includes peripheral nerve blocks as well as neuraxial anesthesia, is an option for some surgical procedures, particularly those involving the extremities. It has the advantage of avoiding the risks of general anesthesia, particularly the need to manage the airway; however, regional anesthesia may need to be converted to general anesthesia when necessary. Sedative medication is often used in conjunction with regional anesthesia, but is not necessary.

Peripheral nerve blocks are managed as they are in nonpregnant patients.

Neuraxial anesthesia is often used for surgery of the lower extremities and may be an option for some procedures of the lower abdomen and pelvis. Management of neuraxial anesthesia for nonobstetric surgery in the pregnant patient is same as for a cesarean delivery. The major concern with neuraxial anesthesia is maternal hypotension, which may reduce placental perfusion.

Doses for neuraxial anesthesia may be decreased in pregnancy. The most common modes in pregnancy are epidural and spinal analgesia. The exaggerated lumbar lordosis of late pregnancy may require an experienced person, and the quantity of medications may decrease compared to a nonpregnant patient. The complications associated with regional neuraxial anesthesia in pregnant women are essentially the same as a nonpregnant woman.

General Anesthesia

Most pregnant women requiring surgery for nonobstetric conditions undergo either laparoscopy or urgent explorative laparotomy and so, require a general anesthesia.

Induction of Anesthesia

Thorough preoxygenation is critical during any stage of pregnancy. In pregnant patients who have not followed fasting guidelines or are felt to be at high risk of aspiration, rapid sequence intubation in the same manner as nonpregnant patients at risk of aspiration should be followed.

Preoxygenation

Compared to a nonpregnant, an apnea leads to more rapid and significant desaturation in pregnant women. Preoxygenation with 100% O_2 by face mask for 3–5 minutes results in effective denitrogenation. During emergencies, eight vital capacity breaths over 60 seconds will get similar effect.

A healthy, fully preoxygenated nonpregnant woman will decrease her saturation level from 100% to <90% in approximately 9 minutes of apnea; whereas, it takes only 3 minutes for a term-pregnant patient to reach the same degree of desaturation and approximately 90 seconds in a morbidly obese pregnant patient. The clinical implications are obvious.

Induction

Propofol is the preferred induction agent in healthy pregnant women. Thiopental, ketamine, and etomidate are also used, and all are reasonably safe. None of these have shown to be teratogenic or to have adverse effects on brain development.

Either succinylcholine or a nondepolarizing neuromuscular blocking agent is used to facilitate endotracheal intubation. These drugs have no direct effect on the fetus, as neuromuscular blocking agents do not cross the placenta.

Intubation

A rapid sequence intubation with cricoid pressure in all pregnant patients is recommended due to concern that decreased lower esophageal sphincter tone leads to increased risk of regurgitation.

Maintenance of Anesthesia

No standard anesthetic agent has been proven teratogenic or to has adverse effects on human brain development. During pregnancy, the minimum alveolar concentration (MAC) for inhalation agents may be decreased.

Hemodynamic and Fluid Management

The goal in all patients is to maintain adequate perfusion and oxygenation to organs and tissue; during pregnancy, this includes placental perfusion also. Hypovolemia, drugs, neuraxial blockade, or aortocaval compression can cause maternal hypotension, leading to a decrease in uteroplacental perfusion.

Anesthetic agents have minimal direct effects on uterine blood flow. However, many anesthetic agents have cardiodepressant or vasodilatory effects that can cause hypotension, which can result in decreased uteroplacental perfusion.

Vasopressors in pregnancy have generally been studied in women undergoing cesarean delivery; these results are assumed to be valid for women having other operations during pregnancy. Both phenylephrine and ephedrine are reasonable choices to treat hypotension. Phenylephrine is generally preferred, but can lead to bradycardia; ephedrine is also effective, but can lead to progression of fetal physiologic acidemia. Controlled hypotension, which is used in some neurosurgical procedures, may be hazardous for the fetus.

Mechanical Ventilation

Mechanical ventilation should be adjusted to maintain the normal physiological chronic respiratory alkalosis of pregnancy. The partial pressure of carbon dioxide ($PaCO_2$) to end-tidal carbon dioxide ($ETCO_2$) gradient decreases during pregnancy; thus, the goal for $ETCO_2$ pressure is around 30 mm Hg. Because CO_2 crosses the placenta relatively easily, higher levels of maternal CO_2 may lead to acidosis and myocardial depression in the fetus; very low maternal CO_2 and severe respiratory alkalosis ($PaCO_2$ < 23 mm Hg and pH > 7.5) caused by maternal hyperventilation can compromise uterine blood flow and fetal oxygenation. Hence, the inspired O_2 of at least 50% should be used to maintain fetal oxygenation.

Recovery from Anesthesia

Recovery from anesthesia requires close monitoring, particularly of the airway and respiratory system, because most severe anesthetic complications occur during this period.

In a review of anesthesia-related maternal mortality in Michigan from 1985 to 2003, no maternal death occurred during induction or maintenance of anesthesia; the majority of deaths resulted from hypoventilation or airway obstruction during emergence, extubation, or recovery.

In the report from the Confidential Enquiries into Maternal and Child Health for 2006–2008 in the United Kingdom, of 7 deaths directly attributed to anesthesia, 4 were postoperative anesthesia-related complications.

Fetal Assessment

The FHR should be monitored in the recovery room, intermittently for the previable fetus and continuously for the viable fetus. Uterine activity should also be monitored, as contractions are most likely to occur soon after the procedure, as tocolytic effect of general anesthetics wears off.

Maternal Position

Left lateral position or uterine displacement should be maintained until the patient is fully awake, alert, and able to adjust her own position.

Postoperative Pain Control

Opioids can be used as needed to control postoperative pain. Epidural analgesia is an option for procedures on the chest, abdomen, or lower extremities, and carries less risk of opioid-induced hypoventilation when compared with intravenous (IV) opioids.

Nonsteroidal anti-inflammatory drugs should be avoided, especially after 32 weeks of gestation, because they may cause premature closure of the fetal ductus arteriosus, if given for more than 48 hours.

Anesthetic Drugs during Pregnancy

The physiologic changes of pregnancy may alter sensitivity to anesthetic medications and may affect drug metabolism. We do not usually change the choice or doses of anesthetic medications during pregnancy.

Anesthetic Medicine Dosages

A reduced dose may be required during pregnancy.

Induction Agents

A study reported 8% reduction in propofol dose needed for loss of consciousness, compared with nonpregnant women. Another similar study found no difference in the concentration required for loss of consciousness! The dose of thiopental required for loss of consciousness was reduced by 17% compared with nonpregnant patients.

Inhalation Anesthetics

Pregnancy appears to reduce the MAC for volatile inhalation agents required for general anesthesia. Studies have reported a 28% reduction in MAC for isoflurane during early pregnancy, and a 30% reduction immediately postpartum, compared with nonpregnant patients. A small study, however, found no difference in the electroencephalography measures of anesthetic effect between pregnant patients during cesarean delivery and gynecologic patients.

Neuromuscular Blocking Agents

Pregnant patients may be more sensitive to the effects of neuromuscular blocking agents (NMBAs) than nonpregnant patients. Therefore, neuromuscular block should be monitored with a "train-of-four twitch monitor" after administration of NMBAs to these patients.

Nondepolarizing NMBAs: Neuromuscular blockade with nondepolarizing NMBAs (i.e., vecuronium and rocuronium) has been studied during anesthesia for cesarean delivery; and they have reported a more rapid onset of neuromuscular block with weight-based administration of vecuronium and rocuronium in patients at time of cesarean delivery, and prolonged duration of action of vecuronium, compared with nonpregnant controls. Applicability of these results to patients earlier during pregnancy is unclear.

Succinylcholine: Succinylcholine is a depolarizing NMBA that is metabolized by plasma pseudocholinesterase, with an action time of 5–10 minutes. The level of pseudocholinesterase is reduced during pregnancy, but the volume of distribution of succinylcholine is gradually increased. Hence, the duration of action of succinylcholine is not predictable. This is mostly clinical insignificant, and a reduction in the dose of succinylcholine for pregnant patients is not recommended despite the reduced pseudocholinesterase. A slightly prolonged neuromuscular block would not have any negative effects on the patient, but an underdose may result in unsatisfactory intubation. Fasciculations after succinylcholine administration is less prominent during pregnancy, with a reduced postoperative myalgia issue.

Fetal Effects of Anesthetics

There is no compelling evidence that any specific anesthetic agents should be avoided during pregnancy.

Fetal Brain Development

Laboratory and animal studies, including in nonhuman primates, have reported neuronal apoptosis, changes in dendritic morphology, and negative effects on neurodevelopment after exposure to anesthetic medications during periods of rapid brain development. These effects occur after exposure to inhalation anesthetics, propofol, and ketamine. Some studies suggest that prolonged or repeated exposure to anesthetics increases risk of neurotoxicity after a continuous exposure of 3 hours+.

Clinical studies in humans have shown mixed results and have involved anesthesia in young children; pregnant women have not been included in clinical studies. These studies suggest that a single, brief exposure to anesthesia may not increase the risk of neurotoxicity. The GAS trial (General Anesthesia compared with Spinal Anesthesia trial), an ongoing prospective randomised control trial will compare neurocognitive outcomes at 5 years of age in approximately 700 children randomly assigned to spinal anesthesia or general anesthesia for inguinal hernia repair as infants. An interim evaluation at age of 2 years showed no difference in Bayley Scales of Infant and Toddler Development III between the groups.

In 2016, the US Food and Drug Administration (FDA) announced warnings about potential risks of negative effects on the developing brain from administration of anesthetics and sedative drugs to pregnant women and children under age 3, especially for repeated exposures or procedures lasting more than 3 hours. The FDA recommends that healthcare providers discuss with pregnant patients and parents of young children the benefits, risks, and appropriate timing of surgery requiring anesthesia that will take longer than 3 hours. However, the degree of risk remains unclear. At present, there is no compelling evidence that any specific anesthetic agent should be avoided during pregnancy, or that necessary surgery should be delayed because of concerns about neurotoxicity. In response to the FDA warning, the ACOG has confirmed the limitations of available data and reaffirmed that necessary surgery should not be delayed during pregnancy.

Teratogenicity

Anesthetic agents have no known teratogenic effects, and multiple large retrospective studies have not shown an increase in congenital defects in infants born to mothers who had surgery and anesthesia during pregnancy, including the 2,252 pregnancies with first trimester exposures. Although many anesthesia drugs were associated with teratogenic effects in animal studies, this may not apply to humans due to species variation and the high dose of agents used in the animal studies.

Early reports suggested that diazepam use in early pregnancy may be associated with a small increase in risk of cleft palate. Most common used benzodiazepines (such as midazolam) have never been associated with congenital malformations.

Neonatal Support with Emergent Delivery

Opioids and all anesthetic agents cross the placenta. But, there is minimal placental transfer because most muscle relaxants are highly ionized with low lipid solubility. Vecuronium crosses the placenta in small amounts, but neonatal outcome does not appear to be affected. The neonate delivered emergently during nonobstetric surgery may require intubation and mechanical ventilation due to the respiratory depressant effects of residual anesthetic agents and opioids. These effects are usually transient, requiring no additional measures other than ventilatory support until the effects of the medications wear off.

Uterine Effects

Potent inhalational agents, such as isoflurane, desflurane, and sevoflurane, decrease uterine tone; thus, they act to inhibit labor during the operative procedure. In the event of emergent delivery, increased amounts of uterotonic agents may be required (e.g., oxytocin, methylergonovine, and carboprost). Inhaled nitrous oxide (N_2O) (alone or as a 50% mixture with O_2) has no effect on uterine tone, maternal hemodynamic status, or FHR variability.

SURGICAL APPROACH

The surgical approach (laparotomy or laparoscopy) should be based on the skills of the surgeon, surgical needs and goals, and the availability of the appropriate staff and equipment. Laparoscopic surgery offers the same advantages to the pregnant woman as to the nonpregnant woman and can be performed safely during pregnancy. If a laparotomy is performed, the type of incision depends on the surgical procedure and gestational age.

POSTOPERATIVE OBSTETRIC MANAGEMENT

Progesterone Supplementation

Postoperative progesterone supplementation is recommended prior to 9 weeks of gestation (progesterone 50–100 mg vaginal suppository every 8–12 hours or a daily 50 mg intramuscular injection). Progesterone in oil and oral progesterone appears to be less effective. Luteal support is shifted from the corpus luteum of ovary to the placenta (called "luteoplacental shift") between 7 and 9 weeks. Hence, it is the placenta and not the CL, which is the source of progesterone to maintain pregnancies after 9 weeks of gestation, and progesterone supplementation is no longer needed. There is no adequate data for efficacy of preoperative progesterone for prevention of possible procedure-related preterm labor in later gestation.

Delivery Route after Surgery during Pregnancy

Cesarean delivery is performed for standard obstetrical indications in patients who have had recent surgery; the presence of a recent abdominal incision should not interfere the pushing in the second stage of labor.

OUTCOME

Outcome of Pregnancy

A number of large studies have investigated outcomes of pregnancy after nonobstetric surgery. A 2005 systematic review evaluated 54 studies of surgery during pregnancy from 1966 to 2001. Most studies were case series without controls, so meta-analysis was not performed, but key findings included:

- The overall rate of miscarriage in pregnant women who were exposed to surgical intervention in the first trimester was 10.5% (n = 43), and was similar to that in general obstetric population.
- The overall rate of major birth defects (2%) was not increased. Major birth defects following first trimester surgery occurred in 3.9%, but this increase was not statistically significant in any individual study and was not felt to be significantly higher in the general obstetrical population.
- The rate of delivery related to surgery was 3.5% (79/2,282); it was impossible to determine whether the cause was the procedure itself or

the underlying condition. The prematurity rate in the reviewed articles was 8.2% (597/7,313).

- The largest study of surgery during pregnancy in this review included 720,000 pregnant Swedish women, of whom 5,405 underwent surgery in the 1970s and 1980s. Major findings from this study were:
  - Specific types of anesthesia or surgical procedures were not associated with an increased incidence of adverse reproductive outcome.
  - Rate of congenital malformations and unexplained stillbirths was similar for women who underwent nonobstetric surgery needing anesthesia (5,405 women; 2,252 during first trimester) and women who did not. This suggests that surgery and anesthesia are not associated with teratogenic effects in early pregnancy.
  - The rates of low birth weight infants (due to prematurity and growth restriction) and early neonatal death (within 7 days of birth) were significantly increased in women who had had surgery with a RR of 2. It is not clear whether this increase resulted from the procedure itself or from an effect of the underlying medical condition necessitating surgery.

After evaluating over 47,000 nonobstetric surgeries identified from nearly 6.5 million pregnancies, the authors estimated that every 287 procedures were associated with one additional stillbirth, every 31 surgeries were associated with one additional preterm birth, every 39 operations were associated with one additional low birth weight infant, and every 25 surgeries were associated with one additional cesarean delivery. Of note, it was not possible to separate out the effects of surgery, anesthesia, or the underlying condition for which surgery was performed.

A later meta-analysis of 10 studies (published between 1990 and 2016, and including 154 women) attempted to define the risk of poor maternal or fetal outcome specific to women undergoing cardiac surgery utilizing cardiopulmonary bypass. Ninety percent of patients underwent urgent or emergency cardiac surgery, and most operations occurred in second trimester. In this meta-analysis, risks of surgery during pregnancy were much greater than in the above retrospective review or in earlier studies, and included an 11% risk of maternal death, 33% risk of pregnancy loss. The fetal loss rate was 2.5% in nonregistry studies and ranged from 0.8 to 1.8% in registry studies.

Appendicectomy patients had higher rates of surgery-related delivery (4.6%) compared with other operations (0.8%). There were also higher rates of fetal loss (2.6%), increasing when peritonitis was present (10.9%) compared with other operations (1.2%).

Specific types of anesthesia or surgical procedures were not associated with an increased incidence of adverse reproductive outcome.

The rate of congenital malformations and unexplained stillbirths was similar for women who underwent nonobstetric surgery requiring anesthesia

(5,405 women; 2,252 during first trimester) and women who did not. These findings suggest surgery and anesthesia are not associated with teratogenic effects in early pregnancy.

Outcome of Surgery

From the woman's perspective, it is unclear if the risk of surgical morbidity or mortality from general surgical procedures is increased for pregnant women compared with nonpregnant women. However, pregnant women who require surgical procedures are advised to proceed and avoid delay, as delaying nonelective surgical intervention increases the risks of complications, especially the risk of infection and venous thromboembolism.

A retrospective cohort study that matched over 2,500 United States pregnant women to non-pregnant controls undergoing general surgical procedures reported no differences in the 30-day mortality rates (0.4 vs. 0.3%) and morbidity rates (6.6 vs. 7.4%). The study indicates that nonelective general surgical procedures can be safely performed in pregnant women and should not be delayed because of pregnancy. In contrast, a different study of 5,500+ pregnant women in Taiwan reported a nearly fourfold increased rate of inhospital maternal mortality, a 2.5-fold increased risk of admission to the ICU, and increased risks of postoperative septicemia, pneumonia, and urinary tract infection for pregnant women undergoing nonobstetric surgery compared with nonpregnant women.

While the available data on the risk of surgery in pregnant women are conflicting, surgical delay has been linked to worsened outcomes, particularly for infectious surgical indications such as appendicitis and cholecystitis. As an example, a study of over 7,100 women with appendicitis in pregnancy reported that conservative medical management was associated with an increased risk of septic shock (adjusted odds ratio—6.3), venous thromboembolism (adjusted odds ratio—2.5), and peritonitis (adjusted odds ratio—1.6) compared with appendectomy. Similarly, in a study of pregnant women with cholecystitis, women managed surgically had lower maternal complication rates (4% vs. 16%) and fetal complication rates (6% vs. 16%) compared with women treated medically.

▌ SUMMARY AND RECOMMENDATIONS

- Physiologic and anatomic changes related to pregnancy require adaptations of anesthetic and surgical techniques.
- Anesthetic agents are not known teratogens; but due to the inability to conclusively rule out adverse effects, exposure to medications should be minimized during pregnancy.

General principles of nonobstetric surgery in pregnant women include:
- Provide mechanical or pharmacologic thromboprophylaxis. For laparoscopic procedure (gynecologic or general surgical) likely to

take >45 minutes, use low molecular weight heparin, and mechanical thromboprophylaxis is a reasonable alternative for shorter procedures.

- Follow standard fasting recommendations; additional aspiration prophylaxis is not necessary in patients not otherwise at risk of aspiration.
- Displace uterus to the left lateral in 2nd half of pregnancy to reduce risk of hypotension.
- Use regional anesthesia, when appropriate, rather than general anesthesia, to minimize drug exposure and the need to manage the airway.
- Minimize disruption of fetal homeostasis by avoiding maternal hypotension, hypoxemia, and hypercarbia or hypocarbia.
- Titrate IV and inhalation anesthetics, and neuromuscular blocking agents to needed efficacy, keeping in mind that pregnancy may alter sensitivity to these medications. Monitor the level of neuromuscular blockade with a "train-of-four twitch" monitor.
- Maintain maternal FiO_2 > 50% and $ETCO_2$ 32–34 mm Hg.
- Minimize uterine manipulation.
- Document the FHR preoperatively and postoperatively. Continuously monitor the FHR intraoperatively and in the recovery room after 23–24 weeks of gestation. Ensure the ability to perform emergency cesarean delivery when required.
- Promptly provide postoperative progesterone supplementation when the corpus luteum is removed prior to 7–9 weeks of gestation.
- We advise to proceed with nonelective nonobstetric surgery whenever clinically indicated. Nonobstetric surgery does not appear to negatively impact obstetric outcomes, including rates of miscarriage, stillbirth, and congenital malformations. While the data on maternal outcomes after nonobstetric surgery are conflicting, the evidence till date is generally reassuring. In addition, surgical delay has been associated with worsened outcomes, particularly for infectious surgical indications such as appendicitis and cholecystitis.

Aswath Kumar, Reshma Joy

■ INTRODUCTION

Pregnancy is one of the most important periods in a women's life. A time of increased questions and many women find themselves in need of information about everything from early pregnancy, physical changes that happen to her, health-related decisions during pregnancy, do's and don'ts during this period, to parenting an infant after delivery and family planning. This need for information can be even more pronounced when pregnancies are complicated by maternal or fetal issues.

Many important learning needs may arise as prospective parents prepare for and adjust to their new role. Currently, women may have access to significant volumes of information about pregnancy, birth, and parenting from a number of sources, including the internet, medical information websites, and smartphone applications (apps), which can be tailored by demographics such as gestational age, maternal age, language or risk factors and social media platforms, family and friends, popular media such as newspapers and television, and written material from professional and commercial entities, childbirth education classes, and discussions with health professionals. The ability of a woman to have her information needs met is impacted by the access she has to different sources of information, and her ability to comprehend that information. Access to large volumes of information does not necessarily equate with understanding and comprehension. The rapid evolution of communication technologies has created new ways for healthcare consumers to manage their health. Pregnant women appreciate information that is immediate, such as information that can quickly be found using an internet search engine or a smartphone.

Pregnant women seek to find the answer to questions and assume the role of active health-information consumers by using Internet search engines. It has been shown that after using the Internet, pregnant women feel more confident in their pregnancy decision-making. The most commonly searched topics by pregnant women include fetal development, body changes during pregnancy, nutrition in pregnancy, safe medications during pregnancy, and pregnancy complications. Women use these information sources to expand upon the knowledge gained from appointments with their healthcare providers.

This is why in the past few years, E-technology has played an important role in antenatal care. Health information technology (HIT) is evolving rapidly with developments that support new ways to communicate with healthcare providers and to support one's health. Appropriate health technology should be effective, safe, and feasible.

Although Internet searching is widely used, one of the difficulties with this medium is an inability to judge the quality and accuracy of retrieved information and many individuals searching online for health advice believe the information and advice they find. This is a concern, as health information provided on the Internet is not always reliable or current. Health professionals, midwives, and antenatal care providers should be aware of this issue and provide more evidence-based information to these women at the time they require it. Future research should address ways to better inform women of the hazards of Internet searching.

How patients can access E-technology?

Smartphone Applications

Antenatal care apps (acAPPs) are a type of smartphone apps that provide prenatal care services and information targeting pre-pregnant and pregnant women. It is a new way of channeling information and interpersonal interaction in the current era of mobile technology development, which has been widely accepted. Due to high demand and adherence, pregnant women have become a key target group for app developers. The use of these apps in health care is worthy of attention. Functions of these apps are diverse. This form of health guidance is superior to traditional methods and can even improve the quality of pregnancy care in areas with scarce medical resources. In this modern era, apps have been an integral part from the preconceptional time onward. What to avoid preconceptionally are menstrual calendar which can predict days of ovulation to calculation of due date, gestational age, measurement of changes in body weight, and calculation of fetal movement. Many apps also have social functions, professional counseling functions, and special tools. These self-monitored health status functions can be used to track pregnant women's health and diet through these apps. These apps can include motivational messages, monitoring, and behavior change tools. Pregnancy apps may also link to a device such as a camera, glucometer, fitness activity tracker, Kegel "exerciser," fetal heartbeat "listener," or other monitoring equipment. Devices associated with an app are marketed directly to consumers and avoid regulatory scrutiny. The popularity of mobile pregnancy apps has increased irrespective of socioeconomic status. At present, existing studies mainly focus on the use of apps for monitoring or intervening mental disorders. Sensors and apps of smartphones have been used to predict daily mood, detect depression, intervene depression, relieve pressure, and treat depression because pregnancy is being associated with a lot of mental disorder.

WhatsApp Groups

Group antenatal care and participatory learning and action cycles (PLA) with women's groups have been cited by the WHO as health systems interventions that can lead to improvements in adherence to care and health outcomes in pregnancy and the postpartum period. Evidence suggests that social support increases resilience to stress; pregnancy groups that help to build social support could therefore plausibly impact health outcomes. WhatsApp-based version of group support with the aim of improving social support during pregnancy without the time and logistical requirements associated with in-person group-based ANC. WhatsApp is increasingly being integrated into the public health space to assist public health workers and improve service delivery. Antenatal women can get registered to hospital WhatsApp group, also pregnant women can be in touch with each other and discuss their problems among themselves and health worker participating in the group. Reminders and general health information can also be shared.

Search Engine Use (Google/Yahoo)

Pregnancy information has been downloaded hundreds of millions of times and is an integral source of information for many pregnant women. In several pregnancy-focused health information studies, more than 90% of pregnant women reported having Internet access, and over 70% described using the Internet to access pregnancy-related information. Studies found that women with a first pregnancy searched for information on the Internet in early pregnancy, and women who were employed and with higher education were more likely to use Internet. Most women perceive Internet information to be useful and reliable. However, few women discuss information found on the Internet with health professional. The reasons why women prefer the internet to other sources of information relate to privacy, accessibility, and scope of information available. It has also been found that women use the internet to enhance their understanding of information provided by their pregnancy care provider, or to determine if they should seek further advice. Complications in pregnancy can place women and their caregivers in an unfamiliar situation where they must quickly learn about an illness or complication and attempt to fully understand its impact or severity before making decisions for themselves and their families in these situations, they use internet. Lack of reliability is well recognized and a systematic meta-analysis of health website evaluations found that many evaluations (70%) concluded that quality of information was a problem on the Internet.

■ HOSPITAL'S USE OF E-TECHNOLOGY (FIG. 1)

To communicate with patients, the most commonly reported form of technology used was automated phone calls to spread general health information, schedule antenatal appointments and the time, and get reminders. Hospital information sites are at easy access to patients. Patients

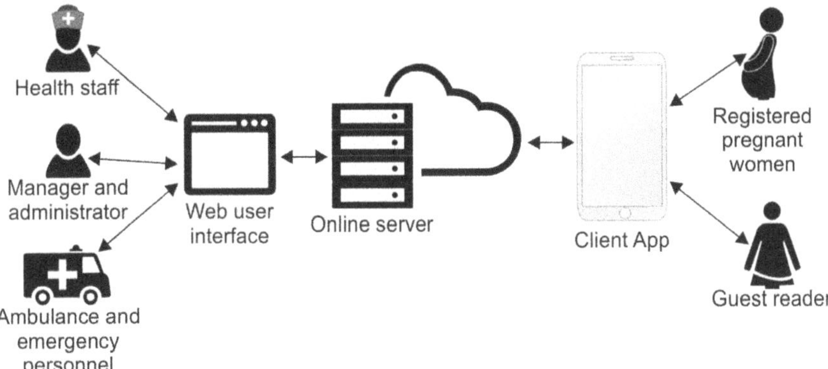

Fig. 1: Use of E-technology in antenatal care.

are made aware of the facilities available at the hospital. Patients can reach out to the medical team on duty via chat. Investigation reports can be analyzed by the patients as well as doctors too.

Health workers can collect offline/online data for registering antenatal women. Women can register for services using toll-free code.

Women with an emergency can alert the hospital GPS system for transportation, which will pick her up and take her to the center. Patients' details can be used for mapping and locating patients. Cell tower triangulation technology functions without internet access so it can also be used for the same purpose.

By improving the patient–provider relationship, antenatal clinic attendance may increase and decrease pregnancy complications.

Connecting to internet has become a daily reflex as we have easy access to it, but the quality and authenticity of information obtained must be thought about. Access to a large information does not mean that it will be understood and assimilated. Hoping that right information obtained by our mothers helped them to gain confidence to enter motherhood smoothly. Recommendation of valid healthcare websites to patients by their treating doctors would be useful to them. Studies are investigating the need for a centralized website giving reliable information to meet the mother's need.

SUGGESTED READING

1. Eriksson-Backa, 2003
2. Lagan BM, Sinclair M, Kernohan WG. Internet use in pregnancy informs women's decision making: a web-based survey. Birth. 2010;37(2):106-15.
3. Lagan, et al., 2010
4. Larsson M. A descriptive study of the use of the Internet by women seeking pregnancy-related information. Midwifery. 2009;25(1):14-20.
5. Lowe, et al., 2009.
6. Pati A, Dehury RK, Dehury P. Birth Preparedness among Women and Factors Associated with Antenatal Care. J Health Manag. 2018;20(3):378-400.
7. Sayakhot P, Carolan-Olah M. Internet use by pregnant women seeking pregnancy-related information: a systematic review. BMC Pregnancy Childbirth. 2016;16(1):65.

CHAPTER 38

Antenatal Screening: Quiz

Sebanti Goswami, Abha Rani Sinha, Seema Hakim

1. **In trisomy 21 pregnancies at 12 weeks maternal serum free beta human chorionic gonadotropin (β-hCG) increased—True/False**

Ans. True

2. **In which trisomy, the heart rate is increased?**

Ans. Trisomy 13

3. **What is triploidy with double paternal contribution known as?**

Ans. Diandric

4. **What are the fetoplacental products measured in the quadruple test?**

Ans.

- Free β-hCG
- α-fetoprotein (AFP)
- Unconjugated estriol (uE3)
- Inhibin A

5. **What is the most common cardiac abnormality in trisomy 21?**

Ans. Atrioventricular septal defect

6. **Dandy–Walker malformation is cystic dilatation of the:**
   - **Lateral ventricle**
   - **Third ventricle**
   - **Fourth ventricle**
   - **Cerebellum**

Ans. Fourth ventricle

7. **What is the full form of FETO?**

Ans. Fetoscopic endoluminal tracheal occlusion

8. **Legal limit of termination of abnormal fetuses is:**
   - **24 weeks**
   - **20 weeks**
   - **28 weeks**
   - **Anytime**

Ans. 20 weeks

INFECTIONS

9. **Risk of congenital rubella, if infection acquired in the 10th week:**
   - **10%**
   - **55%**
   - **75%**
   - **100%**

Ans. 100%

10. **The most common congenital viral infection is:**
    - **Toxoplasma**
    - **Herpes**
    - **Cytomegalovirus (CMV)**
    - **Rubella**

Ans. CMV

11. **Hydrops fetalis is caused by:**
    - **Parvovirus B19**
    - **Toxoplasmosis**
    - **Syphilis**
    - **All of the above**

Ans. All of the above

12. **Current Federation of Obstetric and Gynaecological Societies of India recommendation for influenza vaccine in pregnancy:**
    - **One dose after 20 weeks**
    - **Two doses after 20 weeks**
    - **One dose after 26 weeks**
    - **Two doses after 26 weeks**

Ans. One dose after 26 weeks

13. **What is the contingent screening protocol suggested by Nicolaides (2016) for implementing cell-free DNA (cfDNA) after combined screen test?**
    - **High risk > 1 in 100**
    - **Intermediate risk 1:100–1:2,500**
    - **Low risk > 1:2,500**

Ans.
   - High risk > 1 in 100—invasive testing/cfDNA testing
   - Intermediate risk 1:100–1:2,500—cfDNA or no further testing
   - Low risk > 1:2,500—no further testing

14. **What are the indications for fetoscopy? What is the associated fetal loss with fetoscopy?**

Ans.
   - Fetal skin sampling—genodermatoses
   - Liver, kidney, and muscle biopsies

- Laser photocoagulation of placental vessel anastomosis in severe twin-to-twin transfusion syndrome (TTTS)
- Loss: 3–5%

15. **At what parameters decision for intrauterine transfusion (IUT) is taken? What are the various routes and which one is better?**

Ans.

- *Middle cerebral artery-peak systolic velocity (MCA-PSV) > 1.5 MoM*: Confirm fetal anemia with hCT < 30%
- Intraperitoneal and intravascular
- Intravascular is better—less volume of transfusion needed, more efficacy

16. **Mention indication of skin biopsy in fetus. Which site is recommended?**

Ans.

- *Indications*: Bullous disorders, hyperkeratotic disorders, and oculocutaneous albinism
- Skin over occiput or buttocks

17. **What is the Solomon technique of laser ablation in TTTS?**

Ans. After coagulation of all visible anastomosis, a thin line of tissue at the placental surface at the level of vascular equator is coagulated.

18. **Management for all Quintero stages:**

Ans.

- Quintero stage 1 and 2: Serial amnioreduction
- Quintero stage 3 and 4: Laser

19. **What is the management of fetal goiter diagnosed by ultrasonography (USG)? (Drug, doses, and route)**

Ans. Intra-amniotic thyroxine therapy 150–600 µg of thyroxine/week

20. **What are the second and third line of treatment of supraventricular tachycardia in fetus?**

Ans. Sotalol, flecainide, and amiodarone

21. **A 28-year-old woman is 22 weeks' pregnant. She has long-standing type 1 diabetes mellitus (DM). Her blood sugars have remained well controlled in pregnancy. However, she is concerned about how her DM may cause congenital fetal anomalies in her unborn child. Which single action best addresses her anxiety and why?**

Ans. USG for detecting fetal structural abnormalities, including examination of fetal heart (four chambers, outflow tracts, and three vessels), and fetal ECHO because congenital heart defects is the most common anomaly associated with type 1 DM.

22. **A 32-year-old woman with in vitro fertilization conception comes to your clinic with diagnosis of twin pregnancy at 18 weeks with 1 twin demise, and the placentation is Diamniotic monochorionic. How will you proceed in terms of investigations (any special radiological test), counseling, and timing of delivery?**

Ans. Level-II scan, antenatal MRI should be offered 2–3 weeks after demise.

Counsel regarding increased risk of congenital anomaly in surviving fetus, encephalomalacia, increased theoretical risk of coagulopathy in mother, psychological counseling is needed.

In absence of any other complication, deliver at term.

23. **A 27-year-old woman at 30 weeks' period of gestation (POG) comes with USG report of asymmetric intrauterine growth restriction (IUGR) and reversal of flow in umbilical artery color Doppler. How will you manage the case and when will you terminate?**

Ans.

- Admit
- Steroid cover
- Daily biophysical profile and color Doppler—ductus venosus (DV)
- Weekly abdominal circumference and estimated fetal weight
- Recommend delivery by 32 weeks, if DV flow is normal
- If abnormal DV color Doppler, terminate (RCOG, Green top guidelines)

24. **A 30-year-old woman at 16 weeks' POG came to you with an ultrasound report showing a choroid plexus cyst (CPC) of 6-mm size, what will be the further management and counseling?**

Ans.

- Get detailed genetic sonogram done
- Quadruple screen—special emphasis on trisomy 18
- If isolated CPC, screen negative and age <35 years, no karyotyping recommended (SOGC)

25. **What is the role of transabdominal embryoscopy?**

Ans.

- Identify fetal anomalies not recognizable early in pregnancy by USG (3 weeks)
- Confirm anomalies detected by USG

26. **How early cfDNA can be isolated from maternal blood?**

Ans. 5 weeks

27. What are the side effects of doing early amniocentesis in first trimester?

Ans.

- Increased risk of fetal loss
- Amniotic fluid leakage
- Congenital talipes equinovarus

28. What are the causes of false-negative noninvasive prenatal testing (NIPT)?

Ans.

- Obesity
- Early gestational age
- Suboptimal sample

29. If screening is negative for NIPT, what to do next?

Ans. Follow-up as routine

30. Increased PAPPA is a risk factor for IUGR—(True/False):

Ans. False

31. Amniocentesis is done at which gestational age?

Ans. Early: 11–14 weeks and Late: 15–20 weeks

32. Isolated raised NT > 3.5 mm with normal karyotype of fetus is associated with increased cardiac anomaly—(True/False):

Ans. True

33. *CFTR* gene is located on which chromosome?

Ans. Chromosome 7p

34. Post-transfusion target for fetal hematocrit in IUT in Rh isoimmunization is:

Ans. 48–55%

35. Diagnostic criteria for APLA is known as:

Ans. Sapporo criteria

36. Kell sensitization is clinically less severe than D sensitization—(True/False):

Ans. False; more severe, because it attaches to red cell precursors also in bone marrow.

37. False-positive NIPT is found in:

Ans. Placental mosaicism

38. As per ISUOG (International Society of USG in Obstetrics and Gynecology) guidelines, at what % discordancy in CRL in twin pregnancy, it is recommended to refer the patient to FMU?

Ans. More than or equal to 10%

39. Elaborate PLUTO study.

Ans. Percutaneous shunting in lower urinary tract obstruction

40. MSAFP levels are raised in NTD—(True/False):

Ans. True

41. Gestational age for fetal reduction is:

Ans. 11–13 weeks

42. What is the cut off for fetal hydronephrosis in second trimester?

Ans. 15 mm

43. Inheritance pattern of Lesch Nyhan syndrome:

Ans. X-linked recessive

44. Recurrence risk of TTTS after laser ablation is:

Ans. 14%

45. Elaborate EXIT.

Ans. Ex utero intrapartum treatment

46. Fetal loss rate is more in transcervical chorionic villus sampling (CVS) compared to transabdominal route—(True/False):

Ans. False

47. What is founder effect?

Ans. A rare genetic abnormality found in higher frequency in certain population

48. CLASP trial is associated with:

Ans. Collaborative low-dose aspirin study in pregnancy

49. In lupus anticoagulant-positive antiphospholipid antibody (APLA) women, on anticoagulant therapy, what assay is used to monitor anticoagulation?

Ans. Anti-factor Xa level

50. In trisomy 13, what change occurs in PAPPA value?

Ans. Decrease

51. Cut off level for MCA PSV Doppler for considering cordocentesis:

Ans. 1.5 MoM

52. What is the % incidence of choroid plexus cysts in normal fetuses?

Ans. 1–2%

53. Most common aminoacidopathy is:

Ans. Phenylketonuria

54. Recommended hematocrit % of blood used for IUT in Rh isoimmunization:

Ans. 70–80%

55. What is the disadvantage of polar body biopsy in PGD?

Ans. Only maternal DNA can be checked

56. Most common cause of death in Duchenne muscular dystrophy:

Ans. Respiratory failure

57. Ventriculomegaly is a soft marker of Down's syndrome—(True/ False):

Ans. False

58. Elaborate PRIDE study.

Ans. PR interval and dexamethasone evaluation study

59. Drugs causing SLE like syndrome:

Ans. Procainamide, hydralazine, quinidine, INH, diltiazem, and minocycline

60. Integrated screening combines PAPPA, β-hCG, estriol, inhibin— (True/False):

Ans. False (NT is part of it)

61. Ideal gestational age to perform CVS:

Ans. 11–13 weeks

62. To diagnose echogenic bowel, the echogenicity of bowel is compared with what?

Ans. Bone, preferably iliac wings

63. Clinical features of Hurler's syndrome:

Ans. Coarse facies, macrocephaly, hernias, joint stiffness, corneal clouding, and deafness

64. FETO is done for which congenital defect?

Ans. Congenital diaphragmatic hernia

65. What is the risk of neonatal lupus, if mother is suffering from SLE?

Ans. Less than 5%

66. **American College of Obstetricians and Gynecologists (ACOG) recommends aneuploidy screening to be done, if maternal age > 35 years—(True/False):**

Ans. False (all women irrespective of age)

67. **Upper limit of DFI (DNA fragmentation index):**

Ans. 30%

68. **RADIUS trial stands for:**

Ans. Routine antenatal diagnostic imaging with ultrasound

69. **Fetal skin biopsy is performed at which gestational age?**

Ans. 20 weeks

70. **Full form of NIPT?**

Ans. Noninvasive prenatal genetic testing

SUGGESTED READING

1. Cunningham FG, Leveno KJ, Bloom SL, Dashe JS, Hoffman BL, Casey BM, et al. Williams Obstetrics, 25th edition. New York: McGraw Hill; 2018.
2. Gabbe SG, Niebyl JR, Simpson JL, Landon MB, Galan HL, Jauniaux RM, et al. Gabbe obstetrics: normal and problem pregnancies, 7th edition. Amsterdam: Elsevier; 2016.
3. Gregg AR, Skotko BG, Benkendorf JL, Monaghan KG, Bajaj K, Best RG, et al. Noninvasive prenatal screening for fetal aneuploidy, 2016 update: a position statement of the American College of Medical Genetics and Genomics. Genet Med. 2016;18(10):1056-65.
4. James D, Steer PJ, Weiner CP, Gonik B, Robson SC. High-risk pregnancy: management options, 5th edition. Cambridge UK: Cambridge University Press; 2018.
5. Rafi I, Hill M, Hayward J, Chitty LS. Non-invasive prenatal testing: use of cell-free fetal DNA in Down syndrome screening. Br J Gen Pract. 2017;67(660):298-9.

Index

Page numbers followed by *b* refer to box, *f* refer to figure, *fc* refer to flowchart, and *t* refer to table.

A

Abdomen 87, 91, 111
   acute 152
Abdominal circumference 87*f*, 91, 97, 111, 111*f*
Abdominal cramps 171
Abdominal discomfort 150
Abdominal organs 113*f*
Abdominal pain 150, 154, 156, 162, 171
   causes of 151
   history of acute 153
Abdominopelvic discomfort 152
Aberrant right subclavian artery 73, 76, 77, 77*f*
Abortion
   therapeutic 185
   threatened 185
Absent end diastolic flow 302
Accredited Social Health Activist 4
Acellular pertussis vaccine 10
Acetaminophen 15
Acquire infection 189
Acquired immunodeficiency syndrome 195
Acyclovir 160, 161, 165, 256
Additional therapy 303, 305
Adnexa 120
Advanced fetal deterioration 332
Advanced neurosonogram 93
Alanine
   aminotransferase 134
   transaminase 138
Alcohol 263
Allergic reaction, mild 248
Alloimmunization 185
Allopurinol 257
Alpha-linoleic acid 232
Alpha-methyldopa 299
Amantadine 256
Amenorrhea, period of 152
American Diabetes Association 223
Amikacin 255
Aminoglycosides 255
Aminopterin 262
Amniocentesis 12, 13
Amnionicity, establishment of 122
Amnionitis 168

Amniotic fluid 119
   amount of 97
   evaluation 14
   index 92, 119*f*, 224, 302
Amoxicillin 167, 254
Ampicillin 254
Analgesics 259
Androgens 262, 265
Anemia 43, 44, 47, 158, 283, 284, 305
   aplastic 44
   causes of 284, 286, 294
   chronic 284
   dimorphic 44
   evaluation of 44, 286, 287
   high incidence of 43
   management of 286, 288*fc*, 292, 293*fc*
   maternal 6
   megaloblastic 47
   mild 292
   mild-to-moderate 284, 292
   moderate-to-severe 292
   nutritional 284
   physiologic 284
   risk of 284
   screening of 43, 50*fc*
   severe 9, 286, 292
   sideroblastic 47
   treatment guidelines 286
   type of 45, 286
Anesthesia
   general 389, 390
   induction of 391
   light 390
   maintenance of 391
   management 389
   monitored 390
   recovery from 392
   types of 397
Anesthetic
   fetal effects of 394
   medicine dosages 393
   type of 389
Anesthetic agents 392
   teratogenesis from 385
Aneuploidy 220, 377
   high risk for 12
   screening, ultrasound in 124